Oral Health Care - An Important Issue of the Modern Society

Edited by Lavinia Cosmina Ardelean and Laura Cristina Rusu

Published in London, United Kingdom

Oral Health Care - An Important Issue of the Modern Society
http://dx.doi.org/10.5772/intechopen.95132
Edited by Lavinia Cosmina Ardelean and Laura Cristina Rusu

Contributors
Antonio Garcia, Lara Eltze, Maren Eltze, Pinar Kiymet Karataban, Zuhair Natto, Lavinia Ardelean, Laura Cristina Rusu, Codruta Victoria Tigmeanu, Tracey Lynn Harney, Irma Fabiola Díaz-García, Dinorah Munira Hernández-Santos, Julio Alberto Díaz-Ramos, Neyda Ma. Mendoza-Ruvalcaba, Diego Romario-Silva, Andréa Cristina Barbosa Cristina Barbosa da Silva, Edja Maria Melo de Brito Costa, Otávio Akira Souza Sakaguchi, Francisco Mendonça, Joanylda Raimundo, Bruna Dantas, Frederico Ribeiro, Tahyna Deps, Carlus Santos, David Andrade, Joana Andrade, Maria-João Palha, Cristina Areias, Paula Macedo, Ana Norton, Miguel Palha, Lurdes Morais, Dóris Ruiz, Sônia Groisman, Tetsuo Nakamoto, Alexander U Falster, William B. Simmons Jr, Amornrat Ratanasiri, Thitima Nutravong, Arisara Poosari, Supaporn Chatrchaiwiwatana, Thawalrat Ratanasiri, Kanokporn Wongcharee, Denise Tostes Oliveira, Kellen Cristine Tjioe, Gabriela Lopes Santos, Silas Juvêncio Freitas-Filho, Kaique Preto, Ljiljana Kesic, Milica Petrovic, Marija Bojovic, Radmila Obradovic, Branislava Stojkovic, Simona Stojanovic, Dragoslav Lazic, elif nadide akaypolat, Ichiro Nakajima, Ken-ichiro Ejima, Yoshinori Arai, Kunihito Matsumoto, Kazuya Honda, Hirofumi Aboshi, Marina Hamaguch, Akao Lyvongsa, Bounnhong Sidaphone, Somphone Phanthavong, Chanthavisao Phanthanalay, Souksavanh Vongsa, Martin Grootveld, Benita Percival, Angela Wann, Sophie Taylor, Mark Edgar, Miles Gibson, monisha Khatri, Shreya Kishore, Nagarathinam S, Suvetha Siva, Vanita Barai, Nelli Yildirimyan, David Gillam, Alexandra Roman, Andrada Soanca, Bogdan Caloian, Alexandru Bucur, Gabriela Caracostea, Andreia Preda, Dora Maria Popescu, Iulia Cristina Micu, Petra Surlin, Andreea Ciurea, Diana Onet, Mircea Viorel Ciurea, Dragos Alexandru Termure, Marius Negucioiu, Aparna Narayana, Dhanasekar Balakrishnan, Gayathri Krishnamoorthy

First published in London, United Kingdom, 2022 by IntechOpen
IntechOpen is the global imprint of INTECHOPEN LIMITED, registered in England and Wales, registration number: 11086078, 5 Princes Gate Court, London, SW7 2QJ, United Kingdom
Printed in Croatia

British Library Cataloguing-in-Publication Data
A catalogue record for this book is available from the British Library

Additional hard and PDF copies can be obtained from orders@intechopen.com

Oral Health Care - An Important Issue of the Modern Society
Edited by Lavinia Cosmina Ardelean and Laura Cristina Rusu
p. cm.

This title is part of the Dentistry Book Series, Volume 10
Topic: Oral Health
Series Editor: Sergio Alexandre Gehrke
Topic Editors: Sandra Marinho and Esra Guzeldemir-Akcakanat

Print ISBN 978-1-80355-123-4
Online ISBN 978-1-80355-124-1
eBook (PDF) ISBN 978-1-80355-125-8
ISSN 2631-6218

For EU product safety concerns:
IN TECH d.o.o., Prolaz Marije Krucifikse Kozulić 3, 51000 Rijeka, Croatia,
info@intechopen.com or visit our website at intechopen.com.

IntechOpen Book Series

Dentistry

Volume 10

Aims and Scope of the Series

This book series will offer a comprehensive overview of recent research trends as well as clinical applications within different specialties of dentistry. Topics will include overviews of the health of the oral cavity, from prevention and care to different treatments for the rehabilitation of problems that may affect the organs and/or tissues present. The different areas of dentistry will be explored, with the aim of disseminating knowledge and providing readers with new tools for the comprehensive treatment of their patients with greater safety and with current techniques. Ongoing issues, recent advances, and future diagnostic approaches and therapeutic strategies will also be discussed. This series of books will focus on various aspects of the properties and results obtained by the various treatments available, whether preventive or curative.

Meet the Series Editor

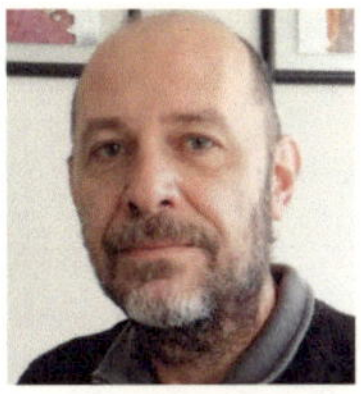

Dr. Sergio Alexandre Gehrke is a doctorate holder in two fields. The first is a Ph.D. in Cellular and Molecular Biology from the Pontificia Catholic University, Porto Alegre, Brazil, in 2010 and the other is an International Ph.D. in Bioengineering from the Universidad Miguel Hernandez, Elche/Alicante, Spain, obtained in 2020. In 2018, he completed a postdoctoral fellowship in Materials Engineering in the NUCLEMAT of the Pontificia Catholic University, Porto Alegre, Brazil. He is currently the Director of the Postgraduate Program in Implantology of the Bioface/UCAM/PgO (Montevideo, Uruguay), Director of the Cathedra of Biotechnology of the Catholic University of Murcia (Murcia, Spain), an Extraordinary Full Professor of the Catholic University of Murcia (Murcia, Spain) as well as the Director of the private center of research Biotecnos – Technology and Science (Montevideo, Uruguay). Applied biomaterials, cellular and molecular biology, and dental implants are among his research interests. He has published several original papers in renowned journals. In addition, he is also a Collaborating Professor in several Postgraduate programs at different universities all over the world.

Meet the Volume Editors

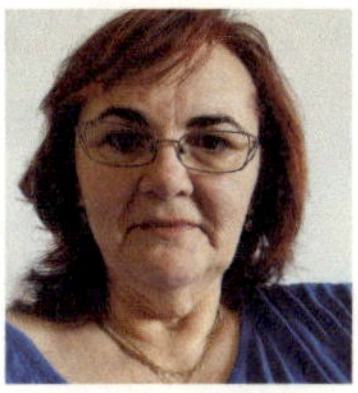

Professor Lavinia Cosmina Ardelean, DMD, Ph.D., is a professor and head of the Department of Technology of Materials and Devices in Dental Medicine, "Victor Babes" University of Medicine and Pharmacy, Timisoara, Romania. She has authored/co-authored 16 books, 10 book chapters, and 120 peer-reviewed papers. She is an editorial board member of numerous journals and a member of reviewer/topic boards of Materials, Prosthesis, Metals, and Polymers, and an academic editor for Scanning. She has guest-edited five special issues in different journals and is an active reviewer, with more than 200 reviews to her credit so far. Her research interest includes most areas of dentistry, with a focus on dental materials/biomaterials, dental alloys, resins, ceramics/bioceramics, CAD/CAM milling, 3D printing/bioprinting in dentistry, laser welding, scanning, and oral health care.

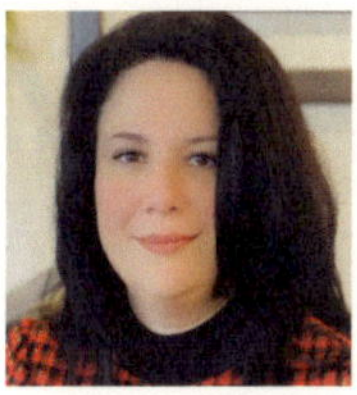

Professor Laura Cristina Rusu, DMD, Ph.D., is the mother of two lovely boys and a full-time professor and head of the Oral Pathology Department, Faculty of Dental Medicine, "Victor Babes" University of Medicine and Pharmacy, Timisoara, Romania. Her Ph.D. thesis was centered on allergens in dental materials. In 2017 she obtained a Dr. Habil and was confirmed as a Ph.D. coordinator in the field of dental medicine. She took part in 10 research projects, including FP7 COST Action MP 1005, and authored 140 peer-reviewed papers. She has published eight books and book chapters as an author and co-author. Her main scientific interests are oral pathology and oral diagnosis in dental medicine, with a focus on oral cancer.

Contents

Preface **XV**

Section 1
Issues Related to the Health of Oral Environment **1**

Chapter 1 **3**
Evaluation of Trans-Resveratrol as a Treatment for Periodontitis
by Tracey Lynn Harney

Chapter 2 **27**
Periodontitis and Heart Disease: Current Perspectives on the Associative Relationships and Preventive Impact
by Alexandra Roman, Andrada Soancă, Bogdan Caloian, Alexandru Bucur, Gabriela Valentina Caracostea, Andreia Paraschiva Preda, Dora Maria Popescu, Iulia Cristina Micu, Petra Șurlin, Andreea Ciurea, Diana Oneț, Mircea Viorel Ciurea, Dragoș Alexandru Țermure and Marius Negucioiu

Chapter 3 **49**
Ulcerative Lesions of the Oral Cavity
by Nelli Yildirimyan

Chapter 4 **63**
Alternative Denture Base Materials for Allergic Patients
by Lavinia Cosmina Ardelean, Laura-Cristina Rusu and Codruta Victoria Tigmeanu

Chapter 5 **81**
White Spot Lesions and Remineralization
by Monisha Khatri, Shreya Kishore, S. Nagarathinam, Suvetha Siva and Vanita Barai

Chapter 6 **99**
Oral Cancer around Dental Implants: Are the Clinical Manifestations and the Oncogenic Mechanisms Unique?
by Gabriela Lopes dos Santos, Kaique Preto Alberto, Silas Antonio Juvêncio de Freitas Filho, Kellen Cristine Tjioe and Denise Tostes Oliveira

Chapter 7 111
Variability of Saliva Viscosity - Potential Impact
by Lara Eltze, Maren Eltze and Antonio Garcia

Chapter 8 121
Metabolomics Distinction of Cigarette Smokers from Non-Smokers Using Non-Stationary Benchtop Nuclear Magnetic Resonance (NMR) Analysis of Human Saliva
by Benita C. Percival, Angela Wann, Sophie Taylor, Mark Edgar, Miles Gibson and Martin Grootveld

Chapter 9 145
Molecular Docking of Phytochemicals against *Streptococcus mutans* Virulence Targets: A Proteomic Insight into Drug Planning
by Diego Romário da Silva, Tahyná Duda Deps, Otavio Akira Souza Sakaguchi, Edja Maria Melo de Brito Costa, Carlus Alberto Oliveira dos Santos, Joanilda Paolla Raimundo e Silva, Bruna Dantas da Silva, Frederico Favaro Ribeiro, Francisco Jaime Bezerra Mendonça-Júnior and Andréa Cristina Barbosa da Silva

Section 2
Oral Health Management and Prevention **165**

Chapter 10 167
Oral Health Knowledge, Attitudes, and Behavior in Young Adults
by Ljiljana Kesic, Radmila Obradovic, Milica Petrovic, Marija Bojovic, Dragoslav Lazic, Branislava Stojkovic and Simona Stojanovic

Chapter 11 183
Upper Airway Expansion in Disabled Children
by David Andrade, Joana Andrade, Maria-João Palha, Cristina Areias, Paula Macedo, Ana Norton, Miguel Palha, Lurdes Morais, Dóris Rocha Ruiz and Sônia Groisman

Chapter 12 203
Oral Health and Prevention in Older Adults
by Irma Fabiola Díaz-García, Dinorah Munira Hernández-Santos, Julio Alberto Díaz-Ramos and Neyda Ma. Mendoza-Ruvalcaba

Chapter 13 223
Oral Aspects and Dental Management of Special Needs Patient
by Pinar Kiymet Karataban

Chapter 14 239
Oral Health Problems of Thai People Reported by Khon Kaen University Staffs during 1984 to 2020
by Amornrat Ratanasiri, Thitima Nutravong, Supaporn Chatrchaiwiwatana, Arisara Poosari, Thawalrat Ratanasiri and Kanokporn Wongchalee

Chapter 15 251
Management and Prevention Strategies for Treating Dentine Hypersensitivity
by David G. Gillam

Chapter 16 267
Preventive Methods and Treatments of White Spot Lesions in Orthodontics
by Elif Nadide Akay

Chapter 17 283
The Dental Implant Maintenance
by Gayathri Krishnamoorthy, Aparna I. Narayana and Dhanasekar Balakrishnan

Chapter 18 301
Herbs and Oral Health
by Zuhair S. Natto

Chapter 19 317
The Contrasting Effects between Caffeine and Theobromine on Crystallization: How the Non-fluoride Dentifrice Was Developed
by Tetsuo Nakamoto, Alexander U. Falster and William B. Simmons Jr

Chapter 20 339
Empirical Study on Medical Information and Communication Technology System in Dentistry in Southeast Asia
by Ichiro Nakajima, Ken-ichiro Ejima, Yoshinori Arai, Kunihito Matsumoto, Kazuya Honda, Hirofumi Aboshi, Marina Hamaguchi, Akao Lyvongsa, Bounnhong Sidaphone, Somphone Phanthavong, Chanthavisao Phanthanalay and Souksavanh Vongsa

Preface

Oral health is an essential part of human health and wellbeing. Oral health issues not only affect basic abilities such as eating, speaking, and smiling, but also self-esteem, school or job performance, and the chance of obtaining employment.

Oral diseases have a high prevalence. According to the World Health Organization, nearly 100% of the adult population has at least one cavity, and 20% suffer from severe gum disease.

Oral health issues, ranging from cavities to oral cancer, cause pain and disability. Edentulism may be considered the ultimate stage of oral suffering. Most oral diseases are preventable and can be treated in the early stages. Preventive methods include proper oral hygiene, regular dental checkups and cleaning, a healthy diet, limited sugar intake, and no smoking. Treatment, depending on the oral health issue, involves using a wide range of materials and techniques. All the materials for dental use are supposed to be biocompatible, their characteristics and properties being strongly dependent on their purpose. The currently available dental materials are in constant development, and techniques such as lasers, microscopy, and 3D-bioprinting are becoming more complex. Nowadays, even edentulism is a condition that can be treated effectively by means of dental implants.

The relationship between oral and general health is obvious, for example, certain medications (painkillers, antihistamines, diuretics, antidepressants, etc.) may reduce saliva flow and lead to oral problems. Alternatively, various diseases and conditions, such as endocarditis, cardiovascular disease, and pneumonia, are linked to oral bacteria and inflammation. Diabetes, AIDS, osteoporosis, eating disorders, and Alzheimer's also have a distinct influence on oral condition.

Lack of appropriate health facilities and limited access to primary oral health services is quite common in certain geographical areas. High costs of dental treatment may represent a major barrier for large categories of people. Targeted health programs and specific approaches are attempted to overcome these issues.

This book, consisting of twenty chapters, focuses on different aspects of oral health issues, including prevention, treatment, and management.

Lavinia Cosmina Ardelean
Department of Technology of Materials and Devices in Dental Medicine,
"Victor Babes" University of Medicine and Pharmacy Timisoara,
Timişoara, Romania

Laura Cristina Rusu
Department of Oral Pathology,
"Victor Babes" University of Medicine and Pharmacy Timisoara,
Timişoara, Romania

Section 1

Issues Related to the Health of Oral Environment

Chapter 1

Evaluation of Trans-Resveratrol as a Treatment for Periodontitis

Tracey Lynn Harney

Abstract

Periodontitis is a globally prevalent inflammation-mediated disease that can result in varying degrees of destruction to the tissues supporting the teeth. The microbial pathogenic dysbiosis, oxidative stress, and deregulated inflammation, found in patients with periodontitis, make it a multifaceted condition that is difficult to fully resolve. Further to this, periodontitis has been associated with other systemic inflammatory conditions. Trans-resveratrol (3,5,4′-trihydroxy-trans-stilbene) is a plant-derived molecule present in many foods, which have been shown to exhibit antimicrobial, antioxidant, anti-inflammatory, and regenerative properties. However, trans-resveratrol has been reported to have physicochemical shortcomings, which make its clinical translation a challenge. This review outlines a critical analysis of identified samples from the scientific literature that was conducted to assess the potential of RES as a viable therapeutic for periodontitis. The potential for the improvement of the limiting pharmacological profile of trans-resveratrol via nanoformulation is also explored.

Keywords: periodontitis, trans-resveratrol, nanotechnology, pharmacognosy, pharmacology

1. Introduction

Periodontal disease (PD) is a chronic condition accompanied by a progressive pathogenic biofilm that continuously triggers inflammation, potentially resulting in the loss of both soft and bony periodontal tissues. Ultimately, in severe cases, edentulism may result (**Figure 1**) [1].

Although aspects such as age, genetics, or sex can affect the chance of developing PD, there are also modifiable risk factors that have been identified. That is, smoking, nutrition (e.g., low vitamin D and calcium), and poorly managed diseases (e.g., diabetes, rheumatoid arthritis, and obesity) as well as stress, have also been found to play a significant role in susceptibility [2–4].

According to several epidemiological reports, the prevalence of PD is increasing over time. In fact, current publications indicate that approximately 10% of the global population presents with severe periodontitis, while almost half of the remaining 90% of all adults present with a less severe form of the disease. By and large, the most conservative estimate places the prevalence of PD at approximately 50% of the adult population worldwide [1, 5–7].

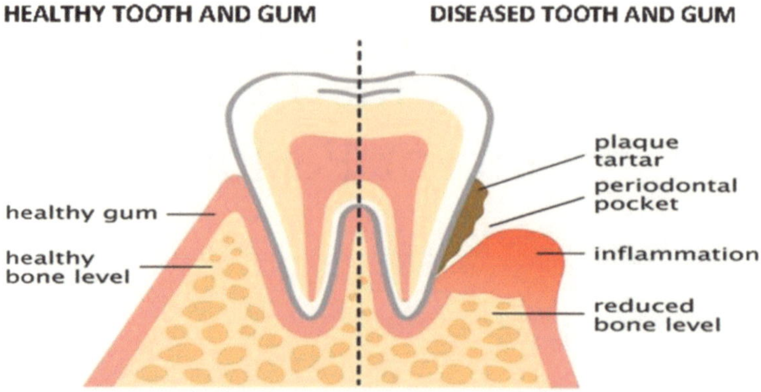

Figure 1.
An illustration of a healthy tooth and periodontal tissue (left side) compared to periodontal disease (right side).

Since people suffering from PD may experience chronic pain and tissue destruction, which can lead to anxiety and depression, the overall loss of quality of life has become an additional area of epidemiological observation. In fact, the deleterious impact of PD on wellness has recently been quantified using the index for Oral Health-Related Quality of Life (OHRQoL) and it was reported that the quality of life significantly decreases proportionally to the severity of PD [8, 9].

Additionally, PD has been found to have a widespread detrimental economic impact. For example, a recent study using accumulated data from the USA and 32 European countries, reported the approximate expenditure due to PD to be $154.06B in the USA, and 158.64B Euros in Europe [10].

Overall, a body of epidemiological evidence has emerged, reporting the increasing prevalence, economic burden, and diminished quality-of-life for a large enough portion of the global population, that PD has gained attention as growing concern of global proportion.

Although compiled review reports pertaining to the epidemiology of PD have been used as a benchmark, the distinction between gingivitis, mild to moderate PD, and more severe disease forms, has been inconsistent, creating a lack of comparability between and within the various epidemiological demographics [11].

Despite these steps towards unified categorisation, the ability to compare studies may still be diminished by the variation in classification of PD between clinicians and investigators [11–13].

2. Other inflammation-mediated conditions associated with PD

The conflicting reports, regarding the extent and severity of PD in the epidemiological literature, do not change the legitimate growing concern around the prevalence of the disease, especially when one considers the many inflammation-mediated systemic diseases with which it has been associated. For example, several reports indicate that PD can potentially increase the chance of developing heart disease [14–20], neurodegenerative disease [21–23], and autoimmune disease [24, 25] (**Figure 2**).

Further to this, chronic PD has been linked to a range of malignancies [26–30] and respiratory diseases [31–34] (**Figure 2**). Accordingly, the necessity for more ways to effectively prevent, manage, and treat PD, remains paramount.

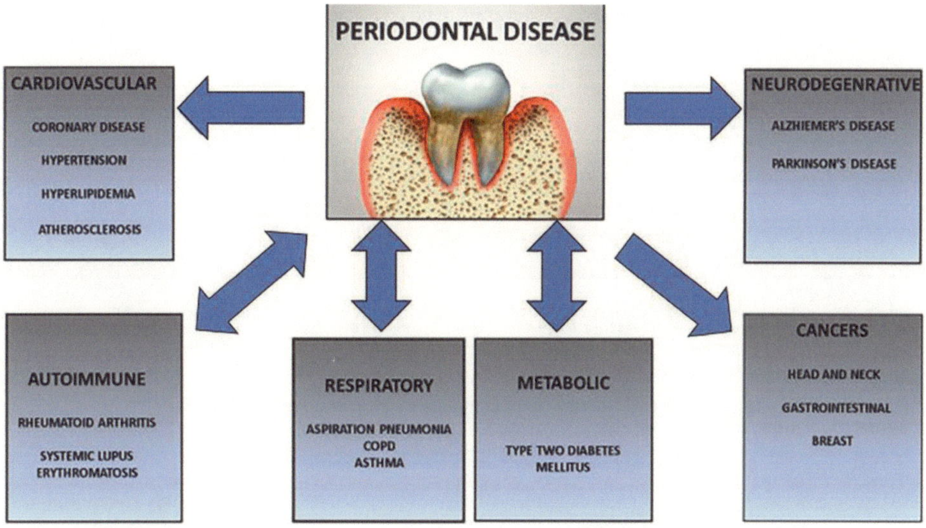

Figure 2.
An overview of some of the diseases that have been associated with PD.

3. Healthy periodontium and the pathogenesis of periodontitis

The periodontium consists of the tooth's surrounding anatomical structures, which include, from superficial to deep, the gingiva, gingival ligament, root cementum, and alveolar bone (**Figure 3**).

In a healthy periodontium, the supportive anatomical structures adhere to the tooth by way of connective and epithelial tissue types [35]. The epithelia exist as different subtypes around the erupted tooth and have been described as the first line of defence, protecting the underlying tissues of the periodontium from microbial infiltration from the oral cavity (**Figure 4**) [35]. The pathogenesis of PD first involves

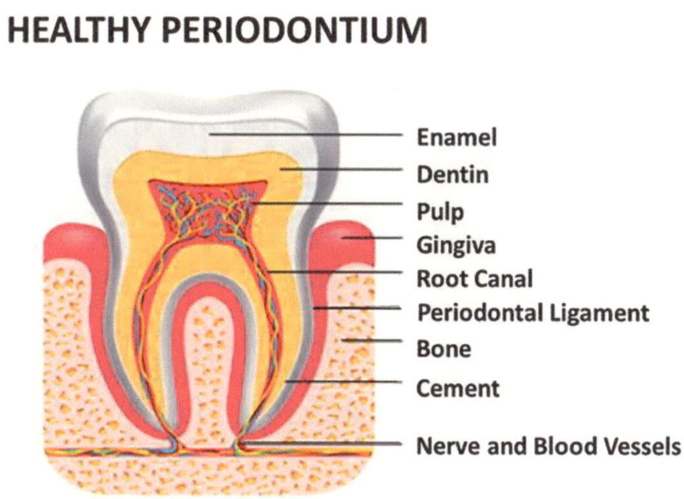

Figure 3.
An illustration of a healthy tooth and its surrounding structures (i.e., periodontium).

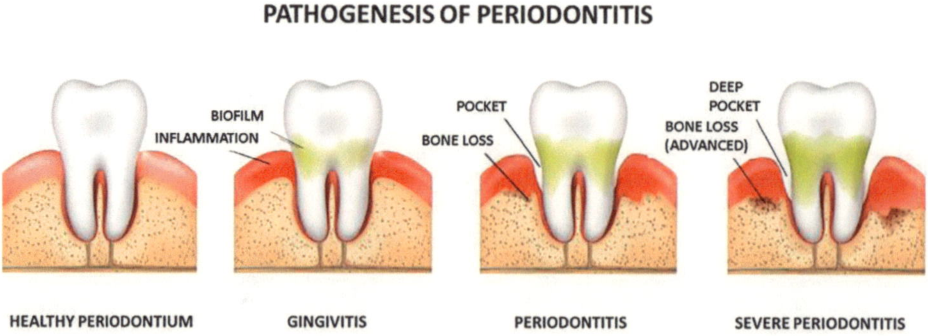

Figure 4.
An overview of the pathogenesis of PD starting with gingivitis progressing to severe PD.

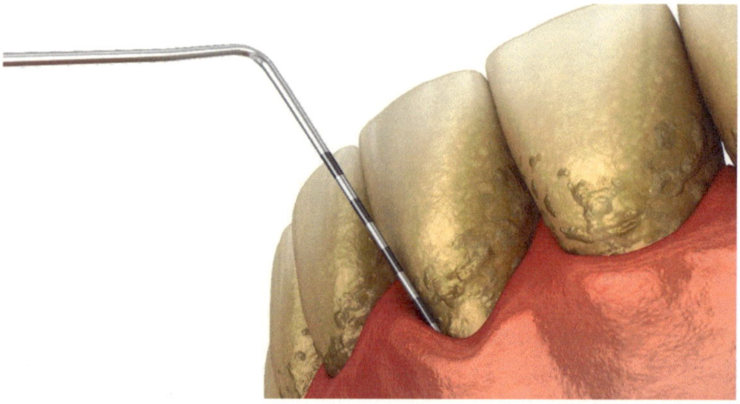

Figure 5.
Measuring of the depth of periodontal pockets with a probe is part of the diagnostic criteria predicting the severity of periodontal disease.

a shift in the oral milieu which optimizes the formation of a dysbiotic microbial biofilm, resulting gingival inflammation, which then progresses to the subgingival region (**Figure 4**) [36].

Clinically, people suffering from PD present with bleeding gingiva upon probing and varying degrees of detachment (i.e., clinical attachment loss [CAL]) of the gingiva from the tooth as measured with a periodontal probe (ada.org) (**Figure 5**).

4. Porphyromonas gingivalis and its central role in the pathogenesis of PD

Understanding further details of the disease process of PD from the perspective of the oral microbiome can assist in the creation of novel preventative and treatment applications.

Overall, bacteria, fungi, viruses, and protozoa are among the estimated 1000 microbial species that make up the oral microbiome. However, more than 700 microbes are bacterial, giving investigators a rationale for focusing on the bacterial taxa of the oral cavity, when examining health status [36–38].

Keystone pathogen, *P. gingivalis* (*Pg*), is a Gram-negative, anaerobic, non-motile, a-saccharolytic bacteria, which is a part of the normal flora of the subgingival region of the oral cavity, becomes an opportunistic pathogen when the microenvironmental factors permit it to thrive [39].

Also of note, is lipopolysaccharide (LPS), a feature found in the cell walls of Gram-negative bacteria, which triggers an inflammatory response as a pathogen-associated molecular pattern (PAMP). inflammation [40].

Detection by the host complement system is avoided due to the capsule, which is seen in most strains of *Pg* [41]. Also, the bacterial virulence factors, FimA and Mfa, which are proteins that make up the bacterial appendages, fimbriae, and pili, allow *Pg* to adhere to the periodontal cells whilst encouraging agglutination between bacteria, thus promoting the formation of a pathogenic biofilm [39, 42–44] (**Figure 6**).

Following adherence to the gingival epithelia, *Pg* can enter into its host cell with ease, due to the secretion of the serine phosphatase, SerB, which enters the host cell and triggers the de-polymerisation of cytoskeletal actin microfilaments [45] (**Figure 6**).

For increased success in gaining an intracellular foothold, *Pg* also employs a sophisticated secretory system (e.g., Type IX Secretory System [T9SS]), which spans the periplasmic space and allows for the passage of its secretory products from the cytoplasm into the extracellular environment [46, 47].

Further to this, gingipains are involved in the manipulation of the host immune system, making them key players in tissue destruction through chronic inflammation. For example, gingipains have been found to degrade many cytokines as well as the CD4 and CD8 integral membrane proteins of T lymphocytes, creating interference within the host's adaptive immune system [46, 48–50].

Moreover, an autoimmune attack on host tissue is assisted by the effector protein, peptidylarginine deaminase (PAD), which post-translationally modifies host proteins through citrullination, setting them up as immune targets [46, 51, 52] (**Figure 6**).

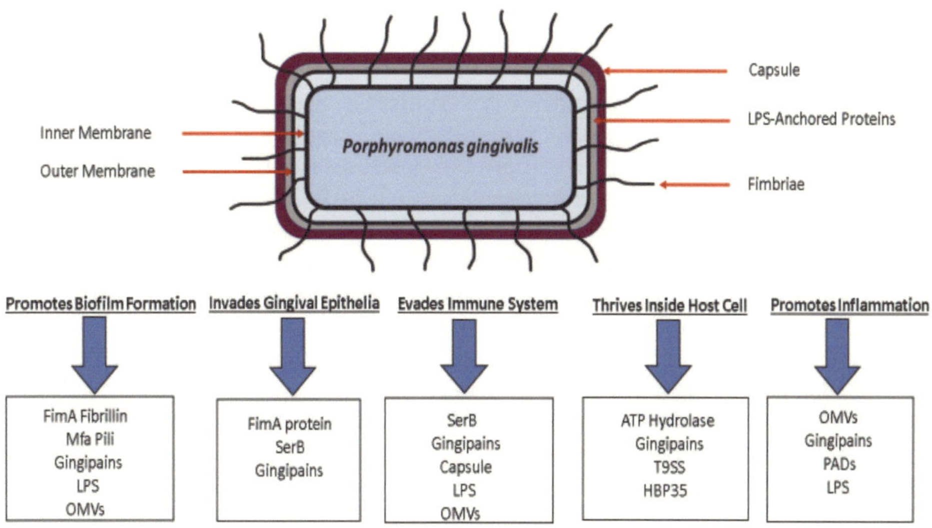

Figure 6.
A schematic of the major virulence factors of Porphyromonas gingivalis and a general overview of their involvement in pathogenicity.

Other significant virulence factors of *Pg* include outer membrane vesicles (OMVs), which are released from most Gram-negative bacteria and can infiltrate places that the bacteria cannot. However, those derived from *Pg*, are armed with an outer membrane layer, consisting of a capsule, LPS, and gingipains, enclosing an internal compartment loaded with effector proteins and other macromolecules such as nucleic acids. Indeed, OMVs are pro-inflammatory agents of cytotoxic destruction aiding in biofilm formation, as well as the manipulation and evasion of the host immune response [46, 53] (**Figure 6**).

5. *Pg* links to PD-related diseases

Common and frequent activities like mastication and oral care, have been found to release oral pathogens and their components into the lymphatic and cardiovascular systems of PD patients. Therefore, periodontal *Pg* infections likely act as pathogenic reservoirs, possibly promoting certain systemic diseases [52, 54].

5.1 Neurodegenerative disease

A 2021 study by Franciotii et al. hypothesised that there is a "bidirectional oral-brain" highway through which neurodegenerative processes are stimulated by pro-inflammatory oral processes and *vice versa* [55].

Most importantly, initiatives towards the innovation of preventative measures for PD have been recommended, especially since the global population is ageing [55].

5.2 Head and neck cancer

The reports regarding *Pg* infection as a risk factor for oral squamous cell and oesophageal carcinoma, align with the emerging perspective in the clinical arena linking chronic systemic inflammation to serious disease states [23, 56–59].

5.3 Cardiovascular disease

Regarding PD as it relates to cardiovascular disease, decades of literature reflect a close association [15, 19, 60]. DNA (i.e., 16S rDNA) from *Pg* has been identified in atheroma isolated from patients with coronary heart disease through PCR analysis [61]. Interestingly, *Pg* may also encourage atherosclerosis by switching HDL properties from antiatherogenic to proatherogenic via the manipulation of monocytes [62].

Further to this, *Pg* has been shown to invade and multiply within coronary endothelia *in vitro*, whilst damaging the smooth muscle cells and possibly distorting the vasodilatory mechanism of the central arterial system [63, 64].

Overall, the literature encourages appreciation of the clinical significance of the assault on the coronary endothelia demonstrated by *Pg*, especially since the vasculature acts as a vital line of defence for the cardiovascular system [63, 65].

5.4 Respiratory disease

Mortality risks from aspiration pneumonia are high in geriatric populations [66]. Of note, *in vitro* studies have identified *Pg* as a potent pro-inflammatory agent in isolated respiratory epithelia cells [67]. Additional *in vitro* studies identified *Pg*-derived OMVs as significant bacterial virulence factors which connect PD to respiratory disease [68].

5.5 Liver disease

It is worth noting that a significant correlation ($P < 0.05$) between non-alcoholic steatohepatitis (NASH) and oral *Pg*, has been reported. Furthermore, following treatment for PD, an improvement of liver function, displayed by the normalisation of AST and ALT, has been demonstrated [54, 69].

5.6 Diabetes mellitus

The relationship between PD and diabetes mellitus (DM) has also been studied with respect to *Pg*. For example, gingipains carried by OMVs derived from oral *Pg*, decreased the insulin sensitivity of hepatocytes whilst hepatocytes invaded by *Pg* were also found to display a decrease in glycogen synthesis *in vitro* (human) and *in vivo* (mouse model) [70].

5.7 Rheumatoid arthritis

DNA sequences from *Pg* have been isolated from the synovial fluid and bloodstream of patients with rheumatoid arthritis (RA). Further to this, the consistently reported relationship between an oral *Pg* infection and RA has encouraged medical clinicians to place more emphasis on the oral health of their patients [71].

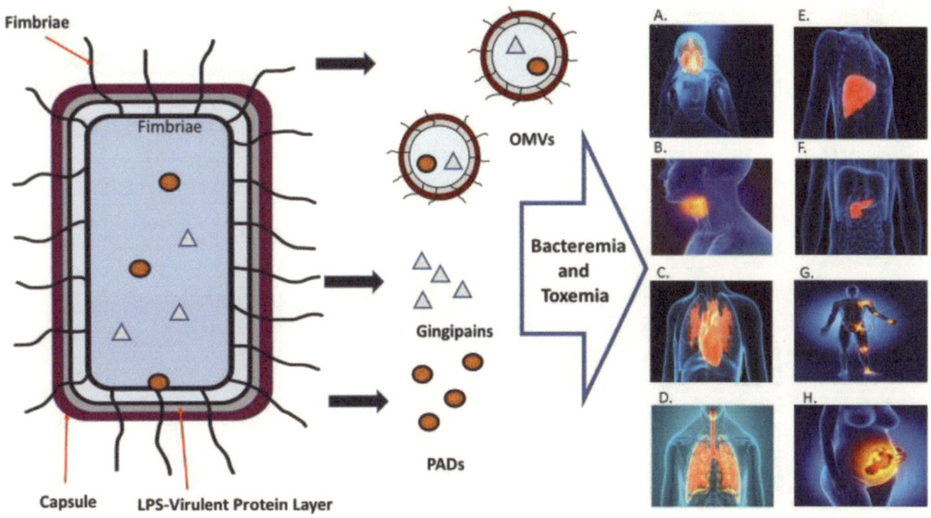

Figure 7.
The virulence factors of Pg and the systemic illnesses with which they have been associated. (A) Alzheimer's disease, Parkinson's disease, depression, (B) head and neck cancers, (C) atherosclerosis, myocardial infarction, aortic aneurism (D) aspiration pneumonia, (E) non-alcoholic fatty liver disease (NASH) (F) diabetes mellitus (G) rheumatoid arthritis (H) adverse pregnancy outcomes.

5.8 Adverse pregnancy outcomes

Pg DNA has also been detected in the amniotic fluid, umbilical cord, and placenta of women who encountered pregnancy complications such as preeclampsia and preterm birth [72]. Additionally, results from animal studies suggest that the mechanism involves the direct invasion and damage of the uterine and placental tissue [65].

The adage that correlation does not mean causation, should be considered, and although *Pg* cannot be the sole etiological agent of all the systemic diseases with which it is associated, there is accumulating evidence demonstrating its value as a modifiable risk factor for the prevention, management, and treatment of PD and other systemic diseases (**Figure 7**) [65].

6. Treatment of PD

Typically, treatment for periodontitis includes physical removal of the biofilm and calculus from under the gingiva by way of scaling and root planning (SRP) followed by comprehensive care (CC) (www.NHS.uk; www.ADA.org) (**Figure 8**). Whereas, in cases where more severe destruction has occurred, flap surgery is performed, which is often accompanied by expensive reconstructive treatments and/or procedures. In all cases of PD, patients are advised to adhere to lifelong CC to mitigate any further destruction [73–76].

Adjunct therapies are often combined to optimise results following SRP [76]. For example, one type of host modulation therapy (HMT) consisting of a sub-antimicrobial dose of doxycycline (SDD), is an internationally approved adjunct treatment for PD. SDD acts through the inhibition of the pathogenic collagenase activity in the host, thus decreasing inflammation and tissue destruction [77].

Interestingly, some naturally occurring phytonutrients also may work through the management of the host inflammatory response. For example, chemically modified curcumin has been shown to be safe and effective for the treatment of PD and other inflammation-mediated diseases in animal models [77–79]. Another bioactive phytonutrient of interest is trans-resveratrol, which in combination with curcumin, has been gaining attention as a supplement for the prevention and treatment of PD and other inflammation-mediated conditions [80].

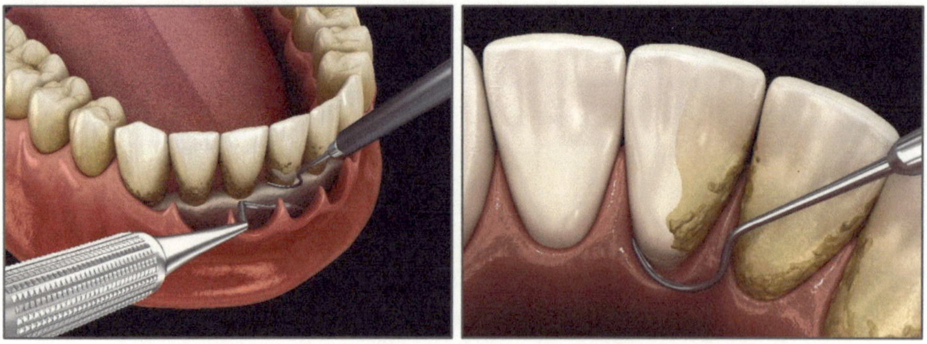

Figure 8.
Scaling and root planning with an open (left) and closed (right) curettage for the treatment of periodontitis.

DOI: http://dx.doi.org/10.5772/intechopen.101477

7. Resveratrol: a bioactive polyphenol with attractive medicinal properties

Trans-resveratrol (trans-3,5,4′-trihydroxystilbene) (RES) is a polyphenol that can be sourced from various edible plants, which has demonstrated antioxidant, anti-inflammatory, antimicrobial, anticancer, and restorative properties [81–84]. Therefore, RES is positioned in alignment with the treatment principles for PD and the diseases with which it has been associated (**Figure 9**).

Even though RES is found in a breadth of plant-based foods (e.g., red wine, berries, peanuts, and dark chocolate), the naturally occurring concentrations of RES are not substantial enough (e.g., 0.1–0.7 mg/L in red wine) to reasonably attain the therapeutic values reported in the scientific literature (e.g., an oral dose of approximately 10 mg/kg body) [86–88].

Consequently, the purified and optimised extracts of RES are often used in research and some products have been made commercially available as wellness supplements (https://megaresveratrol.net; https://biotivia.com/pages/transmax-tr-1).

However, RES is a hydrophobic molecule and therefore, like other promising phytotherapeutics such as curcumin, has poor water solubility (<0.05 mg/mL). RES has also been found to rapidly metabolise *in vivo* and revert to its less stable isomer when exposed to light, demonstrating its instability and photosensitivity, respectively [85].

Additionally, the low oral bioavailability of RES has been considered a significant obstacle to its clinical translation, resulting in the development of drug carrier models. In fact, there is ample evidence indicating that nano-formulation may be a successful strategy to improve the pharmacological indices of RES under physiological conditions [89–91].

Interestingly, the design of functional foods also includes the application of nanotechnology, via the incorporation of liposomal nanocarriers or other nano-encapsulated systems. In this way, the therapeutic potential of customised, effective, and stable fortified foods with specific pharmacokinetic parameters, such as steady time-release, can be investigated [92].

Indeed, both oral and buccal delivery systems, such as those possible via functional food design, have plausible applications regarding PD therapeutics, especially since the primary target area for treatment is in the oral cavity. In fact, many nano-formulations also aim to enhance the delivery and efficacy of targeted therapeutics by engineering combinations of selected bioactive molecules that offer specific properties that promise to optimise the probability of the desired treatment outcome [93].

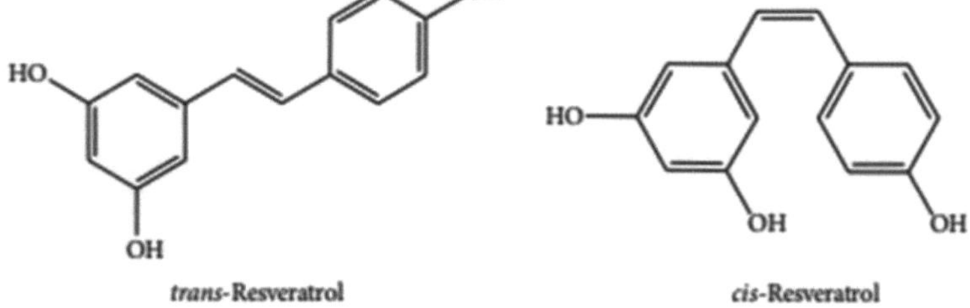

Figure 9.
The molecular structures of trans-resveratrol (trans-3,5,4′-trihydroxystilbene) (RES) (see left), which is the more stable, and therefore bioactive form compared to its isomer, cis-resveratrol (see right) (Gambini et al. [85]).

8. The attenuation of inflammatory processes by RES *in vitro*

The modulation of deregulated inflammation, which has been consistently reported for RES in the *in vitro* reports within the literature, is a central treatment principle for a viable therapeutic for PD. Additionally, *in vitro* studies allow for a breadth of experiment parameter manipulation not afforded by *in vivo* studies. So, although such studies cannot probe disease development and treatment, they can support the elucidation of mechanisms of action, thus identifying potential molecular targets for therapeutic applications.

For example, studies that used LPS-stimulated human gingival fibroblasts (HGFs), found through ELISA, and MTT assays, that RES significantly decreased IL-6 and IL-8, but did not increase cell viability. Interestingly, once RES was combined with the polyphenol silymarin (SIL), the viability increased in combination with the decrease in IL-6, IL-8 as well as TNF-α, suggesting that RES- ± SIL have a more widespread modulatory effect on LPS-induced inflammation [94, 95].

Additionally, in 2014, Fordham et al. examined the effect of RES (plus antioxidants, phloretin, silymarin, hesperetin) on LPS-stimulated peripheral blood mononuclear cells (PBMCs) obtained from healthy human donors. ELISA showed that RES decreased the secretion of IL-1β, IL-6, and IFN-γ in the LPS-induced PBMCs. Further to this, TNF-α was attenuated at the level of mRNA, as determined by RT-PCR. The researchers concluded that hesperetin and RES significantly inhibited ($p < 0.05$) the inflammatory response in LPS-stimulated PBMCs [96].

9. The influence of RES on regenerative processes in periodontal cells

RES has also shown promise regarding the restoration of periodontal tissue, which is a crucial part of the complete treatment of PD. For example, in a complex human *in vitro* and *in situ* study, Wang and colleagues reported that RES preserved cell aggregation and osteo-differentiation of normal human periodontal ligamental stem cells (HPLSCs) treated with TNF-α. In this study, histological analysis confirmed that RES treatment (even pre-implantation) improved regeneration in tissue originating from both healthy and pro-inflammatory microenvironments [97].

In accordance, Yuan and colleagues also found through histochemical analysis, RT-PCR, Western blot, and ELISA, that RES attenuated TNF-α – induced osteogenic suppression in HPLSCs *in vitro* [98].

10. RES as an attenuator of risk factors and conditions associated with PD

It has been well-established that PD is associated, to varying degrees, with a collection of modifiable risk factors as well as a myriad of systemic inflammation-mediated diseases [24, 99]. Hence, studies examining the effect of RES on PD in combination with purported comorbidity, and/or risk factor, could contribute to the argument regarding the breadth of its benefits.

Studies employing the integration of RA, DM, cigarette smoking, or osteoporosis (OP) into the induced-PD model have demonstrated that RES may assist in the mitigation of the periodontal damage contributed by associated risk factors and concomitant conditions. For example, with cigarette smoking added to the animal model, it was found that RES decreased both alveolar bone loss and oxidative stress [100, 101]. Additionally, using a ligature-induced PD model, RES was found to reduce alveolar bone loss and attenuate hyperglycemia in diabetic mice [102, 103].

Another study, which employed an induced-PD and RA animal model, determined immunoenzymatically, that both Ibuprofen and RES reduced the tissue levels of anti-cyclic citrullinated peptide antibody (ACCPA) by 99 and 72%, respectively ($p < 0.05$), and RES alone, was reported to reduce serum rheumatoid factor (RF) ($p < 0.05$) [101].

Interestingly, the results of a study that used an induced-PD model which concurrently induced osteoporosis (OP) by ovariectomising the rats, suggested that RES may reduce alveolar bone loss in oestrogen-deficient rats via the attenuation of nicotinamide adenine dinucleotide phosphate (NADPH) oxidase, making NADPH oxidase a potential drug target for RES [104].

Also of note, an extensive *in vitro* study showed the potential for RES to address *Pg*-related disease, with a particular focus on the prevention of Alzheimer's disease. Using a human *in vitro* model for neuroinflammation, Bahar and Singarao demonstrated that RES successfully modulated the ROS and deregulated inflammation. A total of 96 genes were analysed in *Pg* LPS-induced human neuroblastoma cells via qPCR followed by pathway analysis. In this way, RES was found to diminish NF-κB, neuroinflammatory acute phase pathways [105].

11. Animal studies: the amelioration of ligature-induced PD by RES

Although microbial dysbiosis is a necessary early occurrence in the pathogenesis of PD, the resulting chronic inflammation is the causal factor regarding its progression and continuous tissue destruction [106, 107]. Therefore, an effective therapeutic approach for the mitigation of PD would be to address the pathogenetically deregulated inflammatory pathways, mediators, and markers, encouraging the system to return to balance without deleterious side effects.

In a commonly used animal model, PD is induced by fitting a ligature around the neck of pre-selected molar teeth. Typically, PD that is induced in this way predictably presents with significant alveolar bone loss, accompanied by the increased expression of pro-inflammatory genes such as those for IL-1β, IL-6, and TNF-α. Notably, increased mRNA expression of genes coding for osteoclastogenic proteins and receptor activator of nuclear factor-k B ligand (RANKL) has also been reported when applying this model [108].

Morphometric analysis [27, 100, 101, 103, 109–111] and/or Micro-CT [104, 112–114] has been employed to demonstrate that RES reduced the alveolar bone loss from experimentally induced PD. The micro-CT analyses also reported improved bone density, suggesting that at the very least, RES has therapeutic potential as an adjunct to traditional SRP. This of course is caveated by emphasising the dependence of this data on the relevance of the PD animal model, and the need for validation with human studies.

12. Low bioavailability and stability: an obstacle to the clinical translation of RES

The poor water solubility of RES is well established. However, RES is highly stable in aqueous solutions of acidic pH. Moreover, researchers must consider that RES degrades rapidly in buffers of 7.4 pH or higher [115]. For example, RES incorporated into buffered cell medium was found to degrade to 50% of its original concentration within 24 h of incubation at 37°C [115]. Hence, many of the *in vitro* studies, which assume that the pre-determined RES concentration is consistent for the study duration, are likely to produce misleading results regarding therapeutic dose.

Research has emerged employing novel RES formulations to overcome the pharmacological limitations and optimise therapeutic potential, ultimately improving its clinical translation [116–119].

13. Overcoming therapeutic limitations of RES by the application of nanotechnology

RES has been reported as having notably poor water solubility as well as high sensitivity to heat and pH [115]. Also, since RES is unstable under physiological pH and temperature, *in vivo* assays are challenging to design and *in vitro* assays are likely to have low translatability [92, 120, 121].

Additionally, oral administration of RES has demonstrated unfavourable pharmacokinetics due to its extensive first pass, resulting in the accumulation of potentially recycled conjugates, RES-glucuronides, and RES-sulphates; although these metabolites have also been found to possess biological activity, it may not match that of the parental compound [85].

Previous reports highlighting the physicochemical limitations of RES indicate that meticulous consideration of aqueous solubility, pH, temperature, and light, during the experimental design phase is crucial for the optimisation of clinical translation [122].

Consequently, the search for effective strategies for the improvement of the limited oral bioavailability and stability, is a complex, yet necessary, undertaking for the successful development of RES as a therapeutic.

Regarding RES, improvement of one or more physicochemical and/or pharmacological parameters has been reported when in a nano form, indicating the potential of nanotechnological formulation as a viable strategy for improving its physicochemical stability and pharmacological profile.

Solid lipid nanoparticles (SLNs) and nanostructured lipid carriers (NLCs) are commonly employed to improve the therapeutic potential of hydrophobic drugs such as RES. Furthermore, findings that assessed the pharmacological potential of RES-loaded SLNs and NLCs, indicated their higher stability and sustained release compared to RES in its bulk form [123–128].

Further to this, studies seeking out to fortify and/or functionalise foods with RES, reported that nanoencapsulation substantially increased thermostability and photostability whilst retaining or optimising the desired biological activity. For example, an *in vitro* investigation examining the nano-encapsulation of RES in starch, conducted at pH 7.4 at 37° C, was reported to demonstrate an almost ten-fold increase in drug retention following a food extrusion process, as well as higher anti-diabetic, anti-obesity, and antioxidant effects, compared to bulk RES [129].

Similarly, the sustained release of RES from ZEIN-encapsulated nanoparticles (NPs) under physiological conditions (pH 7.4, 37°C) was reported [130] and casein-encapsulated RES NPs, designed by Penlava et al., were found to be stable through a continuous pH range mimicking those of the gastrointestinal compartments (i.e., pH 1.2 for 2 h and pH 6.8 for 2–24 h). Interestingly, the latter study also demonstrated *in vivo* (using rats), a ten-fold increase in oral availability of casein-nano-encapsulated RES compared to the bulk form as determined by blood plasma assays over a 24 h period following a single oral dose of 15 mg/kg of RES (in ddH_2O and PEG) or casein-encapsulated RES NPs [131].

These studies and others bring to light the prospect of the customisation of functional foods, to serve as both local and systemic delivery system for the effective prevention, management, and treatment of PD.

14. Restoration of tissue damage from PD: potential of current Nano RES formulations

Nano-RES formulations intended specifically for the treatment of PD, are only beginning to emerge. For example, Berta et al., reported a nano-formulated RES-cyclodextrin mouthwash that was found to reduce plaque and bleeding gums in children [132]. Nonetheless, there are several nano RES formulations, intended to treat other conditions, which could, in theory, be studied as potential formulations for PD, with little divergence from the original formula.

For example, in a 2021 study, Li and colleagues produced nano-hydroxyapatite-RES-chitosan (CS) microspheres for bone generation, which could potentially be used to restore bone loss due to PD [133].

Also, electrospun 3-D nano-scaffolds loaded with RES, consisting of a biodegradable polymer (PLA)-biopolymer-gelatin (GEL) nano-scaffold was found to repair cartilage defects in the rat model [134].

Notably, monodispersed, spherical chitosan-zinc oxide-RES (CS-ZnO-RES) nanoparticles (NP) (38 nm) engineered by Du et al., were reported to attenuate gestational DM (GDM) [135].

Moreover, the successful application of nano-RES as a potential treatment for AD has been reported by Sun et al., who designed a RES-loaded mesoporous selenium-Fc-β-cyclodextrin-Borneol nanoparticle that crossed a blood-brain barrier model [136].

15. RES has evolved to be a viable agent for the treatment of PD

RES has been shown to execute biological action that alleviates deregulated inflammation, and restores both soft and bony tissues, *in vitro*, and *in vivo*, via modulation on the genetic, protein, and cellular level, thus strengthening the case for RES as a therapeutic for PD. Further to this, improvement of the pharmacokinetic and physicochemical limitations of RES has been demonstrated via nanoformulation. There is now much work to be done in identifying and optimising the ideal nanoformulation and administration route to achieve optimal benefit from the activities RES has demonstrated.

Author details

Tracey Lynn Harney[1,2,3]

1 Nanotechnology for Medicine and Health Care from University of Oxford, Oxford, England, UK

2 United States of Consciousness Ltd, Paget, Bermuda

3 Biological Sciences at Bermuda College, Paget, Bermuda

*Address all correspondence to: tharney@college.bm

References

[1] Genco R, Sanz M. Clinical and public health implications of periodontal and systemic diseases: An overview. Periodontology 2000. 2020;**83**(1):7-13. DOI: 10.1111/prd.12344

[2] Genco R, Borgnakke W. Risk factors for periodontal disease. Periodontology 2000. 2013;**62**(1):59-94. DOI: 10.1111/j.1600-0757.2012.00457.x

[3] Peruzzo D, Benatti B, Ambrosano G, Nogueira-Filho G, et al. A systematic review of stress and psychological factors as possible risk factors for periodontal disease. Journal of Periodontology. 2007;**78**(8):1491-1504

[4] Reynolds M. Modifiable risk factors in periodontitis: At the intersection of aging and disease. Periodontology 2000. 2013;**64**(1):7-19

[5] Bernabe E, Marcenes W, Hernandez C, Bailey J, et al. Global, regional, and national levels and trends in burden of oral conditions from 1990 to 2017: A systematic analysis for the global burden of disease 2017 Study. Journal of Dental Research. 2020;**99**(4):362-373. DOI: 10.1177/0022034520908533

[6] Frencken J, Sharma P, Stenhouse L, Green D, et al. Global epidemiology of dental caries and severe periodontitis – A comprehensive review. Journal of Clinical Periodontology. 2017;**44**: 94-105. DOI: 10.3390/ma13112631

[7] Tonetti M, Jepsen S, Jin L, Otomo-Corgel J. Impact of the global burden of periodontal diseases on health, nutrition and wellbeing of mankind: A call for global action. Journal of Clinical Periodontology. 2017;**44**(5):456-462

[8] Buset S, Walter C, Friedmann A, Weiger R, et al. Are periodontal diseases really silent? A systematic review of their effect on quality of life. Journal of Clinical Periodontology. 2016;**43**(4): 333-344. DOI: 10.1111/jcpe.12517

[9] Duane B, Reynolds I. Periodontal disease has an impact on patients' quality of life. Evidence-Based Dentistry. 2018;**19**(1):14-15

[10] Botelho J, Machado V, Leira Y, Proença L, et al. Economic burden of periodontitis in the United States and Europe – An updated estimation. Journal of Periodontology. 2021. DOI: 10.1101/2021.01.19.21250090

[11] Papapanou P, Susin C. Periodontitis epidemiology: Is periodontitis under-recognized, over-diagnosed, or both? Periodontology 2000. 2017;**75**(1):45-51

[12] Baelum V, Lopez R. Epidemiology of periodontal diseases. In: Peres MA, Antunes JLF, Watt RG, editors. A Textbook on Oral Health Conditions, Research Topics and Methods. Cham: Springer; 2021. pp. 55-57

[13] Papapanou P. The prevalence of periodontitis in the us. Journal of Dental Research. 2012;**91**(10):907-908

[14] Agarwal S. Impact of periodontitis on cardiovascular diseases. European Journal of Dental and Oral Health. 2021;**2**(2):1-8. DOI: 10.24018/EJDENT.2021.2.2.48

[15] Bengtsson V, Persson G, Berglund J, Renvert S. Periodontitis related to cardiovascular events and mortality: A long-time longitudinal study. Clinical Oral Investigations. 2021;**25**(6):4085-4095. DOI: 10.1007/s00784-020-03739-x

[16] Bodanese L, Louzeiro G, Magnus G, Baptista Â, et al. Association between

periodontitis and myocardial infarction: Systematic review and meta-analysis. International Journal of Cardiovascular Sciences. 2021;**34**(5Supl.1):121-127

[17] Sia S, Jan M, Wang Y, Huang Y, Wei J. Periodontitis is associated with incidental valvular heart disease: A nationwide population-based cohort study. Journal of Clinical Periodontology. 2021;**48**(8): 1085-1092

[18] Surma S, Romańczyk M, Witalińska-Łabuzek J, Czerniuk M, et al. Periodontitis, blood pressure, and the risk and control of arterial hypertension: Epidemiological, clinical, and pathophysiological aspects – Review of the literature and clinical trials. Current Hypertension Reports. 2021;**23**(5). DOI: 10.1007/s11906-021-01140-x

[19] Tiensripojamarn N, Lertpimonchai A, Tavedhikul K, Udomsak A, et al. Periodontitis is associated with cardiovascular diseases: A 13-year study. Journal of Clinical Periodontology. 2021;**48**(3):348-356

[20] Trindade F, Perpétuo L, Ferreira R, Leite-Moreira A, et al. Automatic text-mining as an unbiased approach to uncover molecular associations between periodontitis and coronary artery disease. Biomarkers. 2021;**26**(5):385-394

[21] Abbayya K, Chidambar Y, Naduwinmani S, Puthanakar N. Association between periodontitis and alzheimer's disease. North American Journal of Medical Sciences. 2015;**7**(6): 241. DOI: 10.4103/1947-2714.159325

[22] Cerajewska T, Davies M, West N. Periodontitis: A potential risk factor for Alzheimer's disease. British Dental Journal. 2015;**218**(1):29-34. DOI: 10.1038/sj.bdj.2014.1137

[23] Olsen I, Yilmaz Ö. Possible role of *porphyromonas gingivalis* in oro-digestive cancers. Journal of Oral Microbiology. 2019;**11**(1):1563410. DOI: 10.1080/20002297.2018.1563410

[24] Bae S, Lee Y. Causal association between periodontitis and risk of rheumatoid arthritis and systemic lupus erythematosus: A Mendelian randomization. Zeitschrift für Rheumatologie. 2020;**79**(9):929-936. DOI: 10.1007/s00393-019-00742-w

[25] Bolstad A, Sehjpal P, Lie S, Fevang B. Periodontitis in patients with systemic lupus erythematosus: A nation-wide study of 1990 patients. Journal of Periodontology. 2021:1-8. DOI: 10.1002/JPER.21-0181

[26] Krishnasree R, Jayanthi P, Karthika P, Nandhakumar K, Rathy R. Association of chronic periodontitis and oral cancer: A review on pathogenetic mechanism and clinical implication. Journal of Dr NTR University of Health Sciences. 2020;**9**:209-212

[27] Chen P, Chen Y, Lin C, Yeh Y, et al. Effect of periodontitis and scaling and root planing on risk of pharyngeal cancer: A nested case-control study. International Journal of Environmental Research and Public Health. 2020;**18**(1):8. DOI: 10.3390/ijerph18010008

[28] Ma H, Zheng J, Li X. Potential risk of certain cancers among patients with periodontitis: A supplementary meta-analysis of a large-scale population. International Journal of Medical Sciences. 2020;**17**(16):2531-2543

[29] Vedamanickam S. Microbiological assessment in plaque samples of patients with oral cancer with or without smoking. Annals of the Romanian Society for Cell Biology. 2021;**25**(1):5294-5301

[30] Zhang Y, He J, He B, Huang R, Li M. Effect of tobacco on periodontal disease

and oral cancer. Tobacco Induced Diseases. 2019;**17**(May):1-15. DOI: 10.18332/tid/106187

[31] Candeo L, Rigonato-Oliveira N, Brito A, Marcos R, et al. Effects of periodontitis on the development of asthma: The role of photodynamic therapy. PLoS One. 2017;**12**(11):187945. DOI: 10.1371/journal.pone.0187945

[32] Gomes-Filho I, Cruz S, Trindade S, Passos-Soares J, et al. Periodontitis and respiratory diseases: A systematic review with meta-analysis. Oral Diseases. 2019;**26**(2):439-446. DOI: 10.1111/odi.13228

[33] Marouf N, Cai W, Said K, Daas H, et al. Association between periodontitis and severity of COVID-19 infection: A case-control study. Journal of Clinical Periodontology. 2021;**48**(4):483-491

[34] Soledade-Marques K, Gomes-Filho I, da Cruz S, Passos-Soares J, et al. Association between periodontitis and severe asthma in adults: A case-control study. Oral Diseases. 2017;**24**(3):442-448

[35] Harris S, Rakian A, Foster B, Chun Y, Rakian R. The periodontium. Principles of Bone Biology. 2020:1061-1082. DOI: 10.1016/B978-0-12-814841-9.00043-9

[36] Berger D, Rakhamimova A, Pollack A, Loewy Z, et al. Oral biofilms: Development, control, and analysis. High-Throughput. 2018;7(3):24. DOI: 10.3390/ht7030024

[37] Deo P, Deshmukh R. Oral microbiome: Unveiling the fundamentals. Journal of Oral and Maxillofacial Pathology. 2019;**23**(1):122-128. DOI: 10.4103/jomfp.JOMFP_304_18

[38] Radaic A, Kapila Y. The oralome and its dysbiosis: New insights into oral microbiome-host interactions. Computational and Structural Biotechnology Journal. 2021;**19**:1335-1360

[39] Nagano K, Hasegawa Y, Iijima Y, Kikuchi T, Mitani A. Distribution of *porphyromonas gingivalis* fimA and mfa1fimbrial genotypes in subgingival plaques. PeerJ. 2018;**6**:5581. DOI: 10.7717/peerj.5581

[40] Matsuura M. Structural modifications of bacterial lipopolysaccharide that facilitate gram-negative bacteria evasion of host innate immunity. Frontiers in Immunology. 2013;**4**:1-9. DOI: 10.3389/fimmu.2013.00109

[41] Singh A, Wyant T, Anaya-Bergman C, Aduse-Opoku J, et al. The capsule of *porphyromonas gingivalis* leads to a reduction in the host inflammatory response, evasion of phagocytosis, and increase in virulence. Infection and Immunity. 2011;**79**(11):4533-4542

[42] Gully N, Bright R, Marino V, Marchant C, et al. *Porphyromonas gingivalis* peptidylarginine deiminase, a key contributor in the pathogenesis of experimental periodontal disease and experimental arthritis. PLoS One. 2014;**9**(6):100838. DOI: 10.1371/journal.pone.0100838

[43] Kuboniwa M, Amano A, Hashino E, Yamamoto Y, et al. Distinct roles of long/short fimbriae and gingipains in homotypic biofilm development by *porphyromonas gingivalis*. BMC Microbiology. 2009;**9**(1):105

[44] Ikai R, Hasegawa Y, Izumigawa M, Nagano K, et al. Mfa4, an accessory protein of mfa1 fimbriae, modulates fimbrial biogenesis, cell auto-aggregation, and biofilm formation in *porphyromonas gingivalis*. PLoS One. 2015;**10**(10):0139454

[45] Hajishengallis G, Lamont R. Breaking bad: Manipulation of the host response

byPorphyromonas gingivalis. European Journal of Immunology. 2014;**44**(2):328-338

[46] Lunar Silva I, Cascales E. Molecular Strategies Underlying Porphyromonas gingivalis Virulence. Journal of Molecular Biology. 2021;**433**(7):166836

[47] Vincent M, Canestrari M, Leone P, Stathopulos J, et al. Characterization of the *porphyromonas gingivalis* type IX secretion Trans-envelope por KLMNP core complex. Journal of Biological Chemistry. 2017;**292**(8):3252-3261

[48] Dahlen G, Basic A, Bylund J. Importance of virulence factors for the persistence of oral bacteria in the inflamed gingival crevice and in the pathogenesis of periodontal disease. Journal of Clinical Medicine. 2019;**8**(9):1339. DOI: 10.3390/jcm8091339

[49] de Diego I, Veillard F, Sztukowska M, Guevara T, et al. Structure and mechanism of cysteine peptidase gingipain K (Kgp): A major virulence factor of *porphyromonas gingivalis* in periodontitis. Journal of Biological Chemistry. 2014;**289**(46):32291-32302. DOI: 10.1074%2Fjbc.M114.602052

[50] Jia L, Han N, Du J, Guo L, et al. Pathogenesis of important virulence factors of *porphyromonas gingivalis* via toll-like receptors. Frontiers in Cellular and Infection Microbiology. 2019;**9**:1-14. DOI: 10.3389/fcimb.2019.00262

[51] Aliko A, Kamińska M, Bergum B, Gawron K, et al. Impact of *porphyromonas gingivalis* peptidylarginine deiminase on bacterial biofilm formation, epithelial cell invasion, and epithelial cell transcriptional landscape. Scientific Reports. 2018;**8**(1):1-9. DOI: 10.1038/s41598-018-32603-y

[52] Mulhall H, Huck O, Amar S. *Porphyromonas gingivalis*, a long-range pathogen: Systemic impact and therapeutic implications. Microorganisms. 2020;**8**(6):869. DOI: 10.3390/microorganisms8060869

[53] De Andrade K, Almeida-da-Silva C, Coutinho-Silva R. Immunological pathways triggered by *porphyromonas gingivalis* and fusobacterium nucleatum: Therapeutic possibilities? Mediators of Inflammation. 2019:1-20. DOI: 10.1155/2019/7241312

[54] Zhang Z, Liu D, Liu S, Zhang S, Pan Y. The role of *porphyromonas gingivalis* outer membrane vesicles in periodontal disease and related systemic diseases. Frontiers in Cellular and Infection Microbiology. 2021;**10**:1-12. DOI: 10.3389/fcimb.2020.585917

[55] Franciotti R, Pignatelli P, Carrarini C, Romei F, et al. Exploring the connection between *porphyromonas gingivalis* and neurodegenerative diseases: A pilot quantitative study on the bacterium abundance in oral cavity and the amount of antibodies in serum. Biomolecules. 2021;**11**(6):845. DOI: 10.3390/biom11060845

[56] Gopinath D, Menon R, K Veettil S, Botelho M, et al. Periodontal diseases as putative risk factors for head and neck cancer: Systematic review and meta-analysis. Cancers. 2020;**12**(7):1893. DOI: 10.3390/cancers12071893

[57] Kong L, Qi X, Huang S, Chen S, et al. Theaflavins inhibit pathogenic properties of *P. gingivalis* and MMPs production in *P. gingivalis*-stimulated human gingival fibroblasts. Archives of Oral Biology. 2015;**60**(1):12-22

[58] Liu X, Gao Z, Sun C, Wen H, et al. The potential role of *P. gingivalis* in

gastrointestinal cancer: A mini review. Infectious Agents and Cancer. 2019;**14**(1). DOI: 10.1186/s13027-019-0239-4

[59] Ibáñez L, de Mendoza I, Maritxalar Mendia X, García de la Fuente A, Quindós Andrés G, Aguirre Urizar J. Role of *porphyromonas gingivalis* in oral squamous cell carcinoma development: A systematic review. Journal of Periodontal Research. 2019;**55**(1):13-22

[60] Dorn B, Dunn W, Progulske-Fox A. *Porphyromonas gingivalis* traffics to autophagosomes in human coronary artery endothelial cells. Infection and Immunity. 2001;**69**(9):5698-5708. DOI: 10.1128/IAI.69.9.5698-5708.2001

[61] Rao A, D'Souza C, Subramanyam K, Rai P, Thomas B, Gopalakrishnan M, et al. Molecular analysis shows the presence of periodontal bacterial DNA in atherosclerotic plaques from patients with coronary artery disease. Indian Heart Journal. 2021;**73**(2):218-220

[62] Kim H, Cha G, Kim H, Kwon E, et al. *Porphyromonas gingivalis* accelerates atherosclerosis through oxidation of high-density lipoprotein. Journal of Periodontal & Implant Science. 2018;**48**(1):60

[63] Fiorillo L, Cervino G, Laino L, D'Amico C, et al. *Porphyromonas gingivalis*, periodontal and systemic implications: A systematic review. Dentistry Journal. 2019;7(4):114. DOI: 10.3390/dj7040114

[64] Sun W, Wu J, Lin L, Huang Y, et al. *Porphyromonas gingivalis* stimulates the release of nitric oxide by inducing expression of inducible nitric oxide synthases and inhibiting endothelial nitric oxide synthases. Journal of Periodontal Research. 2010;**45**(3): 381-388

[65] Mei F, Xie M, Huang X, Long Y, et al. *Porphyromonas gingivalis* and its systemic impact: Current status. Pathogens. 2020;**9**(11):944. DOI: 10.3390/pathogens9110944

[66] Pace C, McCullough G. The association between oral microorgansims and aspiration pneumonia in the institutionalized elderly: Review and recommendations. Dysphagia. 2010;**25**(4):307-322. DOI: 10.1007/s00455-010-9298-9

[67] Takahashi T, Muro S, Tanabe N, Terada K, et al. Relationship between periodontitis-related antibody and frequent exacerbations in chronic obstructive pulmonary disease. PLoS One. 2012;**7**(7):40570. DOI: 10.1371/journal.pone.0040570

[68] He Y, Shiotsu N, Uchida-Fukuhara Y, Guo J, et al. Outer membrane vesicles derived from *porphyromonas gingivalis* induced cell death with disruption of tight junctions in human lung epithelial cells. Archives of Oral Biology. 2020;**118**: 104841. DOI: 10.1016/j.archoralbio.2020.104841

[69] Yoneda M, Naka S, Nakano K, Wada K, et al. Involvement of a periodontal pathogen, *porphyromonas gingivalis* on the pathogenesis of non-alcoholic fatty liver disease. BMC Gastroenterology. 2012;**12**(1). DOI: 10.1186/1471-230X-12-16

[70] Seyama M, Yoshida K, Yoshida K, Fujiwara N, et al. Outer membrane vesicles of *porphyromonas gingivalis* attenuate insulin sensitivity by delivering gingipains to the liver. Biochimica et Biophysica Acta (BBA) – Molecular Basis of Disease. 2020;**1866**(6):165731. DOI: 10.1016/j.bbadis.2020.165731

[71] Kriauciunas A, Gleiznys A, Gleiznys D, Janužis G. The influence of

porphyromonas gingivalis bacterium causing periodontal disease on the pathogenesis of rheumatoid arthritis: Systematic review of literature. Cureus. 2019;**11**(5):e4775. DOI: 10.7759/cureus.4775

[72] Chopra A, Radhakrishnan R, Sharma M. *Porphyromonas gingivalis*and adverse pregnancy outcomes: A review on its intricate pathogenic mechanisms. Critical Reviews in Microbiology. 2020;**46**(2):213-236. DOI: 10.1080/1040841X.2020.1747392

[73] Ramanauskaite E, Machiulskiene V. Antiseptics as adjuncts to scaling and root planing in the treatment of periodontitis: a systematic literature review. BMC Oral Health. 2020;**20**:143. DOI: 10.1186/s12903-020-01127-1

[74] Sanz-Martín I, Cha J, Yoon S, Sanz-Sánchez I, Jung U. Long-term assessment of periodontal disease progression after surgical or non-surgical treatment: A systematic review. Journal of Periodontal and Implant Science. 2019;**49**(2):60

[75] Suvan J, Leira Y, Moreno Sancho F, Graziani F, et al. Subgingival instrumentation for treatment of periodontitis. A systematic review. Journal of Clinical Periodontology. 2020;**47**(S22):155-175

[76] Tan O, Safii S, Razali M. Commercial local pharmacotherapeutics and adjunctive agents for nonsurgical treatment of periodontitis: A contemporary review of clinical efficacies and challenges. Antibiotics. 2019;**9**(1):1. DOI: 10.3390/antibiotics9010011

[77] Golub L, Lee H. Periodontal therapeutics: Current host-modulation agents and future directions. Periodontology 2000. 2019;**82**(1):186-204. DOI: 10.1111/prd.12315

[78] Curylofo-Zotti F, Elburki M, Oliveira P, Cerri P, et al. Differential effects of natural curcumin and chemically modified curcumin on inflammation and bone resorption in model of experimental periodontitis. Archives of Oral Biology. 2018;**91**:42-50

[79] Deng J, Golub L, Lee H, Lin M, et al. Chemically modified curcumin: A novel systemic therapy for natural periodontitis in dogs. Journal of Experimental Pharmacology. 2020;**12**:47-60. DOI: 10.2147%2FJEP.S236792

[80] Bisht K, Wagner K, Bulmer A. Curcumin, resveratrol and flavonoids as anti-inflammatory, cyto- and DNA-protective dietary compounds. Toxicology. 2010;**278**(1):88-100. DOI: 10.1016/j.tox.2009.11.008

[81] Gorbunov N, Petrovski G, Gurusamy N, Ray D, et al. Regeneration of infarcted myocardium with resveratrol-modified cardiac stem cells. Journal of Cellular and Molecular Medicine. 2011;**16**(1):174-184

[82] Meng T, Xiao D, Muhammed A, Deng J, et al. Anti-inflammatory action and mechanisms of resveratrol. Molecules. 2021;**26**(1):229. DOI: 10.3390/molecules26010229

[83] Murgia D, Mauceri R, Campisi G, De Caro V. Advance on resveratrol application in bone regeneration: Progress and perspectives for use in oral and maxillofacial surgery. Biomolecules. 2019;**9**(3):94. DOI: 10.3390/biom9030094

[84] Perrone D, Fuggetta M, Ardito F, Cottarelli A, et al. Resveratrol (3,5,4′-trihydroxystilbene) and its properties in oral diseases. Experimental and Therapeutic Medicine. 2017;**14**(1):3-9

[85] Gambini J, Inglés M, Olaso G, Lopez-Grueso R, et al. Properties of resveratrol: In vitro and in vivo studies about metabolism, bioavailability, and biological effects in animal models and humans. Oxidative Medicine and Cellular Longevity. 2015:1-13. DOI: 10.1155/2015/837042

[86] Giovinazzo G, Grieco F. Functional properties of grape and wine polyphenols. Plant Foods for Human Nutrition. 2015;**70**(4):454-462. DOI: 10.1007/s11130-015-0518-1

[87] Salehi B, Mishra A, Nigam M, Sener B, et al. Resveratrol: A double-edged sword in health benefits. Biomedicine. 2018;**6**(3):91. DOI: 10.3390/biomedicines6030091

[88] Weiskirchen S, Weiskirchen R. Resveratrol: How much wine do you have to drink to stay healthy? Advances in Nutrition: An International Review Journal. 2016;**7**(4):706-718

[89] Jose S, Anju S, Cinu T, Aleykutty N, et al. In vivo pharmacokinetics and biodistribution of resveratrol-loaded solid lipid nanoparticles for brain delivery. International Journal of Pharmaceutics. 2014;**474**(1-2):6-13

[90] Pandita D, Kumar S, Poonia N, Lather V. Solid lipid nanoparticles enhance oral bioavailability of resveratrol, a natural polyphenol. Food Research International. 2014;**62**:1165-1174

[91] Summerlin N, Soo E, Thakur S, Qu Z, et al. Resveratrol nanoformulations: Challenges and opportunities. International Journal of Pharmaceutics. 2015;**479**(2):282-290

[92] Singh A, Ahmad I, Ahmad S, Iqbal Z, Ahmad F. A novel monolithic controlled delivery system of resveratrol for enhanced hepatoprotection: Nanoformulation development, pharmacokinetics, and pharmacodynamics. Drug Development and Industrial Pharmacy. 2016;**42**(9): 1524-1536

[93] Jeong H, Samdani K, Yoo D, Lee D, et al. Resveratrol cross-linked chitosan loaded with phospholipid for controlled release and antioxidant activity. International Journal of Biological Macromolecules. 2016;**93**:757-766

[94] Farzanegan A, Shokuhian M, Jafari S, Shirazi F, Shahidi M. Anti-histaminic effects of resveratrol and silymarin on human gingival fibroblasts. Inflammation. 2019;**42**(5):1622-1629. DOI: 10.1007/s10753-019-01023-z

[95] Shahidi M, Vaziri F, Haerian A, Farzanegan A, et al. Proliferative and anti-inflammatory effects of resveratrol and silymarin on human gingival fibroblasts: A view to the future. Journal of dentistry (Tehran, Iran). 2017;**14**(4): 203-211

[96] Fordham J, Raza Naqvi A, Nares S. Leukocyte production of inflammatory mediators is inhibited by the antioxidants phloretin, silymarin, hesperetin, and resveratrol. Mediators of Inflammation. 2014:1-11. DOI: 10.1155/2014/938712

[97] Wang Y, Zhao P, Sui B, Liu N, et al. Resveratrol enhances the functionality and improves the regeneration of mesenchymal stem cell aggregates. Experimental and Molecular Medicine. 2018;**50**(6):1-15

[98] Yuan J, Wang X, Ma D, Gao H, et al. Resveratrol rescues TNF α induced inhibition of osteogenesis in human periodontal ligament stem cells via the ERK1/2 pathway. Molecular Medicine Reports. 2020;**21**:2085-2094. DOI: 10.3892/mmr.2020.11021

[99] Hajishengallis G, Chavakis T. Local and systemic mechanisms linking periodontal disease and inflammatory comorbidities. Nature Reviews Immunology. 2021;**21**:426-440. DOI: 10.1038/s41577-020-00488-6

[100] Ribeiro F, Pino D, Franck F, Benatti B, et al. Resveratrol inhibits periodontitis-related bone loss in rats subjected to cigarette smoke inhalation. Journal of Periodontology. 2017;**88**(8): 788-798

[101] Corrêa M, Pires P, Ribeiro F, Pimentel S, et al. Systemic treatment with resveratrol reduces the progression of experimental periodontitis and arthritis in rats. PLoS One. 2018;**13**(10):204414. DOI: 10.1371/journal.pone.0204414

[102] Ashour A, Xue M, Al-Motawa M, Thornalley P, Rabbani N. Glycolytic overload-driven dysfunction of periodontal ligament fibroblasts in high glucose concentration, corrected by glyoxalase 1 inducer. BMJ Open Diabetes Research and Care. 2020;**8**(2):1458. DOI: 10.1136/bmjdrc-2020-001458

[103] Zhen L, Fan D, Zhang Y, Cao X, Wang L. Resveratrol ameliorates experimental periodontitis in diabetic mice through negative regulation of TLR4 signaling. Acta Pharmacologica Sinica. 2014;**36**(2):221-228

[104] Molez A, Nascimento E, Haiter Neto F, Cirano F, et al. Effect of resveratrol on the progression of experimental periodontitis in an ovariectomized rat model of osteoporosis: Morphometric, immune-enzymatic, and gene expression analysis. Journal of Periodontal Research. 2020;**55**(6):840-849

[105] Bahar B, Singhrao S. An evaluation of the molecular mode of action of trans-resveratrol in the *porphyromonas gingivalis* lipopolysaccharide challenged neuronal cell model. Molecular Biology Reports. 2020;**48**(1):147-156. DOI: 10.1007%2Fs11033-020-06024-y

[106] Delima A, Karatzas S, Amar S, Graves D. Inflammation and tissue loss caused by periodontal pathogens is reduced by interleukin-1 antagonists. The Journal of Infectious Diseases. 2002; **186**(4):511-516. DOI: 10.1086/341778

[107] Könönen E, Gursoy M, Gursoy U. Periodontitis: A multifaceted disease of tooth-supporting tissues. Journal of Clinical Medicine. 2019;**8**(8):1135. DOI: 10.3390/jcm8081135

[108] De Molon R, Park C, Jin Q, Sugai J, Cirelli J. Characterization of ligature-induced experimental periodontitis. Microscopy Research and Technique. 2018;**81**(12):1412-1421. DOI: 10.1002/jemt.23101

[109] Casati M, Algayer C, Cardoso da Cruz G, Ribeiro F, et al. Resveratrol decreases periodontal breakdown and modulates local levels of cytokines during periodontitis in rats. Journal of Periodontology. 2013;**84**(10):58-64. DOI: 10.1902/jop.2013.120746

[110] Corrêa M, Pires P, Ribeiro F, Pimentel S, et al. Systemic treatment with resveratrol and/or curcumin reduces the progression of experimental periodontitis in rats. Journal of Periodontal Research. 2016;**52**(2):201-209. DOI: 10.1111/jre.12382

[111] Corrêa M, Absy S, Tenenbaum H, Ribeiro F, et al. Resveratrol attenuates oxidative stress during experimental periodontitis in rats exposed to cigarette smoke inhalation. Journal of Periodontal Research. 2019;**54**(3):225-232. DOI: 10.1111/jre.12622

[112] Adhikari N, Prasad Aryal Y, Jung J, Ha J, et al. Resveratrol enhances bone formation by modulating inflammation in the mouse periodontitis model. Journal of Periodontal Research. 2021;**56**(4): 735-745. DOI: 10.1111/jre.12870

[113] Bhattarai G, Poudel S, Kook S, Lee J. Resveratrol prevents alveolar bone loss in an experimental rat model of periodontitis. Acta Biomaterialia. 2016;**29**:398-408. DOI: 10.1016/j.actbio.2015.10.031

[114] Tamaki N, Cristina Orihuela-Campos R, Inagaki Y, Fukui M, et al. Resveratrol improves oxidative stress and prevents the progression of periodontitis via the activation of the Sirt1/AMPK and the Nrf2/antioxidant defense pathways in a rat periodontitis model. Free Radical Biology and Medicine. 2014;**75**:22-229. DOI: 10.1016/j.freeradbiomed.2014.07.034

[115] Zupančič Š, Lavrič Z, Kristl J. Stability and solubility of trans-resveratrol are strongly influenced by pH and temperature. European Journal of Pharmaceutics and Biopharmaceutics. 2015;**93**:196-204

[116] Ahmadi Z, Mohammadinejad R, Ashrafizadeh M. Drug delivery systems for resveratrol, a non-flavonoid polyphenol: Emerging evidence in last decades. Journal of Drug Delivery Science and Technology. 2019;**51**:591-604. DOI: 10.1016/j.jddst.2019.03.017

[117] Augustin M, Sanguansri L, Lockett T. Nano- and micro-encapsulated systems for enhancing the delivery of resveratrol. Annals of the New York Academy of Sciences. 2013;**1290**(1): 107-112. DOI: 10.1111/nyas.12130

[118] Aras A, Khokhar A, Qureshi M, Silva M, et al. Targeting cancer with nano-bullets: Curcumin, EGCG, resveratrol and quercetin on flying carpets. Asian Pacific Journal of Cancer Prevention. 2014;**15**(9):3865-3871. DOI: 10.7314/APJCP.2014.15.9.3865

[119] Soo E, Thakur S, Qu Z, Jambhrunkar S, et al. Enhancing delivery and cytotoxicity of resveratrol through a dual nanoencapsulation approach. Journal of Colloid and Interface Science. 2016;**462**:368-374

[120] Smoliga J, Vang O, Baur J. Challenges of translating basic research into therapeutics: Resveratrol as an example. The Journals of Gerontology Series A: Biological Sciences and Medical Sciences. 2011;**67A**(2):158-167

[121] Subramanian L, Youssef S, Bhattacharya S, Kenealey J, et al. Resveratrol: Challenges in translation to the clinic – A critical discussion. Clinical Cancer Research. 2010;**16**(24):5942-5948

[122] Delmas D, Aires V, Limagne E, Dutartre P, et al. Transport, stability, and biological activity of resveratrol. Annals of the New York Academy of Sciences. 2011;**1215**(1):48-59. DOI: 10.1111/j.1749-6632.2010.05871.x

[123] Midha K, Nagpal N, Polonini HC, et al. Nano delivery systems of resveratrol to enhance its oral bioavailability. American Journal of Pharmacy and Health Research. 2015;**3**(7):72-81

[124] Naseri N, Valizadeh H, Zakeri-Milani P. Solid lipid nanoparticles and nanostructured lipid carriers: Structure, preparation and application. Advanced Pharmaceutical Bulletin. 2015;**5**(3):305-313. DOI: 10.15171/apb.2015.043

[125] Poonia N, Kaur Narang J, Lather V, Beg S, Sharma T, Singh B, et al. Resveratrol loaded functionalized

nanostructured lipid carriers for breast cancer targeting: Systematic development, characterization and pharmacokinetic evaluation. Colloids and Surfaces B: Biointerfaces. 2019;**181**: 756-766. DOI: 10.1016/j.colsurfb. 2019.06.004

[126] Qin L, Lu T, Qin Y, He Y, Cui N, et al. In vivo effect of resveratrol-loaded solid lipid nanoparticles to relieve physical fatigue for sports nutrition supplements. Molecules. 2020;**25**(22):5302. DOI: 10.3390/molecules25225302

[127] Soeratri W, Hidayah R, Rosita N. Effect of combination soy bean oil and oleic acid to characteristic, penetration, physical stability of nanostructure lipid carrier resveratrol. Folia Medica Indonesiana. 2019;**55**(3):213

[128] Zu Y, Overby H, Ren G, Fan Z, et al. Resveratrol liposomes and lipid nanocarriers: Comparison of characteristics and inducing browning of white adipocytes. Colloids and Surfaces B: Biointerfaces. 2018;**164**:414-423

[129] Ahmad M, Gani A. Development of novel functional snacks containing nano-encapsulated resveratrol with anti-diabetic, anti-obesity and antioxidant properties. Food Chemistry. 2021;**352**:129-323. DOI: 10.1016/ j.foodchem.2021.129323

[130] Jayan H, Maria Leena M, Sivakama Sundari S, et al. Improvement of bioavailability for resveratrol through encapsulation in zein using electrospraying technique. Journal of Functional Foods. 2019;**57**:417-424

[131] Peñalva R, Morales J, González-Navarro C, Larrañeta E, et al. Increased oral bioavailability of resveratrol by its encapsulation in casein nanoparticles. International Journal of Molecular Sciences. 2018;**19**(9):2816

[132] Berta G, Romano F, Vallone R, Abbadessa G, et al. An innovative strategy for oral biofilm control in early childhood based on a resveratrol-cyclodextrin nanotechnology approach. Materials. 2021;**14**(14):3801. DOI: 10.3390/ma14143801

[133] Li L, Yu M, Li Y, Li Q, et al. Synergistic anti-inflammatory and osteogenic n-HA/resveratrol/chitosan composite microspheres for osteoporotic bone regeneration. Bioactive Materials. 2021;**6**(5):1255-1266

[134] Ming L, Zhipeng Y, Fei Y, Feng R, et al. Microfluidic-based screening of resveratrol and drug-loading PLA/ Gelatine nano-scaffold for the repair of cartilage defect. Artificial Cells, Nanomedicine, and Biotechnology. 2018;**46**(1):336-346

[135] Du S, Lv Y, Li N, Huang X, et al. Biological investigations on therapeutic effect of chitosan encapsulated nano resveratrol against gestational diabetes mellitus rats induced by streptozotocin. Drug Delivery. 2020;**27**(1):953-963. DOI: 10.1080/10717544.2020.1775722

[136] Sun J, Wei C, Liu Y, Xie W, Xu M, et al. Progressive release of mesoporous nano-selenium delivery system for the multi-channel synergistic treatment of Alzheimer's disease. Biomaterials. 2019;**197**:417-431

Chapter 2

Periodontitis and Heart Disease: Current Perspectives on the Associative Relationships and Preventive Impact

Alexandra Roman, Andrada Soancă, Bogdan Caloian, Alexandru Bucur, Gabriela Valentina Caracostea, Andreia Paraschiva Preda, Dora Maria Popescu, Iulia Cristina Micu, Petra Șurlin, Andreea Ciurea, Diana Oneț, Mircea Viorel Ciurea, Dragoș Alexandru Țermure and Marius Negucioiu

Abstract

Due to the important advancement and the accumulation of new evidence on the periodontitis-cardiovascular disease (CVD) relationship as well as the major medical, economic and social burden caused by both diseases this chapter aims to review existing epidemiological and pathogenetic links related to this topic. Also, this chapter aims to highlight the impact of the periodontitis-CVD relationships on clinical practice and on the preventive approaches targeting to decrease the impact of periodontitis on CVD. Periodontitis is an infectious disease eliciting local and general inflammation, which leads to periodontal destruction and systemic involvement. Several pathways could explain the link between periodontitis and CVD such as bacteraemia, chronic persistent systemic inflammation and oxidative stress. The first step in the treatment of periodontitis addresses the elimination of microbial components, which lead to a decrease in local and systemic inflammation. Periodontal therapy seems to positively impact CVD. Specialists should inform patients with CVD on the negative impact of periodontitis on their systemic status and refer patients to the periodontist for an extensive examination as routine management of CVD. Some possible risks of periodontal therapy should be considered in patients undergoing antithrombotic medication.

Keywords: periodontitis, cardiovascular disease, atherosclerosis, hypertension, inflammation, anticoagulants, prevention

1. Introduction

Periodontitis is a noncommunicable infectious disease associated with an important inflammatory component affecting around 50% of the population worldwide and with a prevalence of its severe forms of 11.2% [1]. The Global Burden of Diseases, Injuries, and Risk Factors Study (2017) reported periodontitis as the sixth most prevalent chronic human disease [2].

Periodontitis is characterized by loss of connective tissue attachment that is normally located at the tooth neck (cementoenamel junction) as well as by alveolar bone destruction. Periodontitis is accompanied by the transformation of the shallow gingival sulcus into a deep periodontal pocket and a marked apical diffusion of the dysbiotic subgingival biofilm [3]. In generalized severe periodontitis, the surface area of the epithelial lining of the periodontal pockets is enormous and could favor the direct contact of subgingival bacteria with gingival connective tissue through focal ulcerated areas. Moreover, epithelial ulcerations constitute biological entries for the systemic dissemination of subgingival Gram-negative bacteria and local products eliciting different general biological responses [3, 4].

There is important evidence suggesting periodontitis as a biologically plausible risk factor for the development of other chronic, systemic, inflammatory conditions such as diabetes mellitus, cardiovascular disease (CVD), and adverse pregnancy outcomes [5]. Relationships between periodontitis and chronic obstructive pulmonary disease, rheumatoid arthritis, metabolic syndrome, obesity, cancers, and chronic renal disease have also been reported [6]. An inverse influence of systemic conditions on periodontal status has also been described [7]. Current epidemiological evidence sustains that periodontitis induces an increased risk for future atherosclerotic CVD [8].

The term CVD refers to atherosclerotic conditions such as coronary heart disease, cerebrovascular disease and peripheral vascular disease representing a leading cause of death, impairments, and quality of life alterations [8]. CVDs are the most prevalent noncommunicable diseases globally due to the increasingly aging population as well as to profound alterations of diets and lifestyles. Eurostat, the statistical office of the European Union, reported that in 2016 in UE 1.68 million deaths were resulting from diseases of the circulatory system, which was equivalent to 37.1% of all deaths—considerably higher than the second most prevalent cause of death, cancer (malignant neoplasms 25.8%). They accounted for 50–60% of all deaths in the Baltic Member States and Romania and 65.8% of all deaths in Bulgaria. By contrast, less than one-quarter of all deaths in Denmark (22.6%), France (24.3% 2016 data) and the Netherlands (25.0%) were caused by diseases of the circulatory system [9].

Periodontitis has a negative impact on cardiovascular outcomes. Also, periodontal treatment has been associated with potential risks and complications in patients on anti-thrombotic therapy which must be considered in clinical practice [8].

Due to significant advancement and the accumulation of new evidence on periodontitis-CVD relationships as well as to the major medical, economic and social burden represented by both periodontitis and CVD, this chapter aims to review existing epidemiological and pathogenetic links related to this topic as wells to highlight the impact of the periodontitis-CVD associative relationships on clinical practice and to provide some clinical recommendations for both periodontists and cardiologists on this topic.

2. Pathophysiological links between periodontitis and CVD

2.1 Subgingival microbiota and periodontitis development

A highly organized subgingival microbial community is involved in the transition from a periodontal health condition to a dysbiotic pathogenic status namely periodontitis characterized by a complex shift of the microbiota composition, abundance, and arrangement [10, 11]. Three members of the subgingival consortium included in the "Red complex" have been constantly identified in the subgingival microbiota of periodontitis patients are: *Porphyromonas gingivalis* (*P. gingivalis*), *Treponema denticola* (*T. denticola*), and *Tannerella forsythia* (*T. forsythia*) [12]. Previously viewed as true periodontopathogens, they are now rather considered as pathobiont organisms because these bacteria are normally present in low numbers in the subgingival microbiota of periodontal healthy individuals [13]. *Filifacter alocis* and bacteria of genera *Parvimonas, Fusobacterium*, and *Prevotella* are nowadays considered as pathobionts [14]. Pathobionts expand within the microbial community once ecological changes take place, which initiates and favor periodontitis development [11]. Dynamic and synergistic interactions between subgingival microbiota and the host shape and stabilize dysbiotic communities within their subgingival habitat [15]. Gingival inflammation triggers local tissue destruction that releases subgingivally specific nutriments corresponding to the growth of highly demanding Gram-negative bacteria, which amplify local dysbiosis [16].

A paradox remarqued by the specialists is that dysbiotic microbiota requires inflammation to sustain their nutrition in the context in which localized inflammatory reaction developed by the host is a normal function addressed to reestablish local homeostasis through inhibiting bacterial development [11]. The behavior of *P. gingivalis* could explain this paradox through the manipulation of the periodontal immune reactions [17].

A low proportion of *P. gingivalis* in the subgingival microbiota in both periodontal health and periodontitis has been identified. The bacterium is considered a keystone pathogen in the dysbiotic microbiota creating a pro-inflammatory, antiphagocytic environment favorable to the growth and development of pathobionts [18].

Upregulation of many virulence genes of *P. gingivalis* in healthy sites before progression of the attachment loss has been described. In contrast, *T. denticola* and *T. forsythia* upregulate only very few virulence genes and only in the later stages of periodontitis evolution. It seems that *P. gingivalis* serves as a microbial driver in the transition from periodontal healthy status to periodontitis [16].

Microbiota within the subgingival biofilm is a complex highly dynamic architectural arrangement of bacteria rather than a random static positioning of the microbial cells next to each other. Within the biofilm, biochemical interaction, signaling, and genetic exchanges between bacteria take place. Facultative aerobes within subgingival biofilms can sequester oxygen and create anaerobic niches that favor the expansion of anaerobic protobionts and thus the transition toward dysbiosis [11]. The bacterial load in periodontal pockets is exponentially greater compared to the flora of the sulcus at the expense of the dominant species rather than due to the replacement of early colonizers [16]. Four distinct layers have been described in the subgingival biofilm from periodontitis patients. The basal layer of the subgingival biofilm, located in the proximity of the tooth surface, is formed by *Actinomyces* spp. *Fusobacterium* and *Tannerella* reside in the intermediate layers of the biofilms while *Prevotella* and

Porphyromonas are localized in both the apical and intermediate layers [19]. Bacterial cells of the *Cytophaga-Flavobacterium-Bacteroides* cluster were located in the apical layers and *Treponema* was located above the densely packed biofilm. Microbial cells of the genus *Synergistes* have been described closely arranged to polymorphonuclear leukocytes indicating direct physical interactions between biofilm microbes and host immune cells [19]. However, close relationships between polymorphonuclear leucocytes and subgingival microbes have been previously highlighted through transmission electron micrographs [20].

2.2 Pathogenetic mechanisms linking periodontitis and CVD

Atherosclerosis is a chronic, vascular inflammatory condition being a major cause of CVD. In atherosclerosis, the deposition of lipids in the artery walls results in plaque build-up. Its progression results in the reduction of blood flow and consecutive ischemia of organs and tissues and promotes clot formation [21]. The American Heart Association pointed out the relationships between periodontitis and CVD although causality remains unproven [22, 23].

A wide range of studies has investigated the causal relationships between periodontitis and CVD which have resulted in two essential hypotheses explaining this link. One hypothesis sustains the role of systemically disseminated periodontopathogens and of their by-products to induce atheroma formation through the infection of blood vessels [24]. Disseminated bacteria and their products including lipopolysaccharide (LPS) challenge the immune system inducing systemic inflammatory reactions [3].

Several data communicated over time have reported the ability of bacteria from subgingival plaque to migrate and localize to vascular walls and atheromatous plaques. Recent information provided by a systematic review and a meta-analysis showed that the DNA of periodontopathogens was present in atheromatous plaque samples from patients with myocardial infarction [25]. However, less than 5% of patients receiving surgery for atherosclerotic vascular disease presented bacterial DNA in isolated samples which were not statistically significantly different from patients receiving surgeries for rheumatic heart disease [26].

The second hypothesis considers that longstanding periodontal inflammation overlaps with existing chronic systemic inflammation through the dissemination of locally abundantly produced molecules (pro-inflammatory cytokines, chemokines, and gingiva-derived C-reactive protein CRP) promoting atherosclerosis development and CVD [24, 27].

Moreover, a recent emerging hypothesis considers that periodontopathogens and periodontal inflammation promote modifications in oral and gut microbiome which in turn may influence the evolution of both periodontitis and atherosclerosis [24].

In periodontitis patients, the processing of antigenic structures by the liver induces a systemic acute phase response associated with an increased plasma CRP [3]. Periodontitis patients have statistically significantly higher high sensitivity CRP plasma values compared to periodontally healthy subjects amounting to 1.56 mg/L. This difference is biologically relevant since it could drive patients into the high CRP risk category (>3 mg/L) [28]. IgG antibodies against specific periodontal bacteria were associated with all-cause and CVD mortality [29].

A vascular endothelial activation is a central event for atherosclerosis development and a connecting link to periodontitis [30]. Circulating bacterial LPS, outer membrane vesicles and fimbriae, as well as inflammatory cytokines induce the up-regulation of cell-surface receptors and the expression of adhesion molecules on the vascular endothelium, which recruit peripheral blood monocytes at the surface of the activated endothelium. On the other hand, antibodies targeting specific bacterial proteins behave as auto-antibodies through "molecular mimicry" and induce damage of the vascular endothelium [31]. Monocytes follow a chemoattractant gradient and migrate into the sub-endothelial space, become tissular macrophages, capture oxidized low-density lipoprotein cholesterol (LDL) and develop into foam cells. Apoptosis of the latter favor the accumulation of lipids in the sub-endothelial space forming the atheromatous plaques, which become coated by a fibrous shelter and promote platelet adhesion. Apoptosis of endothelial cell exposes the fibrous cap which in association with the enzymatic destruction of the extracellular matrix induce plaque rupture, exposure of pro-thrombotic plaque components, and subsequent thrombus formation that leads to vascular occlusion and CVD related events (myocardial infarction or stroke) [3].

Periodontitis patients have increased platelet recruitment and platelet hyperactivation as sustained by the augmented plasma concentration of platelet factor 4 (PF4) [32, 33]. Moreover, periodontitis has been frequently accompanied by a prothrombotic state. In patients with mild, moderate, or severe periodontitis D-dimer values were found to be increased by 1.62-fold, 2.06-fold and 2.54-fold, respectively than in healthy patients [34].

3. Epidemiologic relationships between periodontitis and CVD

Although, the relationship between periodontitis and CVD has long been the subject of debate in the scientific literature, the existence of a moderate association between periodontitis and CVD was firstly reported by a systematic review in 2003 [35]. Since then, many other systematic reviews and meta-analyses highlighted this idea. Periodontitis patients had 19%, 15% and 14% increased risk of developing CVD, respectively [36–38].

Individuals with active periodontitis had a nearly 2–2.5-fold higher risk of developing acute myocardial infarction than those without the disease [39, 40].

A positive association between both severe and moderate periodontitis and acute myocardial infarction exists, which suggests a relationship between periodontitis severity and CVD [41].

A significant association was found between calcified carotid artery atheroma and the presence of periodontitis both in acute myocardial infarction (OR, 1.51; 95% CI, 1.09–2.10) and controls (OR, 1.70; 95% CI, 1.22–2.38) [42]. Periodontitis was associated with a 45% higher risk of acute myocardial infarction (OR, 1.45; 95% CI, 1.10–1.91), whilst patients with both periodontitis and calcified carotid artery atheromas had a 75% higher risk for acute myocardial infarction then those without these conditions [42].

An increased CVD burden in patients with significant periodontal destruction had been suggested in different studies. Data from the Oral Infections and Vascular Disease Epidemiology (INVEST) study showed that the number of missing teeth was significantly associated with carotid artery plaque after adjustment for CVD risk factors [43]. Moreover, the Periodontitis and Its Relation to Coronary Artery Disease (PAROKRANK) study reported an increased risk of myocardial infarction in patients with periodontitis (odds ratio of 1.28, 95% confidence interval (CI) 1.03–1.6) after adjustment for some behavioral, social and medical risk factors. The radiographic bone loss was used to quantify periodontal destruction [44]. However, concerns have been raised in relation to the difficulty to control for all possible confounders and the possibility that periodontitis could still be a surrogate for other risk factors not highlighted by these studies [45].

Periodontitis may also represent a risk factor for stroke, especially in ischemic events. However, new studies with a robust design are necessary for a reliable conclusion [46].

4. Periodontitis and hypertension

4.1 Epidemiological associations between periodontitis and hypertension

Hypertension is considered a major risk factor of CVD. Periodontitis has emerged as a new contributor to the complete cardiovascular risk profile of CVD.

The associative relationships between periodontitis and hypertension are important in the context of the high prevalence rates of both diseases that induce important medical and social burden. Besides the fact that periodontitis and hypertension share a group of common risk factors (older age, smoking, low socioeconomic and education status, genetics) an independent association between the two diseases has been reported.

The data provided by prospective and retrospective studies reported a higher prevalence of hypertension in patients with periodontal disease ranging from 7 to 77% as compared with patients without periodontitis with prevalence rates ranging from 4 to 70% [47]. Periodontitis patients had 4.5 mmHg higher systolic and 2.0 mmHg higher diastolic blood pressure than non-periodontitis patients [47]; the systolic component of the blood pressure seemed to be more influenced by periodontitis than the diastolic one [48].

Two meta-analyses provided information sustaining the association between periodontitis and hypertension [47, 49]. The heterogeneity of case definitions of both hypertension and periodontitis prevented the drawing of firm conclusions regarding this topic. The association between the two diseases is open to future analyses of data provided by clinical trials using uniform case definitions for periodontitis and hypertension.

The activity of periodontitis monitored through local inflammation index (bleeding on probing) seems also to play an important role in the complex interplay between periodontal disease and hypertension. Data from the Third US National Health and Nutrition Examination Survey (NHANES III) informed that local gingival inflammation (bleeding on probing) was significantly associated with increased systolic blood pressure (2.6 mmHg higher values compared with noninflamed situations) and increased risk of uncontrolled blood pressure after multivariate adjustments of a large make-up of influencing factors including systemic inflammatory diseases as well as behavioral and social factors [50]. Moreover, data from observational studies reported that even for patients on intensive antihypertensive treatment periodontitis was associated with an increased risk of uncontrolled hypertension [48].

The genetic background has been involved in the development of both periodontitis and hypertension at least partially by the modulation of immune-inflammatory reactions that sustain a proinflammatory milieu [48].

The high-salt diet is a common trigger for hypertension, but data has also shown to alter the microbiome and impair immune systems through salt-induced hyperglucocorticoidism [51, 52].

4.2 Periodontitis and pregnancy hypertensive disorders

It was proven that oral health among vulnerable populations, such as pregnant women is an important determinant regarding the pregnancy outcome. Numerous epidemiological studies have demonstrated an increased risk of adverse pregnancy outcome (APO), including preterm birth, low birthweight and pregnancy-induced hypertension or pre-eclampsia (PE) as well as gestational diabetes (GDM), related to periodontal disease [53]. Therefore, maintaining optimal maternal oral hygiene is regarded as a mandatory standard of care for perinatal medicine [54].

The reported prevalence of periodontitis, during the time period of pregnancy, varies between 10 and 74% and it is highly dependent on the economical level and health policies of each country [55].

Two pathogenic mechanisms described the potential effect of periodontal diseases on pregnancy outcomes. On the one hand, the periodontal bacteria could induce bacteremia and a seeding of the feto-placental unit. On the other hand, inflammatory mediators such as interleukin-1 (IL-1), IL-6, IL-8, tumor necrosis factor-α (TNF-α) or prostaglandin E2 (PGE2), secreted by the subgingival inflammatory site are carried to the feto-placental unit, where an inflammatory response will develop [53].

The influence of the gingival bacterial microbiome on APO is confirmed by the new data that revealed the presence of a unique bacterial load even of the placentar tissue. Gram-positive as well as Gram-negative intracellular bacteria were identified in the basal plate of the human placenta [56]. Moreover, due to metagenomic technology, it was shown that placental microbiome profiles are more related to the oral microbiome than other microbiomes in the human body, such as the gut, nares, skin and urogenital tract [57].

The feto-maternal unit is exposed to oral bacteria during bacteriemia episodes caused by daily oral activities (e.g., tooth brushing and flossing) and dental treatments (e.g., scaling and root planing). Katz et al. identified the presence of *Porphyromas gingivalis* antigens in placental tissues and suggested that the colonization of *Porphyromas gingivalis* in the placenta might contribute to the placental dysfunction, a specific obstetrical feature in severe cases of PE [58]. Moreover, the presence of *Porphyromas gingivalis* in the umbilical cord was highly associated with PE. Several meta-analyses found a risk at least twice higher to develop preeclampsia in women diagnosed with periodontitis [59, 60].

The relationship between hypertensive disorders (including both pregnancy pre-existing hypertension and pregnancy-induced hypertension, also called preeclampsia) and periodontitis was mostly explained in relation to the systemic inflammatory response due to maternal infection. In severe cases of periodontitis, the inflammatory mediators (alarmins) and cytokines found in the gingival mucosa, including IL-1β, IL-6, TNF-α and PGE2, entered systemic circulation and affect the feto-placental unit and myometrium [53].

The adequate invasion of the extravillous trophoblast in the vascular layer of spiral uterine arteries will determine appropriate feto-maternal perfusion. In vitro models showed the local interaction between the placental tissue (human trophoblast cell lines) and periodontal pathogens, bacterial components, or inflammatory mediators. According to the data, the inflammatory milieu may suppress the media layer invasion process, leading to an important vascular remodeling. Eventually, that will trigger the development of pregnancy-induced hypertension or will aggravate the chronic vascular changes in pregnant women with preexisting hypertension. This will further cause placental insufficiency, the physiopathological final step to the development of fetal distress in utero [61].

5. Periodontal therapy and cardiovascular risk

Non-surgical treatment of periodontitis refers to subgingival instrumentation of periodontally affected teeth and addresses the polymicrobial aetiologic factor from the subgingival areas. Full-mouth subgingival instrumentation performed within 24 hours has been proposed to prevent the dissemination of bacteria from non-instrumented pockets to the previously treated areas [62]. It is also worth mentioning that in severe generalized periodontitis, due to the mobilization of a huge mass of bacteria from the periodontal pockets, the full-mouth instrumentation could trigger an acute systemic inflammatory response associated with transient endothelial dysfunction [63]. Delivering subgingival instrumentation conventionally in several short sessions could overcome the systemic response and the theoretical short-term risk of developing a vascular event [64].

Data from observational studies observed no effect or just a minimal elevated risk of "*invasive dental treatment*" [65, 66] in augmenting the ischaemic cardiovascular risk. The report concluding that the "*invasive dental treatment*" had no effect in increasing the risk of myocardial infarction was based on the *Taiwanese National Health Insurance Research Database* and included more than 110,000 myocardial infarction patients and 290,000 ischaemic stroke patients over a period of 14 years. However, a modest risk of myocardial infarction during the first week after treatments has been indicated (OR = 1.31, 95% CI [1.08; 1.58], after 3 days). A self-controlled case series on about 10 million persons from an US insurance database reported that "*invasive*" dental treatments, mostly represented by tooth extractions, were associated with an augmented risk of incident acute cardiovascular events (IR = 1.5, 95% CI [1.09; 2.06]) within 1 month after therapy [66]. A small-scale clinical trial reported no cardiovascular adverse events within 3 months after periodontal subgingival instrumentation in patients with established CVD [67]. Also, a randomized secondary prevention trial showed that subgingival instrumentation in patients with established CVD was not associated with an increased incidence of cardiovascular events in 6 months after periodontitis treatment [68]. Moreover, a study on 5297 subjects, with a median follow-up period of 16.8 years concluded that individuals who did not respond well to periodontal treatment had a 28% increased risk for future CVD, indicating that successful periodontal treatment might influence the progression of subclinical CVD [69].

However, nowadays conclusions on this topic sustain that no association between "*invasive*" periodontal treatments and an increased incidence of myocardial infarction or ischaemic cardiovascular risk has been reported [8, 70].

6. Perioperative bleeding risk associated periodontal procedures

6.1 Bleeding risk of periodontal procedures

The perioperative bleeding risk depends on the extent and invasiveness of the periodontal therapeutic approach. A low bleeding risk has been mentioned for most periodontal interventions such as subgingival instrumentation, conventional surgeries (debridement flaps and regenerative or resective interventions), dental implants placement, or tooth extraction [8]. The bleeding associated with these interventions could be controlled through local haemostatic measures. On the other hand, a moderate bleeding risk is considered for autogenous bone augmentation procedures including block bone harvesting and sinus floor elevation or interventions associated with secondary intention healing such as free gingival graft placement [71, 72]. The frequencies for low and moderate bleeding associated with periodontal therapies have been reported to be less than 1% and between 2 and 5%, respectively [8].

6.2 Patients undergoing antiplatelet and anticoagulant therapy

Single antiplatelet therapy such as acetylsalicylic acid (aspirin), clopidogrel, ticlopidine or ticagrelor did not increased the frequency of bleeding events as compared with control patients [73, 74].

Dual antiplatelet therapy usually using the combination of aspirin and clopidogrel may induce a certain risk for post-operative bleeding, which may be managed with local haemostatic approaches [75, 76].

The discontinuation of single or dual antiplatelet therapy before any kind of periodontal approach including dental implant placement is not recommended by current evidence [8].

"Current American Heart Association, American College of Cardiology, Society for Cardiovascular Angiography and Interventions, American College of Surgeons, and American Dental Association, European Society of Cardiology, American College of Chest Physicians Evidence-Based Clinical Practice (AHA/ACC/SCAI/ACS/ADA/ESC/ACCP) guidelines on perioperative management of antithrombotic therapy do not suggest discontinuation of anti-platelet therapy for low bleeding risk procedures" [77–79].

No increased risk of bleeding has been associated with oral vitamin K antagonist-anticoagulant therapy (warfarine, cumarine) in patients receiving dental extraction, minor dental procedures or dental implant placement when compared to patients discontinuing anticoagulant therapy [80, 81]. However, in comparison with non-vitamin K patients, a higher post-operative bleeding risk in patients continuing vitamin K antagonist-anticoagulant therapy and suffering from minor or higher-risk dental procedures have been reported, although post-operative bleeding could be effectively controlled with local haemostatic agents [80, 82, 83].

As for novel/direct anticoagulants such as apixaban, rivaroxaban, betrixaban, edoxaban, and dabigatran, it seems that the interruption of these drugs is not necessary for most dental-periodontal therapies, due to a low incidence of bleeding events associated with these drugs and which can be successfully managed with local haemostatic measures [84–86]. As a positive advancement in the field, a neutralizing agent (idarucizumab) has been developed for dabigatran. However, a higher incidence of delayed bleeding (2 days and later) has been reported in patients not discontinuing novel/direct anticoagulants in comparison with healthy persons [87]. Although, it has been widely used in the past, especially in the era of anti-vitamin K anticoagulants, the low molecular weight heparins (LMWH) bridging strategy should be avoided in patients treated with novel oral anticoagulants (NOAC) as it increases the risk of bleeding, with no benefit on the risk of cardioembolic events. It is reserved for patients with mechanical valve prostheses at high thrombotic risk [88].

However, in CVD patients receiving complex antithrombotic medication a strict communication with cardiologist is mandatory.

7. Periodontitis and CVD: recommendations for clinicians and patients

7.1 Recommendations for periodontologists treating patients with CVD

a. Patients with medium or severe generalized periodontitis without known CVD should [8]:

- be advised that periodontitis induces a higher risk of CVD and its acute events (myocardial infarction and stroke)
- actively manage all their CV risk factors such as smoking, lack of exercise, excess weight and blood pressure, lipid, and glucose profile
- receive intensive periodontal therapy and tailored oral hygiene education and regimen
- receive a strict scheduled periodontal maintenance
- be referred to the cardiologist for CVD screening if CVD risk factors are present.

b. Patients with periodontitis and CVD should:

- be informed that they may be at higher risk for CVD complications
- receive active periodontal treatment and tailored oral hygiene education and regimen
- be included in periodontitis regular maintenance and secondary preventive regimes.

c. People with CVD should:

- be referred by the cardiologist to the periodontist for a thorough full-mouth oral examination and screening
- receive a tailored oral hygiene education and regimen
- be placed on a preventive care regime if no periodontitis is diagnosed and monitored regularly (at least once a year) for changes in periodontal status
- be managed as for point b) if periodontitis is diagnosed.

d. Subgingival instrumentation in periodontitis patients with CVD should be provided preferably in several 30- to 45-minute sessions to reduce the putative acute systemic inflammation.

e. In patients with CVD, surgical periodontal and implant therapy when indicated should be provided similarly as in patients without CVD.

f. In hypertensive patients, high blood pressure above 180/100 indicates to postpone periodontal surgical procedures until stabilization of blood pressure.

g. In patients with antiplatelet and anticoagulant therapy

- The periodontist should not modify the patient's antiplatelet and anticoagulant medication to perform periodontal and implant surgeries which are associated with a low to medium risk of bleeding.

- A consultation with the cardiologist is advised when doubts are raised.

- Local management of bleeding complications should be considered such as: oxidized cellulose, absorbable gelatine sponges, sutures, tranexamic acid mouthwashes, compressive gauze soaked in tranexamic acid.

- It has been suggested to discontinue vitamin K antagonist-antithrombotic therapy if the Internationalized Normalized Ratio (INR) ≤ 4 for low or medium bleeding risk surgeries, but the decision should be considered in consensus with the cardiologist. For INR ≥ 3.5 the advice of the responsible specialist is mandatory [8, 89].

- For non-vitamin K novel and direct anticoagulant (NOAC/DOAC) and when low bleeding risk periodontal approaches are scheduled, the anticoagulant therapy should not be discontinued [8, 71, 72]. Periodontal procedures should be undertaken within 18–24 hours after the last intake (depending on a renal function assessment for the medication in question) after which medication intake should be resumed after 6 hours following treatment.

- **For all intentions to adjust antithrombotic therapy to perform periodontal surgeries the periodontologist should consult with the responsible cardiologist.**

- **If discontinuation of antithrombotic therapy is planned for medium bleeding risk periodontal approaches, the decision should be made in agreement with the cardiologist.**

- In higher thrombotic and ischaemic risk patients (i.e., chronic atrial fibrillation or after an acute myocardial infarction or recent coronary stenting) receiving combined antiplatelet and anticoagulant therapies, **all periodontal treatments and antithrombotic change intensions (either of low or medium bleeding risk) must be discussed and agreed upon with the responsible cardiologist** [8, 71, 72]. The periodontal interventions should be eventually delayed.

- Patients under **triple therapy** (dual antiplatelet and one anticoagulant) or one **anticoagulant plus one antiplatelet should be individually managed** in consensus with the responsible cardiologist and eventually referred in dental specialized care centres [79, 90].

h. Patients with a risk of endocarditis should be premedicated with antibiotics following current guidelines (such as the European or the American guidelines).

i. People with CVD who have extensive tooth loss should be encouraged to pursue dental rehabilitation to restore adequate mastication for proper nutrition.

j. Diet counseling including low salt consumption could be beneficial for the management of both periodontitis and hypertension.

k. CVD including hypertension could benefit from periodontitis primary and secondary prevention.

7.2 Periodontitis-related recommendations for physicians and cardiologists

a. Cardiologists should know that periodontitis is a highly prevalent disease that has potentially negative influences on CVD development and complications as well as that efficient periodontal treatment may positively impact CV status.

b. **Cardiologists should advise all CVD patients on the above-mentioned topic and to seek periodontal specialized care as part of their ongoing management of CVD.** Even if no periodontitis is diagnosed initially, an annual oral check-up is recommended.

c. For patients already diagnosed with periodontitis, the cardiologist must ensure that the disease has been effectively treated.

d. The cardiologist should assist the periodontist in the management of patients under antithrombotic therapy before the periodontal surgery, to avoid risks of bleeding or ischaemic events.

7.3 Recommendations for patients with CVD or at risk of CVD in relation with periodontitis

a. Patients with CVD should know that:

- periodontitis is a chronic infectious disease having the potential to worsen their systemic condition
- periodontitis is treatable in most cases but requires lifelong personal management and professional supervision
- left untreated periodontitis leads to further bone destruction and finally to tooth loss
- periodontitis is a “silent” disease so regular dental-periodontal check-ups are advised
- periodontitis treatment has a positive impact on CVD and reduces the risk of CV events
- **they need to seek periodontal specialized screening for periodontitis and eventually care as part of their ongoing management of CVD**
- an annual oral check-up is recommended even in the absence of periodontitis.

b. Periodontitis patients are important co-therapists and without their sustained daily involvement, periodontitis resolution is not possible.

c. Patients with CVD and periodontitis, like all the other individuals, must efficiently clean the teeth based on the dental practitioner/periodontist personalized advice. The following oral care recommendations should be practiced:

- Tooth brushing twice a day with an electric or a manual toothbrush is recommended; however, electric toothbrushes seem to be more efficient than manual toothbrushes in a personalized local hygiene routine.

- Cleaning the areas between teeth using auxiliary oral hygiene aids is mandatory since using only conventional toothbrushing is not sufficient for complete plaque removal. Interdental brushes, carefully calibrated to fit the size of the interdental spaces should be used. Dental floss is an interdental cleaning option that can be used whenever the gums fill in the interdental spaces.

8. Conclusions

Periodontitis has been considered a risk factor for CVD, although no causal relationship has been demonstrated to this point. Two potential biological mechanisms (periodontal bacteria and endotoxins systemic dissemination and release of inflammatory molecules from the affected periodontal sites into the blood stream) have been described to link periodontitis and atherosclerosis-induced CVD. Periodontitis may increase the risk for hypertension as well as for acute CV events—myocardial infarction and stroke. In pregnant women, periodontitis may trigger adverse pregnancy outcomes and may worsen the chronic vascular changes in relation with pre-existing hypertension, which carries high maternal and fetal health risks. Periodontal screening in specialized medical care settings should be a component of the management of CVD. Periodontologists, cardiologists, and patients should be informed on the potentially negative influences of periodontitis on CVD development and its complications as well as on the positive impact of periodontitis treatment on CV status. All adjustments in antithrombotic treatment in periodontitis-CVD patients must be discussed and agreed upon with the responsible cardiologist.

Conflict of interest

The authors declare no conflict of interest.

Thanks

We would like to thank Mr. Josip Knapic for his understanding and support.

Author details

Alexandra Roman[1*], Andrada Soancă[1], Bogdan Caloian[2], Alexandru Bucur[3], Gabriela Valentina Caracostea[4], Andreia Paraschiva Preda[4], Dora Maria Popescu[5], Iulia Cristina Micu[6], Petra Şurlin[5], Andreea Ciurea[6], Diana Oneţ[6], Mircea Viorel Ciurea[7], Dragoş Alexandru Ţermure[7] and Marius Negucioiu[8]

1 Faculty of Dental Medicine, Department of Periodontology, "Iuliu Hatieganu" University of Medicine and Pharmacy, Emergency County Clinical Hospital, Cluj-Napoca, Romania

2 Department of Cardiology-Rehabilitation, "Iuliu Hatieganu" University of Medicine and Pharmacy, Clinical Rehabilitation Hospital, Cluj-Napoca, Romania

3 Faculty of Dental Medicine, Department of Oro-Maxillo-Facial Surgery, "Carol Davila" University of Medicine and Pharmacy, "Prof. Dr. Dan Theodorescu" Oro-Maxillo-Facial Clinical Hospital, Bucharest, Romania

4 Faculty of Medicine, Department of Obstetrics and Gynecology, "Iuliu Hatieganu" University of Medicine and Pharmacy, Emergency County Clinical Hospital, Cluj-Napoca, Romania

5 Faculty of Dental Medicine, Department of Periodontology, University of Medicine and Pharmacy, Craiova, Romania

6 Faculty of Dental Medicine, Department of Periodontology, "Iuliu Hatieganu" University of Medicine and Pharmacy, Cluj-Napoca, Romania

7 Faculty of Dental Medicine, Department of Oral and Maxillofacial Surgery, "Iuliu Hatieganu" University of Medicine and Pharmacy, Cluj-Napoca, Romania

8 Faculty of Dental Medicine, Department of Prosthetic Dentistry, "Iuliu Hatieganu" University of Medicine and Pharmacy, Emergency County Clinical Hospital, Cluj-Napoca, Romania

*Address all correspondence to: veve_alexandra@yahoo.com

References

[1] Kassebaum NJ, Bernabé E, Dahiya M, Bhandari B, Murray CJ, Marcenes W. Global burden of severe periodontitis in 1990-2010: A systematic review and meta-regression. Journal of Dental Research. 2014;**93**(11):1045-1053. DOI: 10.1177/0022034514552491

[2] GBD 2017 Disease and Injury Incidence and Prevalence Collaborators. Global, regional, and national incidence, prevalence, and years lived with disability for 354 diseases and injuries for 195 countries and territories, 1990-2017: A systematic analysis for the Global Burden of Disease Study 2017. Lancet. 2018;**392**(10159):1789-1858. DOI: 10.1016/S0140-6736(18)32279-7

[3] Papapanou PN. Systemic effects of periodontitis: Lessons learned from research on atherosclerotic vascular disease and adverse pregnancy outcomes. International Dental Journal. 2015;**65**(6):283-291. DOI: 10.1111/idj.12185

[4] Hujoel PP, White BA, García RI, Listgarten MA. The dentogingival epithelial surface area revisited. Journal of Periodontal Research. 2001;**36**(1): 48-55. DOI: 10.1034/j.1600-0765.2001.00011.x

[5] Papapanou PN, Susin C. Periodontitis epidemiology: Is periodontitis under-recognized, over-diagnosed, or both? Periodontology 2000. 2017;**75**(1):45-51. DOI: 10.1111/prd.12200

[6] Peres MA, Macpherson LMD, Weyant RJ, Daly B, Venturelli R, Mathur MR, et al. Oral diseases: A global public health. Lancet. 2019;**394**(10194):249-260. DOI: 10.1016/S0140-6736(19)31146-8

[7] Roman A, Caracostea GA, Bulboacă AE, Soancă A, Ciurea A, Micu IC, et al. Parodontita și unele condiții patologice sistemice: Impactul medical și recomandări pentru specialiști și pacienți. Vol. 1: Asocieri dintre parodontită, complicații ale sarcinii și carcinogeneză. București: Amaltea; 2021. ISBN 978-973-162-220-0

[8] Sanz M, Marco Del Castillo A, Jepsen S, Gonzalez-Juanatey JR, D'Aiuto F, Bouchard P, et al. Periodontitis and cardiovascular diseases: Consensus report. Journal of Clinical Periodontology. 2020;**47**(3):268-288. DOI: 10.1111/jcpe.13189

[9] Cardiovascular diseases statistics. Deaths from cardiovascular diseases [Internet]. 2021. Available from: https://ec.europa.eu/eurostat/statistics-explained/index.php?title=Cardiovascular_diseases_statistics#Deaths_from_cardiovascular_diseases [Accessed: December 14, 2021]

[10] Hajishengallis G. Immunomicrobial pathogenesis of periodontitis: Keystones, pathobionts, and host response. Trends in Immunology. 2014;**35**(1):3-11. DOI: 10.1016/j.it.2013.09.001

[11] Valm AM. The structure of dental plaque microbial communities in the transition from health to dental caries and periodontal disease. Journal of Molecular Biology. 2019;**431**(16):2957-2969. DOI: 10.1016/j.jmb.2019.05.016

[12] Socransky SS, Haffajee AD, Cugini MA, Smith C, Kent RL Jr. Microbial complexes in subgingival plaque. Journal of Clinical Periodontology. 1998;**25**(2):134-144. DOI: 10.1111/j.1600-051x.1998.tb02419.x

[13] Chow J, Tang H, Mazmanian SK. Pathobionts of the gastrointestinal microbiota and inflammatory disease. Current Opinion in Immunology. 2011;**23**(4):473-480. DOI: 10.1016/j.coi.2011.07.010

[14] Dabdoub SM, Ganesan SM, Kumar PS. Comparative metagenomics reveals taxonomically idiosyncratic yet functionally congruent communities in periodontitis. Scientific Reports. 2016;**6**:38993. DOI: 10.1038/srep38993

[15] Hajishengallis G, Lamont RJ. Beyond the red complex and into more complexity: The polymicrobial synergy and dysbiosis (PSD) model of periodontal disease etiology. Molecular Oral Microbiology. 2012;**27**(6):409-419. DOI: 10.1111/j.2041-1014.2012.00663.x

[16] Lamont RJ, Koo H, Hajishengallis G. The oral microbiota: Dynamic communities and host interactions. Nature Reviews. Microbiology. 2018;**16**(12):745-759. DOI: 10.1038/s41579-018-0089-x

[17] Olsen I, Lambris JD, Hajishengallis G. Porphyromonas gingivalis disturbs host-commensal homeostasis by changing complement function. Journal of Oral Microbiology. 2017;**9**(1):1340085. DOI: 10.1080/20002297.2017.1340085

[18] Darveau RP, Hajishengallis G, Curtis MA. Porphyromonas gingivalis as a potential community activist for disease. Journal of Dental Research. 2012;**91**(9):816-820. DOI: 10.1177/0022034512453589

[19] Zijnge V, van Leeuwen MB, Degener JE, Abbas F, Thurnheer T, Gmür R, et al. Oral biofilm architecture on natural teeth. PLoS One. 2010;**5**(2):e9321. DOI: 10.1371/journal.pone.0009321

[20] ten Napel JH, Theilade J, Matsson L, Attström R. Ultrastructure of developing subgingival plaque in beagle dogs. Journal of Clinical Periodontology. 1985;**12**(7):507-524. DOI: 10.1111/j.1600-051x.1985.tb01386.x

[21] Libby P, Buring JE, Badimon L, Hansson GK, Deanfield J, Bittencourt MS, et al. Atherosclerosis. Nature Reviews. Disease Primers. 2019;**5**(1):56. DOI: 10.1038/s41572-019-0106-z

[22] Lockhart PB, Bolger AF, Papapanou PN, Osinbowale O, Trevisan M, Levison ME, et al. Periodontal disease and atherosclerotic vascular disease: Does the evidence support an independent association?: A scientific statement from the American Heart Association. Circulation. 2012;**125**(20):2520-2544. DOI: 10.1161/CIR.0b013e31825719f3

[23] Febbraio M, Roy CB, Levin L. Is there a causal link between periodontitis and cardiovascular disease? A concise review of recent findings. International Dental Journal. 2022;**72**(1):37-51. DOI: 10.1016/j.identj.2021.07.006

[24] Hajishengallis G, Chavakis T. Local and systemic mechanisms linking periodontal disease and inflammatory comorbidities. Nature Reviews. Immunology. 2021;**21**(7):426-440. DOI: 10.1038/s41577-020-00488-6

[25] Joshi C, Bapat R, Anderson W, Dawson D, Hijazi K, Cherukara G. Detection of periodontal microorganisms in coronary atheromatous plaque specimens of myocardial infarction patients: A systematic review and meta-analysis. Trends in Cardiovascular Medicine. 2021;**31**(1):69-82. DOI: 10.1016/j.tcm.2019.12.005

[26] Gode S, Sarp TZ, Saribas S, Ergin S, Kasnak G, Dinc HO, et al. The prevalence of periodontal pathogenic bacteria in atherosclerotic cardiovascular disease.

Clinical Laboratory. 2020;**66**(5). DOI: 10.7754/Clin.Lab.2020.191146

[27] Lu Q, Jin L. Human gingiva is another site of C-reactive protein formation. Journal of Clinical Periodontology. 2010;**37**(9):789-796. DOI: 10.1111/j.1600-051X.2010.01600.x

[28] Ridker PM. Clinical application of C-reactive protein for cardiovascular disease detection and prevention. Circulation. 2003;**107**(3):363-369. DOI: 10.1161/01.cir.0000053730.47739.3c

[29] Qi J, Zihang Z, Zhang J, Park YM, Shrestha D, Jianling B, et al. Periodontal antibodies and all-cause and cardiovascular disease mortality. Journal of Dental Research. 2020;**99**(1):51-59. DOI: 10.1177/0022034519884012

[30] Kebschull M, Demmer RT, Papapanou PN. "Gum bug, leave my heart alone!"--epidemiologic and mechanistic evidence linking periodontal infections and atherosclerosis. Journal of Dental Research. 2010;**89**(9):879-902. DOI: 10.1177/0022034510375281

[31] Epstein SE, Zhu J, Burnett MS, Zhou YF, Vercellotti G, Hajjar D. Infection and atherosclerosis: Potential roles of pathogen burden and molecular mimicry. Arteriosclerosis, Thrombosis, and Vascular Biology. 2000;**20**(6):1417-1420. DOI: 10.1161/01.atv.20.6.1417

[32] Papapanagiotou D, Nicu EA, Bizzarro S, Gerdes VE, Meijers JC, Nieuwland R, et al. Periodontitis is associated with platelet activation. Atherosclerosis. 2009;**202**(2):605-611. DOI: 10.1016/j.atherosclerosis.2008.05.035

[33] Perumal R, Rajendran M, Krishnamurthy M, Ganji KK, Pendor SD. Modulation of P-selection and platelet aggregation in chronic periodontitis: A clinical study. Journal of Indian Society of Periodontology. 2014;**18**(3):293-300. DOI: 10.4103/0972-124X.134563

[34] Dikshit S. Fibrinogen degradation products and periodontitis: Deciphering the connection. Journal of Clinical and Diagnostic Research. 2015;**9**(12): ZC10-ZC12. DOI: 10.7860/JCDR/2015/14729.6922

[35] Scannapieco FA, Bush RB, Paju S. Associations between periodontal disease and risk for atherosclerosis, cardiovascular disease, and stroke. A systematic review. Annals of Periodontology. 2003;**8**(1):38-53. DOI: 10.1902/annals.2003.8.1.38

[36] Janket SJ, Baird AE, Chuang SK, Jones JA. Meta-analysis of periodontal disease and risk of coronary heart disease and stroke. Oral Surgery, Oral Medicine, Oral Pathology, Oral Radiology, and Endodontics. 2003;**95**(5):559-569. DOI: 10.1067/moe.2003.107

[37] Khader YS, Albashaireh ZS, Alomari MA. Periodontal diseases and the risk of coronary heart and cerebrovascular diseases: A meta-analysis. Journal of Periodontology. 2004;**75**(8):1046-1053. DOI: 10.1902/jop.2004.75.8.1046

[38] Bahekar AA, Singh S, Saha S, Molnar J, Arora R. The prevalence and incidence of coronary heart disease is significantly increased in periodontitis: A meta-analysis. American Heart Journal. 2007;**154**(5):830-837. DOI: 10.1016/j.ahj.2007.06.037

[39] Shi Q, Zhang B, Huo N, Cai C, Liu H, Xu J. Association between myocardial infarction and periodontitis: A meta-analysis of case-control studies. Frontiers in Physiology. 2016;**7**:519. DOI: 10.3389/fphys.2016.00519

[40] Xu S, Song M, Xiong Y, Liu X, He Y, Qin Z. The association between periodontal disease and the risk of myocardial infarction: A pooled analysis of observational studies. BMC Cardiovascular Disorders. 2017;**17**(1):50. DOI: 10.1186/s12872-017-0480-y

[41] Gomes-Filho IS, Coelho JMF, Miranda SS, Cruz SS, Trindade SC, Cerqueira EMM, et al. Severe and moderate periodontitis are associated with acute myocardial infarction. Journal of Periodontology. 2020;**91**(11): 1444-1452. DOI: 10.1002/JPER.19-0703

[42] Gustafsson N, Ahlqvist J, Näslund U, Buhlin K, Gustafsson A, Kjellström B, et al. Associations among periodontitis, calcified carotid artery atheromas, and risk of myocardial infarction. Journal of Dental Research. 2020;**99**(1):60-68. DOI: 10.1177/0022034519885362

[43] Desvarieux M, Demmer RT, Rundek T, Boden-Albala B, Jacobs DR Jr, Papapanou PN, et al. Relationship between periodontal disease, tooth loss, and carotid artery plaque: The Oral Infections and Vascular Disease Epidemiology Study (INVEST). Stroke. 2003;**34**(9):2120-2125. DOI: 10.1161/01.STR.0000085086.50957.22

[44] Rydén L, Buhlin K, Ekstrand E, de Faire U, Gustafsson A, Holmer J, et al. Periodontitis increases the risk of a first myocardial infarction: A report from the PAROKRANK study. Circulation. 2016;**133**(6):576-583. DOI: 10.1161/CIRCULATIONAHA.115.020324

[45] Naderi S, Merchant AT. The association between periodontitis and cardiovascular disease: An update. Current Atherosclerosis Reports. 2020;**22**(10):52. DOI: 10.1007/s11883-020-00878-0

[46] Fagundes NCF, Almeida APCPSC, Vilhena KFB, Magno MB, Maia LC, Lima RR. Periodontitis as a risk factor for stroke: A systematic review and meta-analysis. Vascular Health and Risk Management. 2019;**15**:519-532. DOI: 10.2147/VHRM.S204097

[47] Muñoz Aguilera E, Suvan J, Buti J, Czesnikiewicz-Guzik M, Barbosa Ribeiro A, Orlandi M, et al. Periodontitis is associated with hypertension: A systematic review and meta-analysis. Cardiovascular Research. 2020;**116**(1):28-39. DOI: 10.1093/cvr/cvz201

[48] Del Pinto R, Landi L, Grassi G, Sforza NM, Cairo F, Citterio F, et al. Hypertension and periodontitis: A joint report by the Italian Society of Hypertension (SIIA) and the Italian Society of Periodontology and Implantology (SIdP). High Blood Pressure & Cardiovascular Prevention. 2021;**28**(5):427-438. DOI: 10.1007/s40292-021-00466-6

[49] Martin-Cabezas R, Seelam N, Petit C, Agossa K, Gaertner S, Tenenbaum H, et al. Association between periodontitis and arterial hypertension: A systematic review and meta-analysis. American Heart Journal. 2016;**180**:98-112. DOI: 10.1016/j.ahj.2016.07.018

[50] Tsakos G, Sabbah W, Hingorani AD, Netuveli G, Donos N, Watt RG, et al. Is periodontal inflammation associated with raised blood pressure? Evidence from a National US survey. Journal of Hypertension. 2010;**28**(12):2386-2393. DOI: 10.1097/HJH.0b013e32833e0fe1

[51] Dutzan N, Kajikawa T, Abusleme L, Greenwell-Wild T, Zuazo CE, Ikeuchi T, et al. A dysbiotic microbiome triggers TH17 cells to mediate oral mucosal immunopathology in mice and humans. Science Translational Medicine. 2018;**10**(463):eaat0797. DOI: 10.1126/scitranslmed.aat0797

[52] Jobin K, Stumpf NE, Schwab S, Eichler M, Neubert P, Rauh M, et al. A high-salt diet compromises antibacterial neutrophil responses through hormonal perturbation. Science Translational Medicine. 2020;**12**(536):eaay3850. DOI: 10.1126/scitranslmed.aay3850

[53] Komine-Aizawa S, Aizawa S, Hayakawa S. Periodontal diseases and adverse pregnancy outcomes. The Journal of Obstetrics and Gynaecology Research. 2019;**45**(1):5-12. DOI: 10.1111/jog.13782

[54] No CO. 569: Oral health care during pregnancy and through the lifespan. Obstetrics and Gynecology. 2013;**122** (2 Pt 1):417-422. DOI: 10.1097/01.AOG.0000433007.16843.10

[55] Jiang H, Su Y, Xiong X, Harville E, Wu H, Jiang Z, et al. Prevalence and risk factors of periodontal disease among pre-conception Chinese women. Reproductive Health. 2016;**13**(1):141. DOI: 10.1186/s12978-016-0256-3

[56] Stout MJ, Conlon B, Landeau M, Lee I, Bower C, Zhao Q, et al. Identification of intracellular bacteria in the basal plate of the human placenta in term and preterm gestations. American Journal of Obstetrics and Gynecology. 2013;**208**(3):226.e1-226.e2267. DOI: 10.1016/j.ajog.2013.01.018

[57] Aagaard K, Ma J, Antony KM, Ganu R, Petrosino J, Versalovic J. The placenta harbors a unique microbiome. Science Translational Medicine. 2014;**6**(237):237ra65. DOI: 10.1126/scitranslmed.3008599

[58] Katz J, Chegini N, Shiverick KT, Lamont RJ. Localization of P. gingivalis in preterm delivery placenta. Journal of Dental Research. 2009;**88**(6):575-578. DOI: 10.1177/0022034509338032

[59] Sgolastra F, Petrucci A, Severino M, Gatto R, Monaco A. Relationship between periodontitis and pre-eclampsia: A meta-analysis. PLoS One. 2013;**8**(8):e71387. DOI: 10.1371/journal.pone.0071387

[60] Wei BJ, Chen YJ, Yu L, Wu B. Periodontal disease and risk of preeclampsia: A meta-analysis of observational studies. PLoS One. 2013;**8**(8):e70901. DOI: 10.1371/journal.pone.0070901

[61] Genco RJ, Van Dyke TE. Prevention: Reducing the risk of CVD in patients with periodontitis. Nature Reviews. Cardiology. 2010;**7**(9):479-480. DOI: 10.1038/nrcardio.2010.120

[62] Quirynen M, Bollen CM, Vandekerckhove BN, Dekeyser C, Papaioannou W, Eyssen H. Full- vs. partial-mouth disinfection in the treatment of periodontal infections: Short-term clinical and microbiological observations. Journal of Dental Research. 1995;**74**(8):1459-1467. DOI: 10.1177/00220345950740080501

[63] Orlandi M, Graziani F, D'Aiuto F. Periodontal therapy and cardiovascular risk. Periodontology 2000. 2020; **83**(1):107-124. DOI: 10.1111/prd.12299

[64] Graziani F, Cei S, Orlandi M, Gennai S, Gabriele M, Filice N, et al. Acute-phase response following full-mouth versus quadrant non-surgical periodontal treatment: A randomized clinical trial. Journal of Clinical Periodontology. 2015;**42**(9):843-852. DOI: 10.1111/jcpe.12451

[65] Chen TT, D'Aiuto F, Yeh YC, Lai MS, Chien KL, Tu YK. Risk of myocardial infarction and ischemic stroke after dental treatments. Journal of Dental Research. 2019;**98**(2):157-163. DOI: 10.1177/0022034518805745

[66] Minassian C, D'Aiuto F, Hingorani AD, Smeeth L. Invasive dental treatment and risk for vascular events: A self-controlled case series. Annals of Internal Medicine. 2010; **153**(8):499-506. DOI: 10.7326/0003-4819-153-8-201010190-00006

[67] Montenegro MM, Ribeiro IWJ, Kampits C, Saffi MAL, Furtado MV, Polanczyk CA, et al. Randomized controlled trial of the effect of periodontal treatment on cardiovascular risk biomarkers in patients with stable coronary artery disease: Preliminary findings of 3 months. Journal of Clinical Periodontology. 2019;**46**(3):321-331. DOI: 10.1111/jcpe.13085

[68] Beck JD, Couper DJ, Falkner KL, Graham SP, Grossi SG, Gunsolley JC, et al. The Periodontitis and Vascular Events (PAVE) pilot study: Adverse events. Journal of Periodontology. 2008;**79**(1):90-96. DOI: 10.1902/jop.2008.070223

[69] Holmlund A, Lampa E, Lind L. Oral health and cardiovascular disease risk in a cohort of periodontitis patients. Atherosclerosis. 2017;**262**:101-106. DOI: 10.1016/j.atherosclerosis.2017.05.009

[70] Nordendahl E, Kjellström B, Fored CM, Ekbom A, Svensson T, Norhammar A, et al. Invasive dental treatment and risk for a first myocardial infarction. Journal of Dental Research. 2018;**97**(10):1100-1105. DOI: 10.1177/0022034518767834

[71] Steffel J, Verhamme P, Potpara TS, Albaladejo P, Antz M, Desteghe L, et al. The 2018 European Heart Rhythm Association Practical Guide on the use of non-vitamin K antagonist oral anticoagulants in patients with atrial fibrillation: Executive summary. Europace. 2018;**20**(8):1231-1242. DOI: 10.1093/europace/euy054

[72] Steffel J, Verhamme P, Potpara TS, Albaladejo P, Antz M, Desteghe L, et al. The 2018 European Heart Rhythm Association Practical Guide on the use of non-vitamin K antagonist oral anticoagulants in patients with atrial fibrillation. European Heart Journal. 2018;**39**(16):1330-1393. DOI: 10.1093/eurheartj/ehy136

[73] Doganay O, Atalay B, Karadag E, Aga U, Tugrul M. Bleeding frequency of patients taking ticagrelor, aspirin, clopidogrel, and dual antiplatelet therapy after tooth extraction and minor oral surgery. Journal of the American Dental Association (1939). 2018;**149**(2):132-138. DOI: 10.1016/j.adaj.2017.09.052

[74] Lillis T, Ziakas A, Koskinas K, Tsirlis A, Giannoglou G. Safety of dental extractions during uninterrupted single or dual antiplatelet treatment. The American Journal of Cardiology. 2011;**108**(7):964-967. DOI: 10.1016/j.amjcard.2011.05.029

[75] Napeñas JJ, Hong CH, Brennan MT, Furney SL, Fox PC, Lockhart PB. The frequency of bleeding complications after invasive dental treatment in patients receiving single and dual antiplatelet therapy. Journal of the American Dental Association (1939). 2009;**140**(6):690-695. DOI: 10.14219/jada.archive.2009.0255

[76] Nathwani S, Martin K. Exodontia in dual antiplatelet therapy: The evidence. British Dental Journal. 2016;**220**(5):235-238. DOI: 10.1038/sj.bdj.2016.173

[77] Douketis JD, Spyropoulos AC, Spencer FA, Mayr M, Jaffer AK, Eckman MH, et al. Perioperative management of antithrombotic therapy: Antithrombotic therapy and prevention of thrombosis, 9th ed: American College of Chest Physicians evidence-based clinical practice guidelines. Chest.

2012;**141**(Suppl. 2):e326S-e350S. DOI: 10.1378/chest.11-2298

[78] Grines CL, Bonow RO, Casey DE Jr, Gardner TJ, Lockhart PB, Moliterno DJ, et al. Prevention of premature discontinuation of dual antiplatelet therapy in patients with coronary artery stents: A science advisory from the American Heart Association, American College of Cardiology, Society for Cardiovascular Angiography and Interventions, American College of Surgeons, and American Dental Association, with representation from the American College of Physicians. Journal of the American College of Cardiology. 2007;**49**(6):734-739. DOI: 10.1016/j.jacc.2007.01.003

[79] Kristensen SD, Knuuti J, Saraste A, Anker S, Bøtker HE, Hert SD, et al. 2014 ESC/ESA Guidelines on non-cardiac surgery: Cardiovascular assessment and management: The joint task force on non-cardiac surgery: Cardiovascular assessment and management of the European Society of Cardiology (ESC) and the European Society of Anaesthesiology (ESA). European Heart Journal. 2014;**35**(35):2383-2431. DOI: 10.1093/eurheartj/ehu282

[80] Shi Q, Xu J, Zhang T, Zhang B, Liu H. Post-operative bleeding risk in dental surgery for patients on oral anticoagulant therapy: A meta-analysis of observational studies. Frontiers in Pharmacology. 2017;**8**:58. DOI: 10.3389/fphar.2017.00058

[81] Yang S, Shi Q, Liu J, Li J, Xu J. Should oral anticoagulant therapy be continued during dental extraction? A meta-analysis. BMC Oral Health. 2016;**16**(1):81. DOI: 10.1186/s12903-016-0278-9

[82] Biedermann JS, Rademacher WMH, Hazendonk HCAM, van Diermen DE, Leebeek FWG, Rozema FR, et al. Predictors of oral cavity bleeding and clinical outcome after dental procedures in patients on vitamin K antagonists. A cohort study. Thrombosis and Haemostasis. 2017;**117**(7):1432-1439. DOI: 10.1160/TH17-01-0040

[83] Madrid C, Sanz M. What influence do anticoagulants have on oral implant therapy? A systematic review. Clinical Oral Implants Research. 2009;**20** (Suppl. 4):96-106. DOI: 10.1111/j.1600-0501.2009.01770.x

[84] Kwak EJ, Nam S, Park KM, Kim SY, Huh J, Park W. Bleeding related to dental treatment in patients taking novel oral anticoagulants (NOACs): A retrospective study. Clinical Oral Investigations. 2019;**23**(1):477-484. DOI: 10.1007/s00784-018-2458-2

[85] Lababidi E, Breik O, Savage J, Engelbrecht H, Kumar R, Crossley CW. Assessing an oral surgery specific protocol for patients on direct oral anticoagulants: A retrospective controlled cohort study. International Journal of Oral and Maxillofacial Surgery. 2018;**47**(7):940-946. DOI: 10.1016/j.ijom.2018.03.009

[86] Patel JP, Woolcombe SA, Patel RK, Obisesan O, Roberts LN, Bryant C, et al. Managing direct oral anticoagulants in patients undergoing dentoalveolar surgery. British Dental Journal. 2017;**222**(4):245-249. DOI: 10.1038/sj.bdj.2017.165

[87] Miclotte I, Vanhaverbeke M, Agbaje JO, Legrand P, Vanassche T, Verhamme P, et al. Pragmatic approach to manage new oral anticoagulants in patients undergoing dental extractions: A prospective case-control study. Clinical Oral Investigations. 2017;**21**(7): 2183-2188. DOI: 10.1007/s00784-016-2010-1

[88] Hindricks G, Potpara T, Dagres N, Arbelo E, Bax JJ, Blomström-Lundqvist C, et al. 2020 ESC guidelines for the diagnosis and management of atrial fibrillation developed in collaboration with the European Association for Cardio-Thoracic Surgery (EACTS): The task force for the diagnosis and management of atrial fibrillation of the European Society of Cardiology (ESC) developed with the special contribution of the European Heart Rhythm Association (EHRA) of the ESC [published correction appears in European Heart Journal. 2021;**42**(5):507] [published correction appears in European Heart Journal. 2021;**42**(5):546-547] [published correction appears in European Heart Journal. 2021;**42**(40):4194]. European Heart Journal. 2021;42(5):373-498. DOI:10.1093/eurheartj/ehaa612

[89] Perry DJ, Noakes TJ, Helliwell PS, British Dental Society. Guidelines for the management of patients on oral anticoagulants requiring dental surgery. British Dental Journal. 2007;**203**(7):389-393. DOI: 10.1038/bdj.2007.892

[90] Valgimigli M, Bueno H, Byrne RA, Collet JP, Costa F, Jeppsson A, et al. 2017 ESC focused update on dual antiplatelet therapy in coronary artery disease developed in collaboration with EACTS: The task force for dual antiplatelet therapy in coronary artery disease of the European Society of Cardiology (ESC) and of the European Association for Cardio-Thoracic Surgery (EACTS). European Heart Journal. 2018;**39**(3): 213-260. DOI: 10.1093/eurheartj/ehx419

Chapter 3

Ulcerative Lesions of the Oral Cavity

Nelli Yildirimyan

Abstract

Apart from dental and periodontal diseases, oral mucosal lesions are also frequently encountered by both general dentists and dental specialists in outpatient clinics. Although these soft tissue lesions may only reveal a localized issue, sometimes they may be the only sign of a more serious underlying systemic condition. Thus, oral ulcerations pose a unique diagnostic challenge for healthcare providers and should be cautiously handled when they last for more than two weeks, even after any possible traumatic etiologies are eliminated. There are many different classifications regarding oral ulcerations based on their etiologic or clinical features. In order to provide a logical and simple stepwise guidance to accurate diagnosis, this chapter will categorize and explain these lesions based on their clinical properties.

Keywords: oral ulcer, oral mucosa, oral disease, aphthous stomatitis

1. Introduction

Oral ulcerative lesions are defects in the oral epithelia, its underlying connective tissue or both. The oral mucosa is considered among one of the susceptible areas in the human body to painful ulceration [1, 2]. An oral ulcer is not a disease itself but rather a sign of a different underlying condition, therefore it is usually challenging to diagnose the accurate etiology [1]. It is important to identify the etiologic factor to provide a complete resolution to patients rather than constantly prescribing certain medicines to suppress the symptoms [3].

Regardless of the etiology of these lesions, oral ulcerative lesions may be categorized as minor, major or herpetiform ulcerations. Minor ulcerations are usually less than 1 cm in diameter, and they most commonly present on the labial or buccal mucosa or the ventral surface of the tongue. Less common locations include the dorsum of the tongue, hard palate or the gingiva [4, 5].

Ulcerations that measure more than 1 cm in diameter are referred to as major oral ulcerations and have a lower prevalence than minor ones. Among these three types, the least common type is the herpetiform ulceration, which unlike what its name suggests, is irrelevant to herpetic stomatitis since no vesicle formation is observed in advance [5]. These type of ulcerations are multiple and usually are much smaller in diameter (1–3 mm) [4].

Another helpful classification is based on the duration of these lesions, which may aid clinicians establish a more logical stepwise progression towards an accurate diagnosis. Accordingly, an oral ulcerative lesion is diagnosed as acute if it lasts for less than two weeks, chronic if it persists for more than two weeks or recurrent if it presents with a history ulcerative episode with intermittent periods of healing [1].

2. Acute ulcerative lesions

A short-lived oral ulcerative lesion which resolves in less than two weeks is considered as an acute oral ulcer and is commonly referred to as an "aphtha" [1, 2]. This word itself is attributed to Hippocrates which was used to describe disorders of the mouth in general back in his time (460–370 BC) [3]. In order to accurately diagnose and evaluate patients with acute ulcerative lesions, it is crucial that the physician is aware of the broad spectrum of possibilities that may cause these lesions. It is recommended to assess the history of the lesions first, meaning to question the patient regarding any periodic episodes, in order to exclude conditions which are characterized with recurrent oral ulcerations [2].

Clinically acute oral ulcers usually have an oval shape with an erythematous periphery due to the dilation of the blood vessels. Although commonly these are painful lesions, the pain is relatively weaker when the ulcer bed is layered with a yellowish fibro-membrane [2].

Most common acute oral ulcerations may be related to trauma (i.e., traumatic ulcers), chemotherapy (i.e. chemotherapy induced ulcers), necrotizing sialometaplasia, primary herpetic gingivostomatitis, herpes zoster infection, herpangina, hand-foot mouth disease, erythema multiforme, necrotizing ulcerative gingivitis, oral hypersensitivity reactions or plasma cell stomatitis [1, 6, 7].

Traumatic ulcerations are one of the most common oral ulcerative lesions [8]. If a traumatic ulceration is due to the mucosal irritation of natal or neonatal teeth at the ventral surface of the tongue, then it is called "Riga-Fede disease". Ulcerations due to thermal and electrical injuries most commonly occur in children and affect the lip and commissure areas. On the contrary, malformed or fractured teeth, ill-fitting dentures or overheated food are usually encountered in adults (**Figure 1**) [1, 9]. Traumatic ulcerations tend to heal within ten days once the etiologic factor is discarded [8].

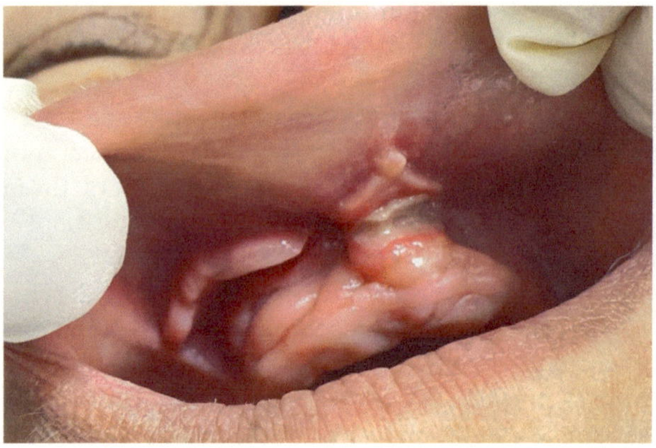

Figure 1.
Irritation fibroma of the right vestibular sulcus and an acute traumatic ulceration of the maxillary frenulum due to ill-fitting dentures.

Chemotherapy induced ulcers are commonly observed in oral mucositis, which is one of the most frequent complications of chemotherapy in oncologic patients [10]. These erythematous and painful ulcerative lesions are due to the detrimental effects of chemotherapy on oral mucosal epithelial cells. Patients receiving chemotherapy for a malignancy have a 24.8–67% incidence rate for oral ulcerations [11]. This rate increases to almost 90% in patients with head and neck cancer, who receive both chemotherapy and radiotherapy for their oncologic condition. Cisplatin, 5-fluoruracil, docetaxel, paclitaxel, everolimus, tenserolimus, ridaforolimus, cetuximab, panitunumab, erlotinib, gefinitib, afatinib, lapatinib and dacomitinib are among the most common chemotherapeutic agents associated with chemotherapy induced oral ulcers [12–15]. The risk to develop mucositis rises when a patient receives both chemotherapy and radiotherapy. The incidence and the severity of oral ulcerative lesions vary in patients with different agents and therapeutic regimen [15]. Besides the overall clinical manifestations such as mucosal congestion, edema, and severe pain, co-infection may affect these patients' oral intake and disturb the smooth progress of chemotherapy. Co-infection may progress into a more severe systemic infection and cumulatively threaten the lives of the patients [11]. Treatments using granulocyte colony-stimulating factor, keratinocyte growth factor, honey intake or low-level laser therapy have been proposed as preventive measures for chemotherapy induced ulcers however a consensus regarding the most effective preventive option is still not established [10]. Among these preventive options, the only drug approved both by Food and Drug Agency (FDA) and European Medical Agency (EMA) is palifermin, and it is a keratinocyte growth factor. It is advised to administer to patients undergoing high doses chemotherapy and radiotherapy prior to their oncologic treatment. Once oral ulcerations develop, it is important to prevent serious nutritional deficiencies due to inadequate food intake and consider parenteral nutrition options [15]. Current guidelines suggest morphine to provide analgesia for pain in these patients [16]. Moreover "magic" mouthwashes have also been formulated containing anesthetics, antacids and diphenhydramine. Formulations with steroids and anti-mycotics are also available [17].

Necrotizing sialometaplasia is a solitary benign condition due to an inflammatory reaction of salivary glands. The true etiology is still unknown however local infarction due to ischemia of the salivary tissue is blamed. Mostly these lesions occur on the posterior palate but may rarely observed on the lower lip, retromolar pad, sublingual region, tongue and the larynx. Clinically necrotizing sialometaplasia manifests as a crater like ulcer with indurated borders. Although it is a self-limiting condition, complete healing may take up to 7 weeks [1]. During this period, patients may aid supportive treatments focused on pain control. Necrotizing sialometaplasia may mimic salivary gland tumors, thus physicians should always question the evolution time since in most cases salivary gland tumors do not present such short evolution times like necrotizing sialometaplasia [18].

Primary herpetic gingivostomatitis is a viral condition due to Herpes Simplex Virus (HSV). It usually occurs in children younger than five years. Oral ulcerative lesions associated with primary herpetic gingivostomatitis develop as multiple pin-headed vesicles which rupture. These small lesions may merge and manifest as larger ulcerations. Systemic symptoms such as fever, nausea, anorexia, submandibular lymphadenopathy, halitosis and dysphagia are also noted [1]. Bed rest, fluids, soft diet and antipyretics are suggested for the systemic manifestations of primary herpetic gingivostomatitis. In order to reduce the spread of infection to other sites, patients must be discouraged from touching the ulcerative areas. Systemic antiviral therapies may be considered in severe cases or for immunocompromised patients [19].

Herpes zoster infection is a secondary viral condition due to Varicella Zoster Virus (VZV). Clinically it is a painful condition with vesicular eruptions both on the skin and the mucosa. Symptoms are unilateral with extreme pain along the course of the nerve [20]. The involvement of the trigeminal nerve is rare but painful, with clustered ulcers of less than 5 mm in diameter. Depending on the involvement of specific nerves, these ulcers may appear on the hard palate, buccal gingivae or tongue in a characteristic unilateral pattern. Antiviral medicine may be required to manage the herpes zoster infection whereas the oral ulcerations are self-limiting and usually heal within two weeks [1].

Herpangina and hand-foot-mouth disease are both self-limiting and mild viral conditions caused by coxsackievirus commonly affecting children. Herpangina clinically manifests with sore throat, fever, blisters and ulcers involving the palate, oropharynx and tonsillar pillars [1, 8]. Posterior involvement of the oral cavity may help alarm the physicians in diagnosing herpangina. Hand-foot-mouth disease differs from other lesions since it simultaneously involves the extremities and oral cavity [8]. Ulcerative lesions related to hand-foot-mouth disease usually involve the tongue, hard and soft palate, and the buccal mucosa. Both diseases are similarly managed targeting analgesia and fever control. Currently, there are no available medical treatments against coxsackievirus infections [1].

Erythema multiforme is an autoimmune mucocutaneous condition with varying etiologic factors. Although oral ulcerative lesions are not the only oral symptoms, several oral manifestations such as macules and bullae are observed in almost 70% of patients with erythema multiforme [1, 21]. Similar to viral infections, erythema multiforme also presents with generalized symptoms like fever, lymphadenopathy, headache, malaise, cough, and sore throat. Oral ulcerative lesions associated with erythema multiforme are usually large, multiple and confluent. Management depends on the severity of the condition. Mild forms usually heal within 10–20 days. Liquid diet is suggested, analgesics or antipyretics are prescribed, and local wound care is applied if necessary [1].

Acute necrotizing ulcerative gingivitis (ANUG) is a bacterial opportunistic infection. The most common etiological factors are *Fusobacterium* and *Prevotella* species [22]. It is a painful and destructive gingival condition that specifically affects the interdental gum tissue. Clinically three essential findings help physicians in an accurate diagnosis which are (a) halitosis, (b) rapid onset, and (c) ulceration and necrosis of the interdental papillae that look like punched out, crater-like lesions. ANUG is often associated with poor oral hygiene, low immune system, nutritional deficiency, smoking or psychological stress [23]. Proper ANUG treatment should focus on the management of the acute symptoms and the prevention of further tissue destruction. Debridement of superficial gingival plaques and calculi at the necrotic lesions along with a prescription for 0.12% chlorhexidine gluconate mouth rinse twice daily should be considered initially. Signs of systemic involvement are fever, malaise or lymphadenopathy [22]. Due to its anaerobic activity, the first drug choice is metronidazole 250 mg, three times daily; however, penicillin, tetracyclines, clindamycin, amoxicillin, and amoxicillin with clavulanate also show acceptable results and may be considered. On the contrary, topical antimicrobials are not recommended [23]. Simultaneous antifungal agents should be considered in immunosuppressed patients along with the antibiotic therapy. Once the acute phase is managed, scaling and root planning along with proper oral hygiene maintenance should be established. Management of any predisposing factors should not be disregarded. Additional periodontal surgical procedures such as gingivectomy or gingivoplasty may be considered on a case-by-case basis [22].

Oral hypersensitivity reactions may be associated with a range of allergens including food, medications, mouthwashes, gums, toothpastes, restorative or cosmetic materials. Clinically these reactions may manifest as mucosal ulcerations or lichenoid reactions (**Figure 2**). Ulcerations usually have irregular borders and a red halo. Other oral symptoms may include erythema and edema of the oral structures or white patches and plaques [24]. Itching of the oral and pharyngeal tissues may or may not be present [1]. Clinical data recording is crucial in these patients. In order to accurately identify the allergens, the patch test is considered the gold standard. It is recommended to order a patch test for all patients when a hypersensitivity reaction is suspected to spot the true etiological factor [25]. Once the etiology is revealed, elimination of this causative agent often results in the resolution of the symptoms usually within two weeks [24]. Patients may aid from topical corticosteroids either as an ointment or mouthwash during this period especially if they present with severe symptoms [26].

Plasma cell stomatitis or *plasma cell mucositis* is a rare benign condition. Although its true etiology is still debatable, several theories consider this entity also as a hypersensitivity reaction but with polyclonal plasma cell infiltration [27]. Clinically epithelial sloughing, desquamation and swelling may be observed besides ulcerations (**Figure 3**). It may affect anywhere on the oral mucosa but the gingivae is the most affected site [1]. Chewing gums, cinnamon, qat (a native plant in eastern Africa and Arabia), toothpaste or flavored mints have been suggested as possible etiologic factors but a specific causative agent is seldom identified [27–29]. Plasma cell

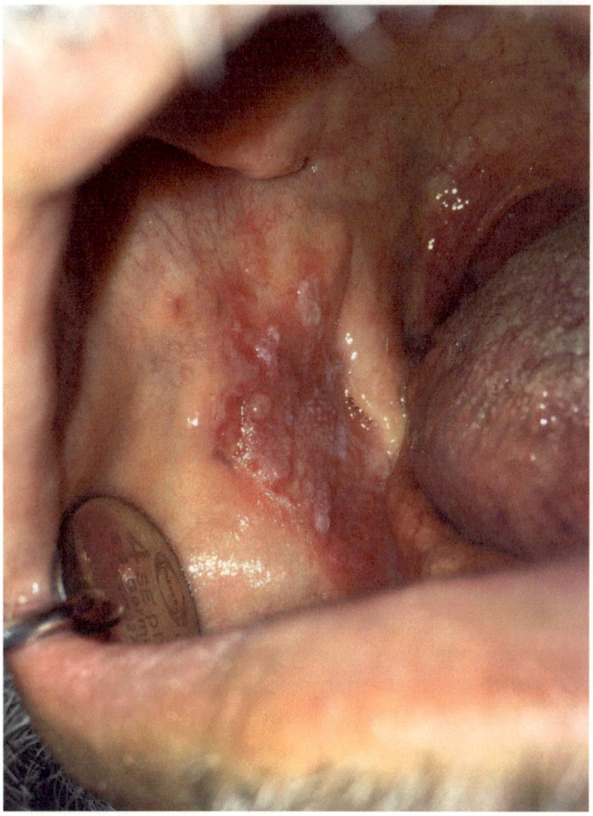

Figure 2.
Oral hypersensitivity reaction, three days after switching to a new brand of toothpaste.

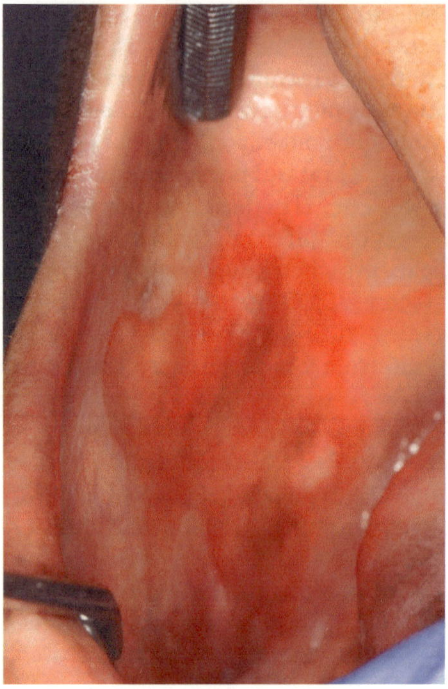

Figure 3.
Severe epithelial sloughing and erythema on a patient with plasma cell stomatitis.

stomatitis is managed with corticosteroids, either topical, intralesional or systemic, with additional antimicrobial medications depending on the systemic symptoms of the patients. Although complete regression is rare, most patients experience disease stabilization. Plasma cell stomatitis is a rare condition however clinically it may easily be confused more common benign and neoplastic conditions of oral cavity.

3. Chronic ulcerative lesions

Chronic ulcerative lesions have a slower onset than acute ulcers and last for more than two weeks. Several vesiculobullous entities, lupus erythematosus, tuberculosis, some mycoses, eosinophilic ulcers and oral cancer are among the most common conditions associated with chronic oral ulcerative lesions [6].

Drug induced oral ulcers are associated with mycophenolate (immunosuppressant), tiotropium (anticholinergic bronchodilator), clopidogrel (platelet aggregation inhibitor), nicorandil (vasodilator), bisphosphonates, protease inhibitors, some antimicrobials and analgesics, antirheumatics and several antihypertensives such as labetalol, enalapril or captopril [30]. This type of ulcerations usually presents with single, isolated ulcers with an erythematous halo. Most commonly the lateral side of the tongue is affected. Once the drug is discontinued, the lesions tend to disappear however it is not always achievable. Drug induced ulcers are also resistant to usual treatments [6].

Erosive lichen planus is a subtype lichen planus, a chronic condition which affects both the skin and the mucosal tissues. It is associated with the attack of cytotoxic T-cells on basal keratinocytes, which results in the areas of atrophy, erosion or ulcerations [6]. The World Health Organization considers lichen planus as a premalignant lesion with 1–5% chance of malignant transformation to oral squamous cell carcinoma. Erosive and atrophic forms are particularly considered at high-risk [31]. The most characteristic presentation of lichen planus is the Wickham's striae, which are white, lace-like keratotic mucosal configurations, commonly found bilaterally on the buccal mucosa (**Figure 4**) [32]. Several subtypes of lichen planus may simultaneously manifest in the oral cavity. Erosive lichen planus is one of the painful subtypes due to the ulcerations. These ulcerative lesions are usually covered with a pseudo-membrane and are erythematous (**Figure 5**) [1]. Once lichen planus is confirmed with a biopsy, corticosteroids are prescribed as an initial treatment. Drug resistance is common particularly in erosive lichen planus, thus topical immunosuppressant therapies, such as tacrolimus, aid in the management of this condition via inhibiting cytotoxic T-cell mediated response [6].

Pemphigus vulgaris is an autoimmune vesiculobullous mucocutaneous disease due to an IgG reaction against desmogleins which are specific proteins in desmosomes [6]. Almost 90% of the patients experience oral symptoms and in more than half of the cases these are the initial signs of the disease [8]. Clinically oral lesions in

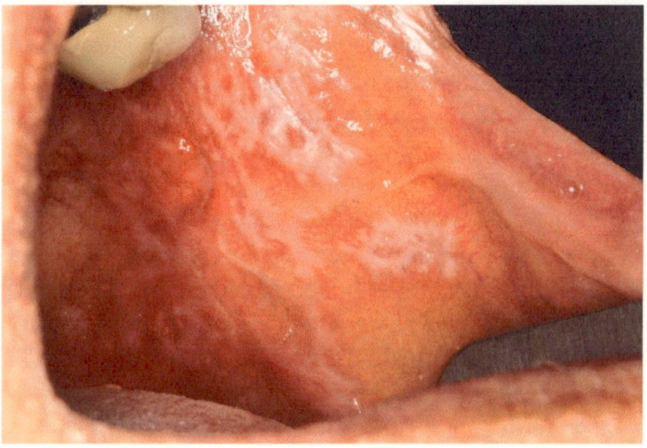

Figure 4.
Wickham's striae: The characteristic white, lace-like keratotic configurations seen in lichen planus.

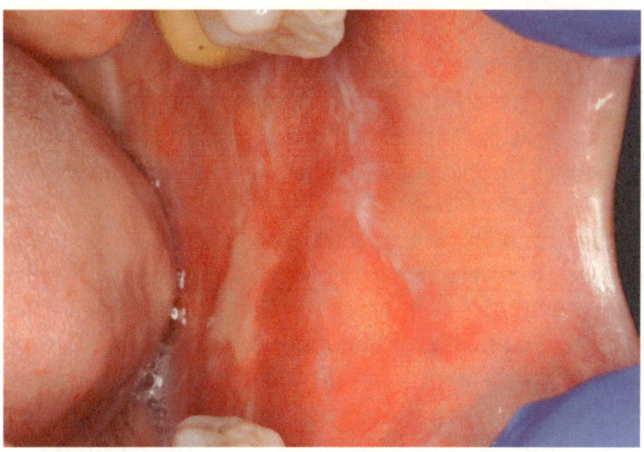

Figure 5.
Erosive lichen planus with an ulcerative area covered with a yellowish white pseudomembrane.

pemphigus vulgaris start as a bulla which quickly raptures in even a slight insult and results in a shallow irregular ulcerative lesion which endures for a long period of time and ultimately involves larger areas of the oral cavity [1, 8]. Ulcerative lesions of pemphigus vulgaris are painful and sometimes bleeding, and they heal with difficulty [8]. Buccal mucosa, palate and the gingival tissues are most commonly affected, and gingival involvement usually manifests as desquamative gingivitis [1]. Biopsy, and direct or indirect immunofluorescence studies confirm the diagnosis. Intraepithelial presence of Tzanck cells is a useful diagnostic sign for pemphigus vulvaris [6]. High dose systemic corticosteroids are used in the treatment of pemphigus vulgaris [1].

Mucous membrane pemphigoid or *cicatricial pemphigoid* is another autoimmune vesiculobullous disease that presents with subepithelial bullae which evolve spontaneously and rupture easily, resulting in painful ulcerative areas [6]. Bleeding into bullae results in blood blisters which are among the diagnostic features of mucous membrane pemphigoid [1]. Skin, ocular mucosa, esophagus, nasopharynx and larynx may also be involved besides the oral mucosa. Lesions of mucous membrane pemphigoid are chronic and persistent, thus often heal with a scar (cicatrix) which is particularly observed in lesions of the eye [33]. Contrary to pemphigus vulgaris, palatal mucosa is the most affected area within the oral cavity [6]. Buccal mucosa and the gingiva may also be affected. Gingival lesions in form of desquamative gingivitis may present as the only symptom of mucous membrane pemphigoid in some patients. Depending on the severity of the disease, mucous membrane pemphigoid is initially treated with either topical or systemic corticosteroids, and with dapsone in case of ocular involvement [1].

Lupus erythematosus is another autoimmune disorder of the connective tissue. Clinically oral lesions of lupus erythematosus may include areas of well-demarcated erythema, erosion or ulcerations, which tend to bleed. Whitish striae, similar to those seen in the oral manifestations of lichen planus, may also be present on the oral mucosa. Striae in lupus typically involves the hard palate, whereas in lichen planus these lesions are often bilaterally found on the buccal mucosa [6, 32]. Literature contains reports of oral lupus lesions transforming to oral squamous cell carcinoma, therefore it is crucial to regularly monitor and record the symptoms of these patients [34]. Therapeutic options for lupus erythematosus range from antimalarials to non-steroidal anti-inflammatory drugs and glucocorticoids, which may be combined with conventional immunosuppressive agents. Lately targeted therapies such as belimumab or rituximab are also gaining attention [35].

Linear IgA disease is also an autoimmune mucocutaneous condition that affects the sub-epithelium. Most patients with linear IgA disease are between 60 and 70 years old, but it may also affect the children. Oral lesions vary from vesicles to painful ulcerations or erosions mostly on the hard or soft palate. Topical or systemic corticosteroids or dapsone may be prescribed depending of the resistance and severity of the lesions [1].

Tuberculosis is a bacterial chronic granulomatous disease. Although rare, some tuberculosis patients may experience oral lesions which clinically manifest as solitary, deep, irregular and painful ulcers commonly on the lateral side of the tongue. These ulcers have a rounded rolled border. Final diagnosis is made via a tissue biopsy [1, 6].

Mycosis-related ulcerative lesions generally affect immunocompromised or uncontrolled diabetes patients, and present secondary to other infections. Clinical manifestations of different kinds of fungi may vary from painless or painful ulcers with indurated borders, areas of erythema, nodules, granuloma formation or areas of necrosis [1, 6, 36]. It is important to make a histologic evaluation via biopsy with

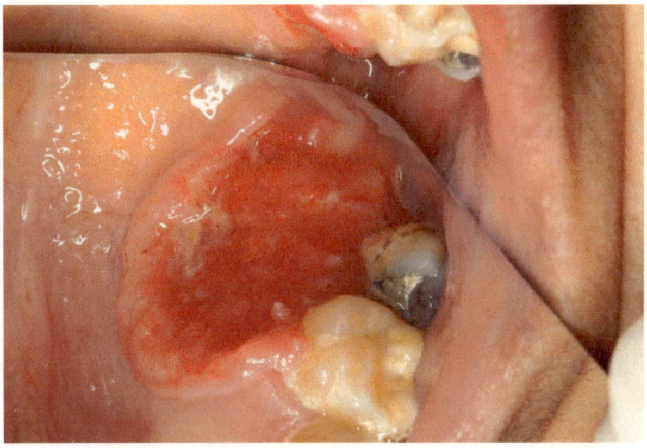

Figure 6.
Typical "crater like lesion with rolled borders"-look on a malignant ulcerative lesion of the hard palate.

specific stains to accurately diagnose mycoses because the oral symptoms of fungal infections may easily be confused with malignancies. The choice of treatment depends on the type of mycosis and may include antifungal medications with or without surgical intervention [36].

Eosinophilic ulcer or *traumatic ulcerative granuloma with stromal eosinophilia* is a benign, solitary ulcer which usually affects patients between fourth and sixth decades of life [1]. Its etiology is not well determined but it is associated with trauma in nearly half of the patients [6]. Viral and toxic agents, eosinophilic cytokines or chemotactic factors, mast cells or other cell-mediated immunity-related factors have also been suggested in the literature. Clinically an eosinophilic ulcer develops rapidly and has elevated borders with a white-yellow fundus [37]. Although it is a self-limiting condition, it heals very slowly and may easily mimic malignancies clinically. Eosinophil-rich inflammatory cell infiltrate also consisting of lymphocytes and mast cells help exclude the possibility of a malignancy [6, 37]. These solitary lesions usually respond to surgical excision with a rare recurrence rate. Other treatment modalities include intralesional or oral corticosteroids, topical antibiotics or cryotherapy [1].

Malignant ulcers may include epithelial neoplasms, solid tumors like lymphomas or minor salivary gland malignancies. Oral squamous cell carcinoma is the most common malignancy in the oral cavity [8]. It may present as a red white, exophytic, endophytic or ulcerative lesion [6]. Ulcerative lesions are usually asymptomatic and progressive, with a crater-like appearance and rolled, indurated borders (**Figure 6**) [1]. Biopsy is the only reliable method of diagnosis, and the treatment options vary depending on the severity of the disease. Smoking is one of the main risk factors for oral squamous cell carcinoma, therefore these patients must be educated properly and monitored closely for any suspicious lesion [6].

4. Recurrent ulcerative lesions

Recurrent aphthous stomatitis (RAS) is painful condition of the non-keratinized mucosa of the oral cavity. It is the most common inflammatory disease of the oral mucosa [1]. RAS has three forms: minor, major and herpetiform. Minor type consists of ulcers with less than 1 cm diameter, whereas the ulcers are larger than 1 cm, long-lasting and they heal with scarring in the major type. Herpetiform type consists of ulcers with less than 2 mm diameter, but the lesions are numerous and extremely painful [1, 3]. Clinically, round and shallow ulcerations occur repeatedly. These ulcers may be solitary or multiple, covered by fibrin and with an erythematous border [1, 8]. Although the true etiology is still unclear, it has been associated with stress, hormonal imbalances, several systemic diseases, certain vitamin or mineral deficiencies [3]. In order to provide a cause-based treatment rather than palliative and temporary management options, it is essential to determine the true cause of RAS. Among the most common causes, iron, zinc, vitamin B12 and folic acid deficiencies, immune disturbances such as either HIV or non-HIV immunodeficiencies, gastrointestinal diseases such as celiac, gluten-sensitive enteropathies, Crohn's or ulcerative colitis, or periodic fever-aphthae-pharyngitis-adenitis syndrome should be questioned, and medical tests should be ordered accordingly. Pain management may be achieved using topical, intralesional or systemic corticosteroids, immunosuppressants or pentoxifylline [3].

Recurrent herpetic stomatitis is an oral infection caused by herpes simplex virus and may either manifest as *recurrent herpes labialis*, which affects the lips, or *recurrent intraoral herpes*, which is confined mainly to the keratinized mucosa, especially the hard palate [38]. Low immunity, stress, ultraviolet light, cold weather, hormonal fluctuations or trauma may trigger these lesions [1]. Recurrent intraoral herpes starts as vesicles on the oral mucosa which often rupture and lead to ulcerative lesions. Patient history and clinical examination are important to achieve a correct diagnosis. Once the diagnosis is made, patients should be educated on the contagious nature of the disease. Palliative treatments include ice or lanolin applications, topical or systemic antiviral medications. Prophylactic use of sunscreen with sun protection factor (SPF) 15 or higher may be considered for patients suffering from recurrent herpes labialis [38].

Herpes-associated erythema multiforme is a challenging diagnosis which requires a through patient history and clinical evaluation. Erythema multiforme (EM) is a reactive mucocutaneous disorder usually due to hypersensitivity to drugs or other allergens [39]. It may also be induced by other infectious agents like the herpes simplex virus [1, 40]. Herpes-associated erythema multiforme makes up almost the quarter of patients with EM. Herpes-associated EM may proceed simultaneously with or within several weeks after herpes simplex infection [41]. Hemorrhagic crusts on the lips and target lesions on the skin are pathognomonic signs that help make a diagnosis of erythema multiforme [39]. Oral lesions present with macules, blisters or ulcerations. Bleeding and the involvement of the non-keratinized mucosae are common [40]. EM, with mild symptoms, is managed by local wound care, topical anesthetic or analgesic agents, whereas patients with more severe symptoms require oral antihistaminic medications and topical corticosteroids. Herpes-associated EM may successfully be managed with systemic antivirals, if prescribed early. Recurrences are seen in almost 20–25% of patients with a rate of 2–24 recurrences per year [41].

Cyclic neutropenia is a lethal condition due to defects in neutrophil maturation which lead to a periodic decrease in neutrophil counts. Gene mutations have been blamed in the etiology of cyclic neutropenia [8, 42]. Recurrent cycles of neutropenia may range from 14 to 35 days and the duration of symptoms also vary between patients [42]. Fever, sore throat, cervical lymphadenopathy, gingivitis, oral ulcerations, tonsillitis, fatigue, otitis media or skin infections are among the most common manifestations of cyclic neutropenia. Ulcers in cyclic neutropenia may either be solitary or multiple, and they heal with scarring [8, 42].

Behçet's disease is a systemic immune-mediated vasculitis. The classic triad of Behçet's disease includes oral and genital ulcers, ocular lesions such as uveitis or retinal vasculitis, and skin lesions mostly consisting of folliculitis-like rashes, ulcers or erythema nodosum [1, 43]. Recurrences occur at least three times a year. Oral ulcers are present in more than 90% of patients and may sometimes precede other symptoms. The ulcers may be shallow or deep, with slightly raised erythematous borders. They may appear anywhere within the oral cavity and heal spontaneously [44]. Proper management of Behçet's disease should focus on improving the quality of life and maintain the remission of lesions. In case of oral ulcers, pain relief and anti-inflammatory applications are aimed. Although there is no gold standard treatment or management method for oral ulcers in Behçet's disease, antimicrobial mouthwashes, laser treatments, topical corticosteroids, or systemic treatment options including colchicine, azathioprine or thalidomide may be considered [45].

5. Conclusions

Cause-based treatment options are more beneficial than palliative management options. Therefore it is crucial for physicians to make a sound clinical examination and take a through patient history [3]. Biopsy should be considered if an ulcerative lesion with an unknown etiology shows no signs of healing after two weeks, or if the lesions is not responsive to a treatment aimed at a probable known etiology. Ulcers of less than 5 mm diameter are advised to undergo an excisional biopsy, whereas for larger ones an incisional biopsy is suggested [6].

Conflict of interest

The author declares no conflict of interest.

Author details

Nelli Yildirimyan
Istanbul Medipol University School of Dentistry, Department of Oral and Maxillofacial Surgery, Istanbul, Turkey

*Address all correspondence to: nyildirimyan@gmail.com

References

[1] Mortazavi H, Safi Y, Baharvand M, Rahmani S. Diagnostic features of common oral ulcerative lesions: An updated decision tree. International Journal of Dentistry. 2016;**2016**:7278925

[2] Lehman JS, Rogers RS III. Acute oral ulcers. Journal of Clinical Dermatology. 2016;**34**(4):470-474

[3] Yıldırımyan N, Özalp Ö, Şatır S, Altay MA, Sindel A. Recurrent aphthous stomatitis as a result of zinc deficiency. Oral Health & Preventive Dentistry. 2019;**17**(5):465-468

[4] Crispian S. Aphthous ulceration. New England Journal of Medicine. 2006;**355**(2):165-172

[5] Meiller TF, Garber K, Scheper M. A review of common oral pathology lesions, with a focus on periodontology and implantology. The Journal of Evidence-Based Dental Practice. 2012;**12**(3):254-262

[6] Muñoz-Corcuera M, Esparza-Gómez G, González-Moles M, Bascones-Martínez A. Oral ulcers: Clinical aspects. A tool for dermatologists. Part II. Chronic ulcers. Journal of Clinical & Experimental Dermatology. 2009;**34**(4):456-461

[7] Muñoz-Corcuera M, Esparza-Gómez G, González-Moles M, Bascones-Martínez A. Oral ulcers: Clinical aspects. A tool for dermatologists. Part I. Acute ulcers. Journal of Clinical & Experimental Dermatology. 2009;**34**(3):289-294

[8] Minhas S, Sajjad A, Kashif M, Taj F, Waddani HA, Khurshid Z. Oral ulcers presentation in systemic diseases: An update. Open Access Macedonian Journal of Medical Sciences. 2019;**7**(19): 3341-3347

[9] Dhanrajani P, Cropley P. Oral eosinophilic or traumatic ulcer: A case report and brief review. National Journal of Maxillofacial Surgery. 2015;**6**(2): 237-240

[10] Zhang J, Feng J, Liu Y. Preventive effect and safety of Chinese herbal medicine mouthwash in chemotherapy-induced oral mucositis: A protocol for systematic review and meta analysis. Journal of Medicine. 2020;**99**(49):1-5

[11] Bo L, Zhang Y, Wu X, Ma A, Zhao Y, Liu H, et al. Effect and mechanism of Kangfuxin liquid on oral ulcer in patients with chemotherapy treated hematologic malignancies: Network pharmacology study and clinical observations. Informatics in Medicine Unlocked. 2021;**25**:100693

[12] Abdel-Rahman O, Fouad M. Risk of oral and gastrointestinal mucosal injury in patients with solid tumors treated with everolimus, temsirolimus or ridaforolimus: A comparative systematic review and meta-analysis. Expert Review of Anticancer Therapy. 2015;**15**(7): 847-858

[13] Vigarios E, Epstein JB, Sibaud V. Oral mucosal changes induced by anticancer targeted therapies and immune checkpoint inhibitors. Support Care Cancer. 2017;**25**(5):1713-1739

[14] Basile D, Di Nardo P, Corvaja C, Garattini SK, Pelizzari G, Lisanti C, et al. Mucosal injury during anti-cancer treatment: From pathobiology to bedside. Cancers. 2019;**11**(6):857

[15] Pulito C, Cristaudo A, La Porta C, Zapperi S, Blandino G, Morrone A, et al. Oral mucositis: The hidden side of cancer therapy. Journal of Experimental & Clinical Cancer Research. 2020; **39**(1):1-15

[16] Lalla RV, Bowen J, Barasch A, Elting L, Epstein J, Keefe DM, et al. MASCC/ISOO clinical practice guidelines for the management of mucositis secondary to cancer therapy. Cancer. 2014;**120**(10):1453-1461

[17] Blakaj A, Bonomi M, Gamez ME, Blakaj DM. Oral mucositis in head and neck cancer: Evidence-based management and review of clinical trial data. Oral Oncology. 2019;**95**:29-34

[18] Fernandes PM, Pedroso EG, Santos-Silva AR, Vargas PA, Lopes MA. Non-ulcerated necrotizing sialometaplasia may mimic a salivary gland tumor. Autopsy & Case Reports. 2021;**11**:1-6

[19] Van Heerden WFP. Oral manifestations of viral infections: CPD. South African Family Practice. 2006; **48**(8):20-24

[20] Santosh ABR, Muddana K. Viral infections of oral cavity. Journal of Family Medicine and Primary Care. 2020;**9**(1):36

[21] Légeret C, Furlano R. Oral ulcers in children—A clinical narrative overview. Italian Journal of Pediatrics. 2021;**47**(1):144

[22] Malek R, Gharibi A, Khlil N, Kissa J. Necrotizing ulcerative gingivitis. Contemporary Clinical Dentistry. 2017;**8**(3):496-500

[23] Aaron SL, DeBlois KW. Acute Necrotizing Ulcerative Gingivitis. Treasure Island, FL: StatPearls Publishing LLC. 2021

[24] Ramachandran A, Varma B, Jose R, Shanmugham AM, Sam LM. Allergic contact stomatitis (stomatitis venenata): A case report of oral hypersensitivity reaction to toothpaste. Indian Journal of Case Reports. 2021;**5**(1):47-49

[25] Cifuentes M, Davari P, Rogers RS III. Contact stomatitis. Clinics in Dermatology. 2017;**35**(5):435-440

[26] Lawrence LM, Farquharson A, Brown RS, Vatanka HO. Oral tissue irritants in toothpaste: A case report. The Journal of Clinical Pediatric Dentistry. 2013;**38**(1):75-78

[27] Arun K, Ambooken M, Varghese SS, Varghese T, Mathew JJ. A rare case of plasma cell mucositis in a young patient. Journal of Indian Society of Periodontology. 2017;**21**(1):63-65

[28] Tailor A, Pemberton MN, Murphy R, Hegarty AM. Plasma cell mucositis related to qat chewing: A report of 2 cases and review of the literature. Oral Surgery, Oral Medicine, Oral Pathology, Oral Radiology. 2021;**131**(3):e65-e70

[29] Sollecito TP, Greenberg MS. Plasma cell gingivitis. Report of two cases. Oral Surgery, Oral Medicine, and Oral Pathology. 1992;**73**(6):690-693

[30] Abdollahi M, Radfar M. A review of drug-induced oral reactions. The Journal of Contemporary Dental Practice. 2003;**4**(1):10-31

[31] Cheng S, Kirtschig G, Cooper S, Thornhill M, Leonardi-Bee J, Murphy R. Interventions for erosive lichen planus affecting mucosal sites. Cochrane Database of Systematic Reviews. 2012;**2**:CD008092

[32] Gonsalves WC, Chi AC, Neville BW. Common oral lesions: Part I. Superficial mucosal lesions. American Family Physician. 2007;**75**(4):501-507

[33] Erugula SR, Singaraju DK, Govada J, Rajajee K, Sudheer M, Sudharshan A, et al. Vesiculobullous lesions of the oral cavity. International Archives of Integrated Medicine. 2016;**3**(11):154-163

[34] Menzies S, O'Shea F, Galvin S, Wynne B. Oral manifestations of lupus. Irish Journal of Medical Science. 2018;**187**(1):91-93

[35] Benli M, Batool F, Stutz C, Petit C, Jung S, Huck O. Orofacial manifestations and dental management of systemic lupus erythematosus: A review. Oral Diseases. 2021;**27**(2):151-167

[36] Rajendra Santosh AB, Muddana K, Bakki SR. Fungal infections of oral cavity: Diagnosis, management, and association with COVID-19. SN Comprehensive Clinical Medicine. 2021;**3**(6):1373-1384

[37] Sah K, Chandra S, Singh A, Singh S. Eosinophilic ulcer of the tongue masquerading as malignant ulcer: An unexplored distinct pathology. Journal of Oral and Maxillofacial Pathology. 2017;**21**(2):321

[38] Stoopler ET, Kuperstein AS, Sollecito TP. How do I manage a patient with recurrent herpes simplex? Journal of the Canadian Dental Association. 2012;**78**:c154

[39] Thongprasom K. Treatment of a pregnant patient with herpes associated erythema multiforme (HAEM): A case report. Acta Stomatologica Croatica. 2016;**50**(3):265-268

[40] Mtiri A, Bouslama G, Messouad NB, Abidi I, Youssef SB, Sriha B. Erythema multiforme attributable to herpes simplex virus: Clinical aspects and treatment. Case Reports in Dentistry. 2021;**2021**:6692495

[41] Güven AG, Keskin S, Çiftçi N, Taşar MA, Alioğlu B. A case of erythema multiforme due to herpes simplex infection. Medical Journal of Ankara Training and Research Hospital. 2019;**52**(1):87-89

[42] Coates TD, Schrier SL, Landaw SA. Cyclic neutropenia. UpToDate. 2018. Available from: https://www.uptodate.com/contents/cyclicneutropenia

[43] Ida Y, Takeuchi M, Ishihara M, Shibuya E, Yamane T, Hasumi Y, et al. An open-label, prospective, single-arm study of switching from infliximab to cyclosporine for refractory uveitis in patients with Behçet's disease in long-term remission. Japanese Journal of Ophthalmology. 2021;**65**(6):843-848

[44] Senusi A, Kang A, Buchanan JAG, Adesanya A, Aloraini G, Stanford M, et al. New mouthwash: An efficacious intervention for oral ulceration associated with Behçet's disease. The British Journal of Oral & Maxillofacial Surgery. 2020;**58**(8):1034-1039

[45] Scherrer MAR, Rocha VB, Garcia LC. Behcet's disease: Review with emphasis on dermatological aspects. Anais Brasileiros de Dermatologia. 2017;**92**: 452-464

Chapter 4

Alternative Denture Base Materials for Allergic Patients

Lavinia Cosmina Ardelean, Laura-Cristina Rusu and Codruta Victoria Tigmeanu

Abstract

Traditionally, a denture base is manufactured using a heat-cured acrylic resin. This type of resin was first used in dental labs in 1936, being a great step forward. Because of the many disadvantages as increased porosity, high water sorption, polymerization shrinkage, allergenic potential and citotoxicity due to the residual monomer, awkward flasking and packaging, and difficult processing, alternatives were continuously searched. Monomer-free and high-impact acrylics were developed, and gold plating of the denture base was experienced, in order to provide an alternative to allergic patients. Once polymers developed, new types of resins, such as polyamides (nylon), acetal, epoxy resins, styrene, polycarbonate, vinyl, urethane, polyether ether ketone (PEEK), became available on the dental market, accompanied by modern technologies, such as injection. CAD/CAM milled and 3D printed denture bases represent the present state of the art in this domain. Our chapter aims to present these alternative materials, which are safe to use in cases of allergic patients and guarantee a healthy oral environment and a high degree of comfort.

Keywords: denture base, acrylic resin, polymers, polyamides, acetal resin, PEEK, allergy, CAD/CAM milling, 3D printing

1. Introduction

Acrylic resins, which represented an important step forward in dentistry, have been used in manufacturing denture bases, artificial teeth, orthodontic appliances, maxillofacial prostheses, single-tooth or provisional restorations, as well as veneering materials, since the middle of the twentieth century [1].

Characterized by low density and thermal conductivity, good resistance to chemical solvents, acrylic resins became the most popular material for denture base fabrication because of the low fabrication cost, easy repair/reline, low weight, and aesthetical properties [2].

The most frequently used acrylic resins in dentistry are heat-cured. They seemed very promising at first, but, in time, it turned out that heat-cured acrylics had various shortcomings, such as poor resistance, dimensional stability issues, polymerization shrinkage, high degradation rate in wet environment, allergenic potential and citotoxicity due to the residual monomer, difficult processing, due to the awkward flasking and packing procedure (**Figure 1**) [3–6].

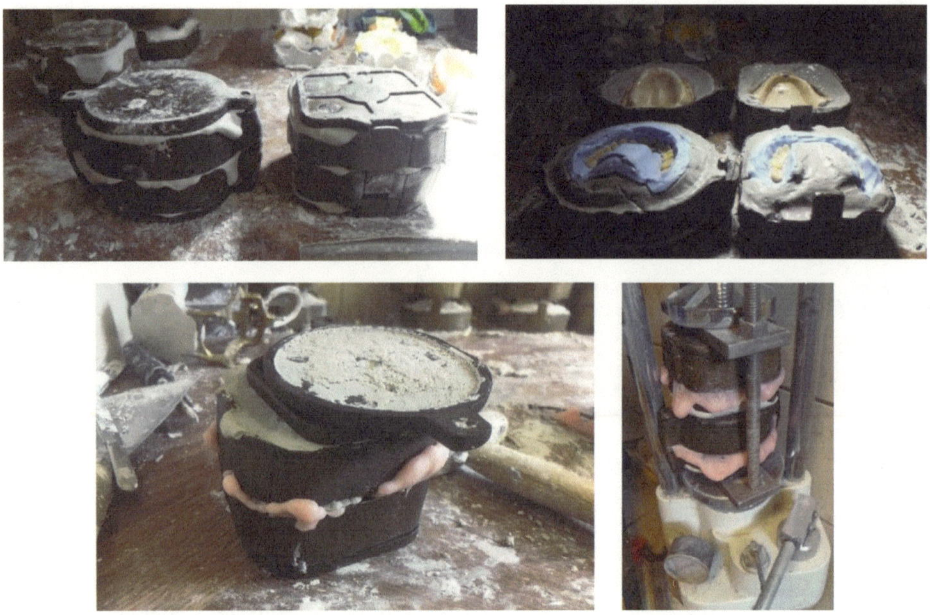

Figure 1.
Flasking and packing of heat-cured acrylic dentures.

Acrylic resin becomes porous and permeable after prolonged use in the mouth wet environment, also being prone to discoloration [7].

The consequence may be denture base fracture, allergic reactions, and improper seating [8].

The fracture of the acrylic denture base is a very common clinical problem, partly due to its complex geometry, which favors stress concentration in certain areas [9]. Most of upper denture base fractures are caused by fatigue and impact, whereas in case of the lower denture base, impact and low fracture toughness are the main causes [10]. One of the primary problems of acrylics is the impact failure when the denture is accidentally dropped on a hard surface and fatigue failure when the unfit denture base deforms repeatedly through occlusal forces [11].

According to literature data, 68% of the acrylic dentures break within a few years after fabrication [12].

Acrylics are also well known for their allergenic potential, their citotoxicity being mainly due to the residual monomer [13, 14].

The adverse reactions of the oral mucosa, in case of conventional acrylic resins, may also be induced by porosity (**Figure 2**), poor hygiene, degradation due to water sorption [15–17].

Inadequately cleaned dentures are subject to quick formation of a biofilm on their surface [18].

The anaerobic environment, characteristic under poorly cleaned denture bases, is associated with the proliferation of certain bacterial species, consequently leading to a pathogenic biofilm composition and inducing denture stomatitis by plaque accumulation (**Figure 3**) [19].

The often contaminated dentures of elderly patients may finally result in affecting the general health condition [20].

The high relative humidity of the oral environment, constant contact of the denture with saliva, cold and hot food and drinks, enzymes, bacteria, and the varying pH

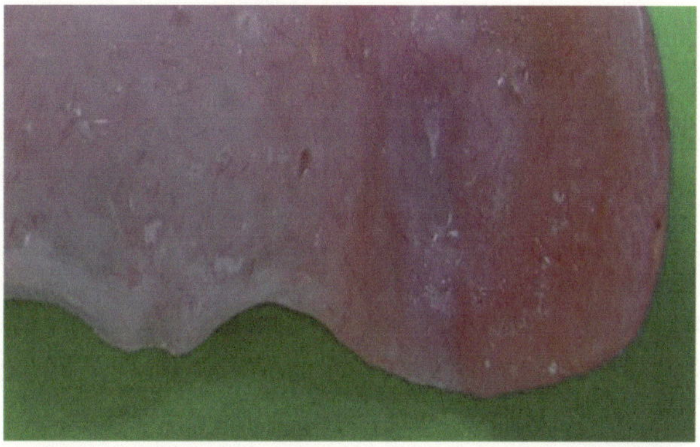

Figure 2.
Porous acrylic denture base.

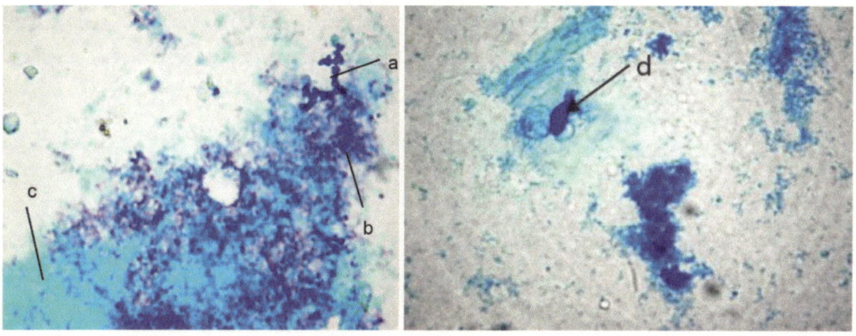

Figure 3.
Microbial flora found on the denture base surface: a. candida hyphae, b. cocci, c. mucinous conglomerate, d. trichomonas tenax (ATP Dragan coloration Ob. Im).

levels can severely affect the physical and mechanical properties of the denture [21]. Dental base materials, and especially acrylic resins, are prone to water sorption, as they tend to form hydrogen bonds with water molecules, which also leads to deteriorated physical and mechanical properties [22].

In order to overcome these disadvantages, various attempts have been made. One of the methods considered was gold plating, which has proved to increase the retention and overcome plaque accumulation. However, the method did not prevail, as the adhesion between the acrylic resin and the gold plated layer deteriorates and abrades.

Later on, reinforced acrylic resins, characterized by better resistance and low/none residual monomer, became available. Alternative polymer systems, such as polyamide, epoxy, styrene, acetal, polycarbonate, polyether ether ketone (PEEK), or vinyl resins, have been experimented, with promising results [23]. However, the desired denture base material has not been developed yet.

2. Alternative materials and techniques

There has been ongoing effort to enhance the strength and fatigue resistance of acrylic resins, by means of: reinforcement with the addition of filling materials, altering the chemistry of acrylic resins, and manufacturing alternative denture base materials [24, 25].

2.1 Reinforced acrylic resins

Previous studies have shown that favorable results in improving mechanical properties such as impact and transverse strength were overcome using various types of fillers such as glass, carbon, polylactic fiber, plyometric polyamide, ultra-high-molecular-weight polyethylene, aramid, rayon, ceramic particle (barium titanate, zirconium dioxide, silicon dioxide, hydroxyapatite, titanium dioxide, and calcium carbonate), and metal plates or wires [26–33].

There are numerous studies focusing on the effect of glass fibers on the mechanical qualities of acrylic resins, which reported improvement of tensile and flexural strength and esthetic results [34–39].

Different other materials have been used for reinforcement, such as viscose fibers, mica, juta, or vegetable fibers [40–42].

2.2 Alternative types of acrylic resins

Alternative manufacturing technologies for acrylic resins, which aimed at obtaining high-quality dentures, were constantly developed, using dedicated materials. These technologies including casting, injection, light curing, microwave polymerization, CAD/CAM milling, 3D printing have been more or less utilized [43].

Thermoplastic and CAD/CAM milled acrylates have a high impact rating resistance, long-term stability, being characterized by a dense and smooth surface. It's highly biocompatible, due to the absence of residual monomer, and has very good long-term stability because of limited water retention [44].

Acrylic resins have been one of the most common commercial materials used for the manufacture of 3D printed denture bases. However, there were some technical challenges that hinder the application of polymethyl methacrylate (PMMA), such as large shrinkage, low degree of one-time curing, poor mechanical strength, low bacterial resistance, etc., limiting their clinical applications [45].

Nevertheless, great progress has been made in manufacturing alternative resin materials with outstanding properties.

2.3 Light-cured urethane-based resins

Urethane-based resins have no allergic potential, due to the absence of methyl, ethyl, propyl, and butyl groups. Manufactured by light curing, full and partial urethane dentures do not need flasking, packing, and heat curing, which are time-consuming. The system is extremely efficient and consists of three wax-like types of resins: baseplate resin, setup resin, contour resin. A full denture base needs no more than 30 minutes to process, starting with complete setting of the master model. The "wax-up" is practically made on the denture's light-cured base, and after try-in, esthetic and phonetic approval, the final conditioning and light curing are carried out (**Figures 4–7**) [46].

2.4 Thermoplastic resins

Thermoplastic denture base materials include different types of hypoallergenic resins: polyamide (nylon), acetal, PEEK, epoxy, styrene, polycarbonate, vinyl, their most prominent advantages being higher elasticity, toxicological safety, and use of heat molding instead of chemical polymerization, which prevents polymerization shrinkage and related deformation [47, 48].

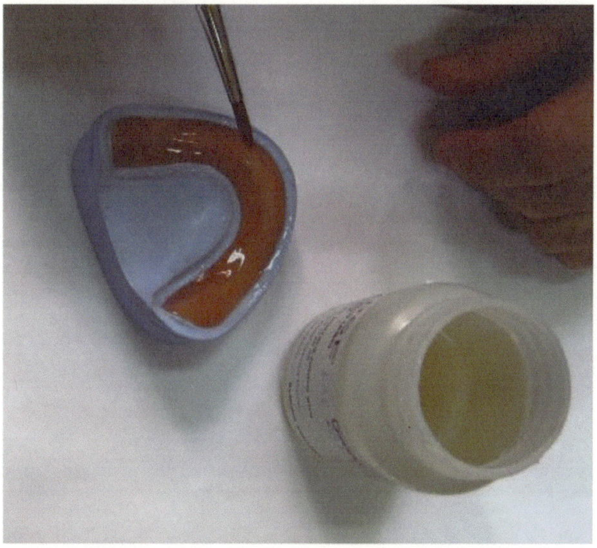

Figure 4.
Baseplate resin before light curing.

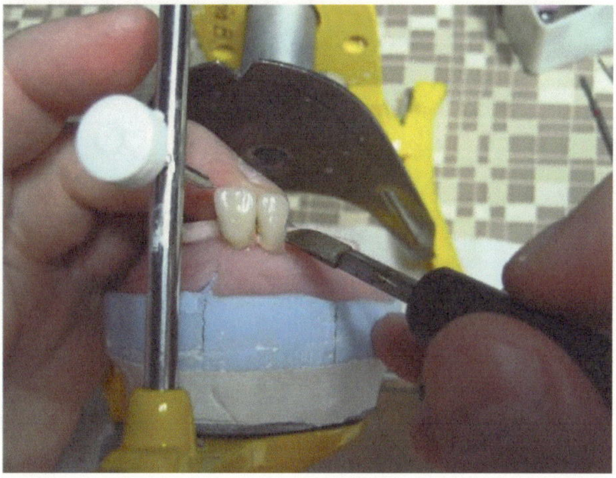

Figure 5.
Attaching the teeth to the cured baseplate, by using the setup resin.

Thermoplastic resins are monomer-free and consequently nontoxic and non-allergenic, with high biocompatibility. They provide better resistance, esthetic appearance, and lower weight, being much more comfortable for the patient [8, 49, 50].

Their manufacture implies injection by special devices (**Figure 8**), after preheating the material (at a temperature of 200–250°C), in granular form, wrapped in special cartridges (**Figure 9**), which prevents dosage errors. The technology excludes any chemical reaction [51].

Thermoplastic materials are suitable for the manufacturing of removable partial dentures, which totally or partially eliminate the metallic framework and clasps, resulting in the so-called "metal-free removable partial dentures." If desired, any combination of the metallic framework or clasps with thermoplastic resin saddles and clasps is possible (**Figure 10**) [52, 53].

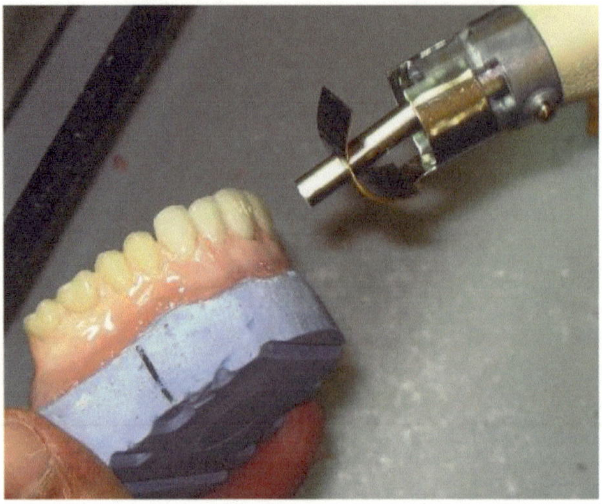

Figure 6.
Contour resin, overlaid on the baseplate, exposed setup resin and necks of the teeth, processed using the warm air gun to create a smooth surface.

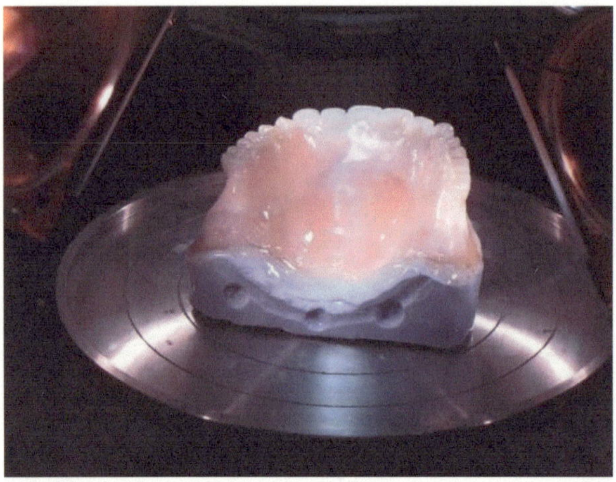

Figure 7.
Final light curing.

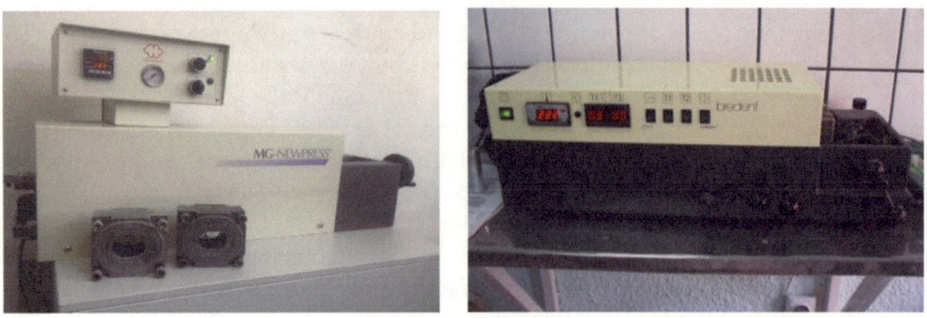

Figure 8.
Injection devices for thermoplatic resins.

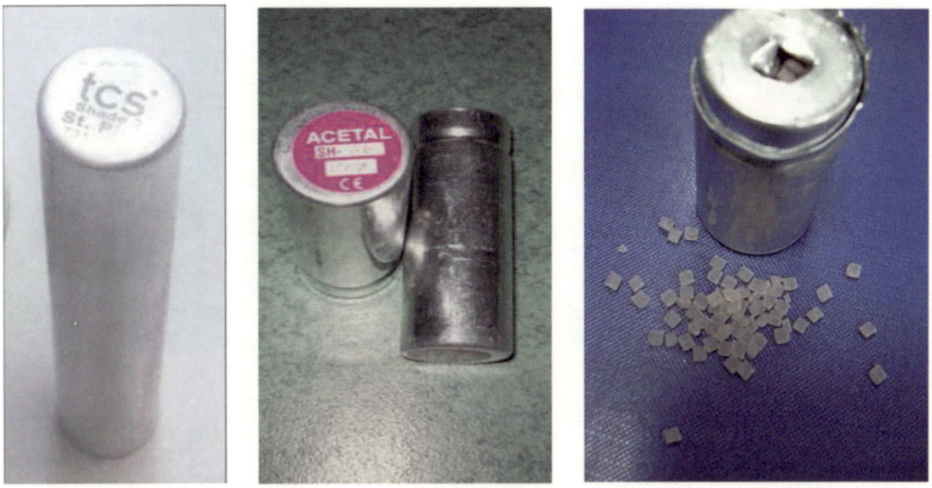

Figure 9.
Thermoplastic grain-like resins, wrapped in cartridges.

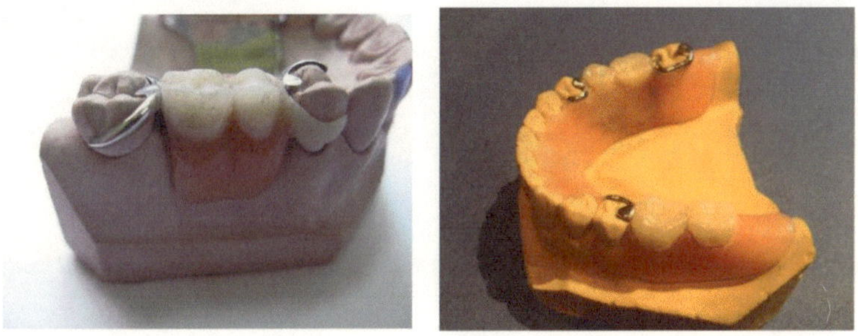

Figure 10.
Combination between thermoplastic resin saddle, metallic and acetal clasps.

Their indications include: removable partial dentures, preformed clasps, removable partial denture frameworks, temporary or provisional crowns and bridges, full dentures, orthodontic appliances, anti-snoring devices, mouthguards and splints [54].

2.4.1 Polyamides

Polyamides (nylon) are the condensation result of a diamine and a dibasic acid [55].

In 1950, they were introduced in dentistry, as an alternative to denture acrylic base, and are being characterized by different degrees of flexibility, depending on the type of polyamide. Their main indications include patients with tissue allergies, cases of retentive dental fields (which are normally problematic for the insertion and disinsertion of the removable partial denture), and repeated denture fracture, as they are unbreakable [56, 57]. A polyamide denture may be bounced off the floor without cracking its base.

The types of polyamides include superflexible polyamide (**Figure 11**), extremely elastic, and medium-low flexibility polyamide, a half-soft comfortable material.

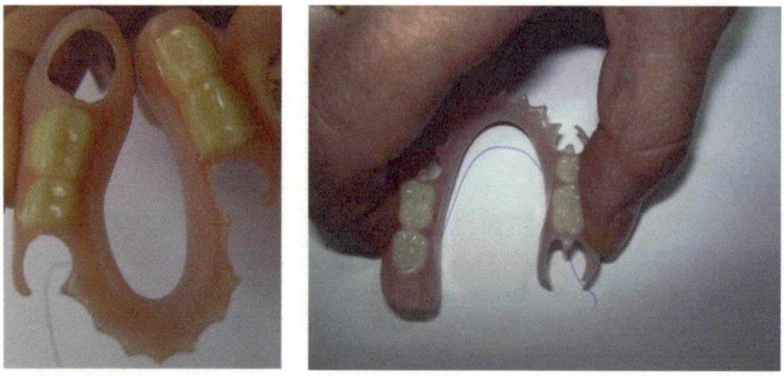

Figure 11.
Metal-free superflexible polyamide removable partial dentures.

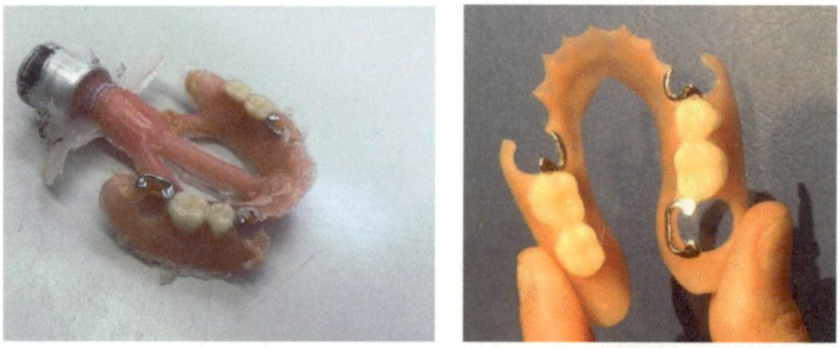

Figure 12.
Superflexible polyamide removable partial denture with metal clasps (right after injection and ready-to-go).

The clasps may be manufactured of the same material as the denture base. In the case of medium-low flexibility polyamide, ready-made clasps may be used. Metal clasps are also an option. (**Figure 12**).

2.4.2 Acetal resins

Acetal resins, also known as polyoxymethylene, are formed by the polymerization of formaldehyde. They have been used in dentistry since 1986, as alternative materials for denture base and clasps (**Figure 13**). Characterized by superior esthetics, acetal resins have been useful for low-weight removable partial dentures framework manufacturing in allergic patients [58]. They show high impact strength and elasticity [59]. Acetal resins are also indicated for Kemeny-type single unilateral partial dentures, provisional bridges, splints, and orthodontic appliances (**Figure 13**).

2.5 Polyether ether ketone

PEEK is a ketone-based semi-crystalline thermoplastic with excellent mechanical and chemical resistance properties, used in dentistry since 2002, for crowns, implant superstructures, fixed partial dentures, and removable partial denture frameworks and clasps (**Figure 14**) [60–63].

PEEK is highly biocompatible, insoluble, lightweight, with superior resistance to wear and fracture and elasticity comparable to bone. It may be optimized by adding

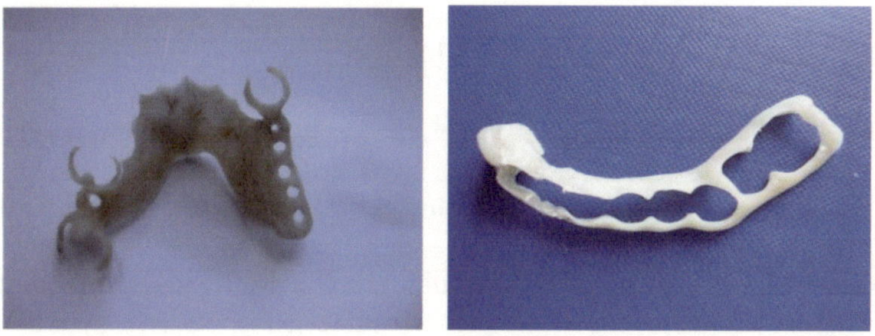

Figure 13.
Acetal framework and clasps; acetal splint.

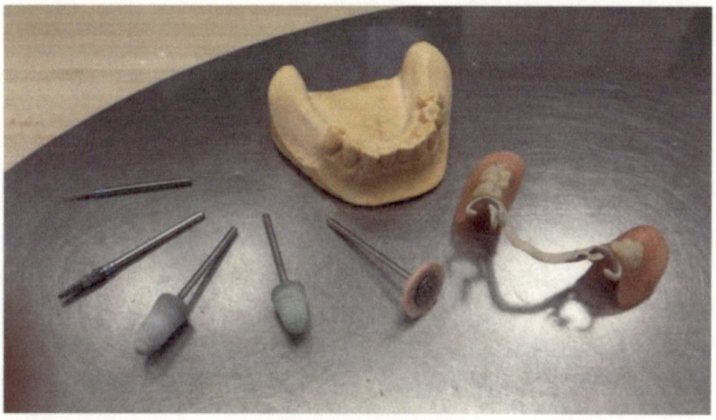

Figure 14.
Removable partial denture with PEEK framework and clasps.

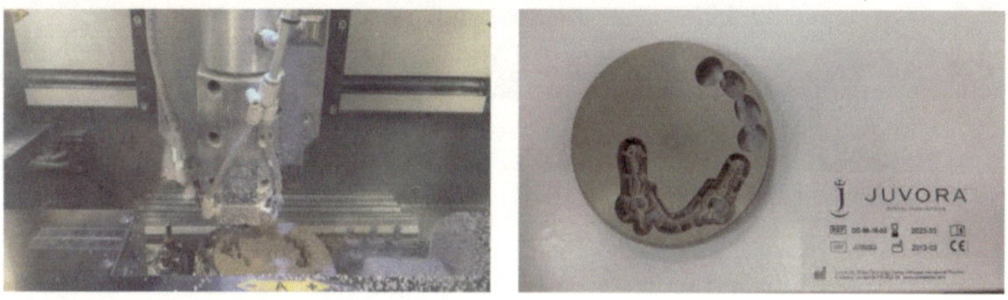

Figure 15.
CAD/CAM milled PEEK framework.

ceramic nanoparticles. The material may be injected (grains) at 400°C or milled (disks) using a CAD/CAM system (**Figure 15**) [44]. Recently, 3D printing using PEEK materials has been utilized. Direct-ink writing 3D printing uses soluble epoxy-functionalized PEEK (ePEEK) and fenchone, but the most widely used technique is fused deposition modeling (FDM), which requires increases in the nozzle and heating bed temperatures for PEEK materials [64–66].

2.6 CAD/CAM milled and 3D printed removable dentures

CAD/CAM systems, which enable manufacturing 3D objects, have been used in dentistry since 1980, at first for fixed prosthodontic restorations [67].

In the 1990s, the fabrication of removable prosthodontic restorations was attempted, using both 3D printing and milling technologies [68, 69].

They offer many advantages to both dentists and patients, such as reduced number of appointments and easily available spare dentures, as digital data are saved [70–72].

Compared with the traditional methods, the lab work can be completed more conveniently and cost-effectively. The high initial cost of the milling machine may be overcome by referring the data to a milling center, which will handle the actual manufacturing.

Currently, both CAD/CAM methods: substractive milling and additive printing, are being used for removable dentures manufacturing [73, 74]. By milling, the denture may be obtained as one item, teeth and denture base in a single body [75], or separate pieces, the artificial teeth requiring subsequent bonding to the denture base [76]. The latter is the most frequently used at present, as it allows using commercially available artificial teeth, with better esthetics and physical properties [77, 78].

In case of 3D printing, the light-curing resin used is quickly converted from a liquid to a solid under the action of ultraviolet or visible light. The emergence of nanomaterials provides a new way to improve the performance of 3D printed acrylics [79]. By incorporating TiO2, antibacterial effects have been obtained [80].

Cellulose nanocrystals were attempted to reinforce acrylic resins for 3D printing, with improved mechanical and antibacterial properties and no significant cytotoxic effect [81].

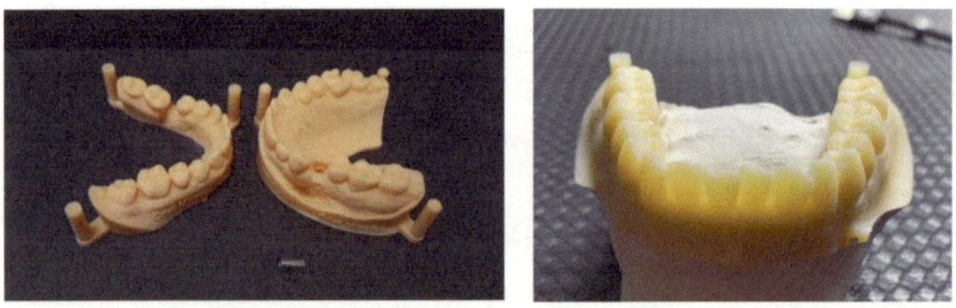

Figure 16.
3D printed high-precision models.

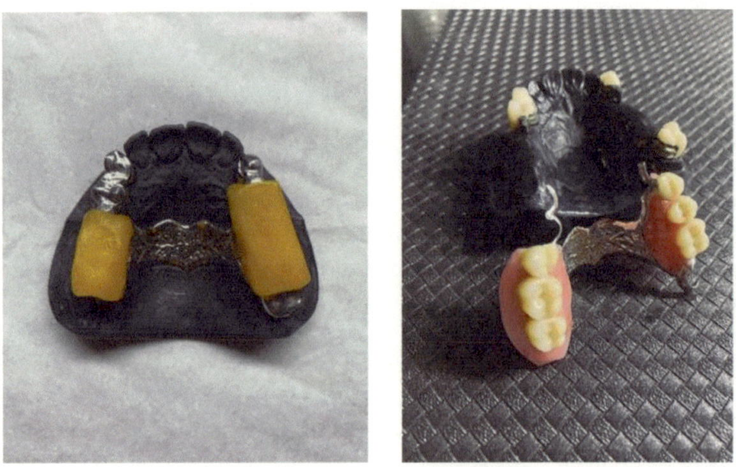

Figure 17.
3D printed working model for manufacturing a removable partial denture.

Light curing is a green technology and the main molding method involved in 3D printing of resin-based dental materials. When irradiated with light, the photosensitive resin undergoes stacking and curing [82].

It consists of three main technologies: stereolithogaphy, digital light processing (DLP), and fused deposition modeling (FDM). The distinctive feature of DLP technology is the diversity of materials, from thermoplastics to resins and ceramics, even zirconia paste. FDM, one of the cheapest and most popular 3D printing technologies in dentistry, enables using polylactic acid, polycarbonate, polyamide, acrylonitrile-butadiene-styrene copolymers [83].

Besides full dentures and frameworks for removable partial dentures, 3D printing dental resins are also indicated for crowns and bridges, high-precision working models (**Figures 16** and **17**), splints, custom trays.

3. Conclusion

Long-term deterioration of acrylic dentures in the oral environment is still an unsolved problem. Their allergic potential, mainly due to the residual monomer, is well known. New choices of resins, with better properties compared with acrylics, have been constantly developed for dental applications. Alternative processing technologies, such as casting, injection, light curing, CAD/CAM milling, and 3D printing, have been aiming to improving their qualities.

Choosing the right material for manufacturing full or removable partial dentures is very important because it has direct effect on their characteristics and lifetime, especially in case of allergic patients.

Acknowledgements

The authors would like to thank Professor Cristina-Maria Bortun for her valuable contribution and support.

Conflict of interest

The authors declare no conflict of interest.

Author details

Lavinia Cosmina Ardelean[1*], Laura-Cristina Rusu[2] and Codruta Victoria Tigmeanu[1]

1 Department of Technology of Materials and Devices in Dental Medicine, Multidisciplinary Center for Research, Evaluation, Diagnosis and Therapies in Oral Medicine, "Victor Babeş" University of Medicine and Pharmacy, Timisoara, Romania

2 Department of Oral Pathology, Multidisciplinary Center for Research, Evaluation, Diagnosis and Therapies in Oral Medicine, "Victor Babeş" University of Medicine and Pharmacy, Timisoara, Romania

*Address all correspondence to: lavinia_ardelean@umft.ro

References

[1] Ardelean L, Rusu LC, Bratu DC, Bortun CM. Diacrylic composite resins as veneering materials. Revista Materiale Plastice. 2013;**50**:93-96

[2] Patil SB, Naveen BH, Patil NP. Bonding acrylic teeth to acrylic resin denture bases: A review. Gerodontology. 2006;**23**:131-139

[3] Kedjarune U, Charoenworaluk N, Koontongkaew S. Release of methyl methacrylate from heat-cured and autopolymerized resins: Cytotoxicity testing related to residual monomer. Australian Dental Journal. 1999; **44**:25-30

[4] Machado C, Sanchez E, Azer SS, et al. Comparative study of the transverse strength of three denture base materials. Journal of Dentistry. 2007;**35**:930-933

[5] Koroglu A, Ozdemir T, Pamir AD, Usanmaz A. Residual acrylic monomer content of denture base resins with different fiber systems. Journal of Applied Polymer Science. 2012; **125**:471-476

[6] Cheng YY, Cheung WL, Chow TW. Strain analysis of maxillary complete denture with three-dimensional finite element method. The Journal of Prosthetic Dentistry. 2010;**103**:309-318

[7] Singh S, Palaskar JN, Mittal S. Comparative evaluation of surface porosities in conventional heat polymerized acrylic resin cured by water bath and microwave energy with microwavable acrylic resin cured by microwave energy. Contemporary Clinical Dentistry. 2013;**4**:147-151

[8] Nakhaei M, Dashti H, Barazandeh R, et al. Shear bond strength of acrylic denture teeth to PMMA and polyamide denture base material. JDMT. 2018;**7**:19-23

[9] Alhareb AO, Akil HBM, Ahmad ZAB. Poly(methyl methacrylate) denture base composites enhancement by various combinations of nitrile butadiene rubber/treated ceramic fillers. Journal of Thermoplastic Composite Materials. 2017;**30**:1069-1090. DOI: 10.1177/0892705715616856

[10] Darbar UR, Huggett R, Harrison A. Denture fracture – a survey. British Dental Journal. 1994;**176**:342-345

[11] Kim SH, Watts DC. The effect of reinforcement with woven e-glass fibers on the impact strength of complete dentures fabricated with high-impact acrylic resin. The Journal of Prosthetic Dentistry. 2004;**91**:274-280

[12] Vojdani M, Bagheri R, Khaledi AAR. Effect of aluminium oxide addition on the flexural strength, surface hardness, and roughness of heat-polymerized acrylic resin. Journal of Dental Sciences. 2012;**7**:238-244

[13] de Araújo AM, Alves GR, Avanço GT, Parizi JLS, Nai GA. Assessment of methyl methacrylate genotoxicity by the micronucleus test. Brazilian Oral Research. 2013;**27**:31-36

[14] Rusu LC, Urechescu H, Ardelean L, Levai MC, Pricop M. Comparative study for oral reaction produced by polymethylmethacrylate. Materiale Plastice. 2015;**52**:413-415

[15] Olms C, Yahiaoui-Doktor M, Remmerbach TW, Stingu CS. Bacterial colonisation and tissue compatibility of denture base resins. Dental Journal. 2018;**6**:20. DOI: 10.3390/dj6020020

[16] Gungor H, Gundogdu M, Duymus ZY. Investigation of the effect of different polishing techniques on the surface roughness of denture base and repair materials. The Journal of Prosthetic Dentistry. 2014;**112**:1271-1277

[17] Takahashi Y, Yoshida K, Shimizu H. Fracture resistance of maxillary complete dentures subjected to long term water immersion. Gerodontology. 2012;**29**: e1086-e1091

[18] Sachdeo A, Haffajee AD, Socransky SS. Biofilms in the edentulous oral cavity. Journal of Prosthodontics. 2008;**17**:348-356

[19] Gendreau L, Loewy Z. Epidemiology and etiology of denture stomatitis. Journal of Prosthodontics. 2011;**20**: 251-260

[20] O'Donnell LE, Smith K, Williams C, et al. Dentures are a reservoir for respiratory pathogens. Journal of Prosthodontics. 2016;**25**:99-104. DOI: 10.1111/jopr.12342

[21] Dogan OM, Bolayır G, Keskin S, Doğan A, Bek B, Boztuğ A. The effect of esthetic fibers on impact resistance of a conventional heat-cured denture base resin. Dental Materials Journal. 2007;**26**:232-239

[22] Soygun K, Bolayir G, Boztug A. Mechanical and thermal properties of polyamide versus reinforced PMMA denturebase materials. The Journal of Advanced Prosthodontics. 2013;**5**: 153-160

[23] Phoenix RD, Mansueto MA, Ackerman NA, Jones RE. Evaluation of mechanical and thermal properties of commonly used denture base resins. Journal of Prosthodontics. 2004;**13**:17-27

[24] Chen SY, Liang WM, Yen PS. Reinforcement of acrylic denture base resin by incorporation of various fibers. Journal of Biomedical Materials Research. 2001;**58**:203-208

[25] Singh JP, Dhiman RK, Bedi RP, Girish SH. Flexible denture base material: A viable alternative to conventional acrylic denture base material. Contemporary Clinical Dentistry. 2011;**2**:313-317

[26] Asar NV, Albayrak H, Korkmaz T, et al. Influence of various metal oxides on mechanical and physical properties of heat-cured poly methyl methacrylate denture base resins. The Journal of Advanced Prosthodontics. 2013; **5**:241-247

[27] Ayad NM, Badawi MF, Fatah AA. Effect of reinforcement of high impact acrylic resin with zirconia on some physical and mechanical properties. Revista de Clínica e Pesquisa Odontológica. 2008;**4**:145-151

[28] Elshereksi NW, Mohamed SH, Arifin A, et al. Effect of filler incorporation on the fracture toughness properties of denture base poly(methyl methacrylate). Journal of Physical Science. 2009;**20**:1-12

[29] Sanchez JLA, Gomez ML, Bon RR, et al. Mechanical behavior of hybrid SiO2-PMMA coating measured by nanoindentation. Advances Technology Materials and Material Process Journal. 2006;**8**:81-86

[30] Alla RK, Sajjan S, Alluri VR, et al. Influence of fiber reinforcement on the properties of denture base resins. Journal of Biomaterials and Nanobiotechnology. 2013;**4**:91-97

[31] Dogan OM, Bolayir G, Keshin S, Dogan A, Bek B. The evaluation of some flexural properties of a denture base resin reinforced with various aesthetic

fibers. Journal of Materials Science. Materials in Medicine. 2008;**19**: 2343-2349

[32] Calamote C, Coelho C, Silva AS, Esteves JL, Moreira L, Correia Pinto A, et al. Comparison of the masticatory force (with 3D Models) of complete denture base acrylic resins with reline and reinforcing materials. Materials. 2021;**14**:3308. DOI: 10.3390/ma14123308

[33] Cheng YY, Li JY, Cheung WL, Chow TW. 3D FEA of high-performance polyethylene fiber reinforced maxillary dentures. Dental Materials. 2010; **26**:e211-e219

[34] Nakamura M, Takahashi H, Hayakawa I. Reinforcement of denture base resin with short-rod glass fiber. Dental Materials Journal. 2007; **26**:733-738

[35] Kanie T, Fujii K, Arikawa H, Inoue K. Flexural properties and impact strength of denture base polymer reinforced with woven glass fibers. Dental Materials. 2000;**16**:150-158

[36] Jagger D, Harrison A, Vowles R, Jagger R. The effect of the addition of surface treated chopped and continuous poly (methyl methacrylate) fibres on some properties of acrylic resins. Journal of Oral Rehabilitation. 2001;**28**:865-872

[37] Tsue F, Takahashi Y, Shimizu H. Reinforcing effect of glass-fiber-reinforced composite on flexural strength at the proportional limit of denture base resin. Acta Odontologica Scandinavica. 2007;**65**:141-148

[38] Yu S-H, Cho H-W, Oh S, Bae J-M. Effects of glass fiber mesh with different fiber content and structures on the compressive properties of complete dentures. The Journal of Prosthetic Dentistry. 2015;**113**:636-644

[39] Kanie T, Arikawa H, Fujii K, Ban S. Impact strength of acrylic denture base resin reinforced with woven glass fiber. Dental Materials Journal. 2003;**22**: 30-38

[40] Mansour MM, Wagner WC, Chu TG. Effect of MICA reinforcement on the flexural strength and microhardness of polymethyl methacrylate denture resin. Journal of Prosthodontics. 2013;**22**: 179-183

[41] Xu J, Li Y, Yu T, Cong L. Reinforcement of denture base resin with short vegetable fiber. Dental Materials. 2013;**29**:1273-1279

[42] Yu S-H, Lee Y, Oh S, Cho H-W, Oda Y, Bae J-M. Reinforcing effects of different fibers on denture base resin based on the fiber type, concentration, and combination. Dental Materials Journal. 2012;**31**:1039-1046

[43] El Bahra S, Ludwig K, Samran A, Freitag-Wolf S, Kern M. Linear and volumetric dimensional changes of injection-molded PMMA denture base resins. Dental Materials. 2013;**29**:1091-1097. DOI: 10.1016/j.dental.2013.07.020

[44] Ardelean L, Bortun CM, Podariu AC, Rusu LC. Acrylates and their alternatives in dental applications. In: Reddy BSR, editor. Acrylic Polymers in Healthcare. London: IntechOpen; 2017. pp. 3-24. DOI: 10.5772/66610

[45] Gautam R, Singh RD, Sharma VP, Siddartha R, Chand P, Kumar R. Biocompatibility of polymethylmethacrylate resins used in dentistry. Journal of Biomedial Materials Research Part B Applied Biomaterials. 2012;**100B**:1444-1450

[46] Kurtzman GM, Melton AB. Full arch removable prosthetics with Eclipse. Spectrum Denturism. 2008;**2**:1-8

[47] Rickman LJ, Padipatvuthikul P, Satterthwaite JD. Contemporary denture base resins: Part 1. Dental Update. 2012;**39**:25-30

[48] Singh K, Aeran H, Kumar N, Gupta N. Flexible thermoplastic denture base materials for aesthetical removable partial denture framework. Journal of Clinical and Diagnostic Research. 2013;7:2372-2373

[49] Fueki K, Ohkubo C, Yatabe M, Arakawa I, Arita M, et al. Clinical application of removable partial dentures using thermoplastic resin-part I: Definition and indication of non-metal clasp dentures. Journal of Prosthodontic Research. 2014;**58**(1):3-10

[50] Fueki K, Ohkubo C, Yatabe M, Arakawa I, Arita M, Ino S, et al. Clinical application of removable partial dentures using thermoplastic resin. Part II: Material properties and clinical features of non-metal clasp dentures. Journal of Prosthodontic Research. 2014;**58**(2):71-84

[51] Ardelean L, Bortun C, Podariu A, Rusu L. Manufacture of different types of thermoplastic. In: El-Sonbati AZ, editor. Thermoplastic - Composite Materials. Rijeka: InTech; 2012. pp. 25-48

[52] Ardelean L, Bortun CM, Podariu AC, Rusu LC. Thermoplastic resins used in dentistry. In: Das CK, editor. Thermoplastic Elastomers. Synthesis and Applications. Rijeka: InTech; 2015. pp. 145-167. DOI: 10.5772/59647

[53] Ardelean LC, Bortun CM, Podariu AC, Rusu LC. Polymeric alternatives in manufacturing removable partial dentures. Materiale Plastice. 2017;**54**:754-756

[54] Ardelean L, Bortun CM, Podariu AC, Rusu LC. Some alternatives for classic thermopolymerisable acrylic dentures. Materiale Plastice. 2012;**49**:30-33

[55] Uçar Y, Akova T, Aysan I. Mechanical properties of polyamide versus different PMMA denture base materials. Journal of Prosthodontics. 2012;**21**:173-176

[56] Yunus N, Rashid AA, Azmi LL, Abu-Hassan MI. Some flexural properties of a nylon denture base polymer. Journal of Oral Rehabilitation. 2005;**32**:65-71

[57] Soygun K, Bolayir G, Boztug A. Mechanical and thermal properties of polyamide versus reinforced PMMA denture base materials. The Journal of Advanced Prosthodontics. 2013;**5**: 153-160

[58] Meenakshi A, Gupta R, Bharti V, Sriramaprabu G, Prabhakar R. An evaluation of retentive ability and deformation of acetal resin and cobalt-chromium clasps. Journal of Clinical and Diagnostic Research. 2016; **10**:ZC37-ZC41. DOI: 10.7860/JCDR/2016/15476.7078

[59] Arda T, Arikan A. An in vitro comparison of retentive force and deformation of acetal resin and cobalt-chromium clasps. The Journal of Prosthetic Dentistry. 2005;**94**:267-274. DOI: 10.1016/j.prosdent.2005.06.009

[60] Ichikawa T, Kurahashi K, Liu L, Matsuda T, Ishida Y. Use of a polyetheretherketone clasp retainer for removable partial dentures: A case Report. Dental Journal. 2019;7:4. DOI: 10.3390/dj7010004

[61] Zoidis P, Papathanasiou I, Polyzois G. The use of a modified Poly-Ether-Ether-Ketone (PEEK) as an alternative framework material for removable dental prostheses. A clinical report. Journal of Prosthodontics. 2016;**140**:580-584

[62] Najeeb S, Zafar MS, Hurshid Z, Siddiqui F. Applications of polyetheretherketone (PEEK) in oral implantology and prosthodontics. Journal of Prosthodontic Research. 2016;**60**:12-19

[63] Rahmitasari F, Ishida Y, Kurahashi K, Matsuda T, Watanabe M, Ichikawa T. PEEK with reinforced materials and modifications for dental implant applications. Dental Journal. 2017;**15**:35. DOI: 10.3390/dj5040035

[64] Vaezi M, Yang S. Extrusion-based additive manufacturing of PEEK for biomedical applications. Virtual and Physical Prototyping. 2015;**310**:123-135

[65] Zalaznik M, Kalin M, Novak S. Influence of the processing temperature on the tribological and mechanical properties of poly-ether-ether-ketone (PEEK) polymer. Tribology International. 2016;**94**:92-97

[66] Lee CU, Vandenbrande J, Goetz A, Ganter M, Storti D, Boydston A. Room temperature extrusion 3D printing of poly-ether ether ketone using a stimuli-responsive binder. Bulletin Am. 2019;**28**:430-438

[67] Han SY, Moon YH, Lee J. Shear bond strength between CAD/CAM denture base resin and denture artificial teeth when bonded with resin cement. The Journal of Advanced Prosthodontics. 2020;**12**:251-258. DOI: 10.4047/jap.2020.12.5.251

[68] Maeda Y, Minoura M, Tsutsumi S, Okada M, Nokubi T. A CAD/CAM system for removable denture. Part I: Fabrication of complete dentures. The International Journal of Prosthodontics. 1994;7:17-21

[69] Kawahata N, Ono H, Nishi Y, Hamano T, Nagaoka E. Trial of duplication procedure for complete dentures by CAD/CAM. Journal of Oral Rehabilitation. 1997;**24**:540-548. DOI: 10.1046/j.1365-2842.1997.00522.x

[70] Pereyra NM, Marano J, Subramanian G, Quek S, Leff D. Comparison of patient satisfaction in the fabrication of conventional dentures vs. DENTCA (CAD/CAM) dentures: A case report. Journal of the New Jersey Dental Association. 2015;**86**:26-33

[71] Park JH, Cho IH, Shin SY, Choi YS. The treatment of an edentulous patient with Denta™ CAD/CAM denture. The Journal of Korean Academy of Prosthodontics. 2015;**53**:19-25. DOI: 368 10.4047/jkap.2015.53.1.19. 369

[72] Kim MJ, Kim KH, Yeo DH. Fabrication of computer-aided design/computer-aided manufacturing complete denture and conventional complete denture: Case report. Journal of Dental Rehabilitation and Applied Science. 2016;**32**:141-148. DOI: 10.14368/jdras.2016.32.2.141

[73] Kattadiyil MT, Goodacre CJ, Baba NZ. CAD/CAM complete dentures: A review of two commercial fabrication systems. Journal of the California Dental Association. 2013;**41**:407-416

[74] Kattadiyil MT, Al Helal A, Goodacre BJ. Clinical complications and quality assessments with computer-engineered complete dentures: A systematic review. The Journal of Prosthetic Dentistry. 2017;**117**:721-728

[75] Bidra AS, Farrell K, Burnham D, Dhingra A, Taylor TD, Kuo CL. Prospective cohort pilot study of 2-visit CAD/CAM monolithic complete dentures and implant-retained overdentures: Clinical and patient-centered outcomes. The Journal of Prosthetic Dentistry. 2015;**115**:578-586.e1. DOI: 10.1016/j.prosdent.2015.10.023

[76] Goodacre BJ, Goodacre CJ, Baba NZ, Kattadiyil MT. Comparison of denture base adaptation between CAD-CAM and conventional fabrication techniques. The Journal of Prosthetic Dentistry. 2016;**116**:249-256. DOI: 10.1016/j.prosdent.2016.02.017

[77] Kim TH, Varjao F. 3D printed complete dentures. In: Duarte S. Jr, editor. Quintessence of Dental Technology. Quintessence Publishing; 2016. p. 141-149

[78] Chung YJ, Park JM, Kim TH, Ahn JS, Cha HS, Lee JH. 3D printing of resin material for denture artificial teeth: Chipping and indirect tensile fracture resistance. Materials. 2018;**11**:1798. DOI: 10.3390/ma11101798

[79] Anne G, Oliganti SHB, Atla J, Budati S, Manne P, Chiramana S. The effect of aluminum oxide addition on the flexural strength of heat activated acrylic resin: An in vitro study. Journal of Dr Ntr University of Health Sciences. 2015;**4**: 21-23. DOI: 10.4103/2277-8632.153307

[80] Totu EE, Nechifor AC, Nechifor G, Aboul-Enein HY, Cristache CM. Poly(methyl methacrylate) with TiO nanoparticles inclusion for stereolitographic complete denture manufacturing - the fututre in dental care for elderly edentulous patients? Journal of Dentistry. 2017;**59**:68-77

[81] Chen S, Yang J, Jia YG, Lu B, Ren L. A study of 3D-printable reinforced composite resin: PMMA modified with silver nanoparticles loaded cellulose nanocrystal. Materials. 2018;**11**:2444. DOI: 10.3390/ma11122444

[82] Rehbein T, Johlitz M, Lion A, Sekmen K, Constantinescu A. Temperature-and degree of cure-dependent viscoelastic properties of photopolymer resins used in digital light processing. Progress in Additive Manufacturing. 2021;**6**:743-756. DOI: 10.1007/ s40964-021-00194-2

[83] Tian Y, Chen C, Xu X, Wang J, Hou X, Li K, et al. A review of 3D printing in dentistry: Technologies, affecting factors, and applications. Scanning. 2021;**202**:9950131. DOI: 10.1155/2021/9950131

Chapter 5

White Spot Lesions and Remineralization

Monisha Khatri, Shreya Kishore, S. Nagarathinam, Suvetha Siva and Vanita Barai

Abstract

As all practitioners are aware, the prevalence and incidence of dental caries keep increasing constantly and therefore early diagnosis and cessation of further progression would greatly help in maintaining the sound tooth structure. One of the earliest signs of dental caries is a white spot lesion, which is mostly missed, and only treated when the condition worsens. WSL are areas of demineralized enamel that occur due to a prolonged period of retained microbial biofilms most commonly associated in patients with poor oral hygiene and fixed orthodontic appliances. If caught early and intervened, WSLs can be reversed. Therefore, the diagnosis and treatment of WSL are of outmost importance, and this chapter will explain in detail various methods of diagnosing WSLs, its treatment protocol with the significance of remineralization of the same.

Keywords: dental caries, demineralization, fluorosis, remineralization, white spot lesions

1. Introduction

White spot lesion (WSL) is the demineralization of the enamel surface and subsurface that is devoid of cavitation [1–3]. They are a result of the imbalance between mineralisation and demineralization, which if not intervened, may further lead to irreversible damage [1, 2]. In early lesions the mineral content in the affected area is reduced, which in turn affects the translucent feature of the enamel, and the colour of these areas appear more opaque white, hence, they are termed as white spot lesions. They are the first visible findings in caries formation and are considered as initial lesions by many clinicians. However, it should be remembered that, for demineralization to be visible, it must have a minimum depth of 300–500 μm implying that a considerable amount of damage to sound tooth structure has already begun [4–7].

These lesions are commonly associated with poor oral hygiene and increased plaque accumulation. In addition to the above other risk factors such as poor dietary habits, high DMFS (Decayed, Missing or Filled Surfaces) index, and lack of preventive measures during orthodontic treatment always prevail.

A white spot may be intrinsic or extrinsic in origin [2], enamel defects such as fluorosis, hypomineralisation, hypomaturation of enamel, hypoplastic defects can lead to noncarious intrinsic white spots of the enamel. These developmental anomalies are greatly influenced by genetic aberrations, environmental variations, metabolic diseases, drug abuse, use of chemicals, radiation and trauma [4]. The differential diagnosis is imperative to the treatment plan.

An early enamel lesion can easily be identified as a white opaque spot when air-dried and is the most efficient way to detect it [5]. What may appear to be a smooth, shiny, non-carious lesion under light may be a rough, opaque and porous lesion on cleaning and drying [6]. It is challenging for a clinician to detect these in a regular check-up, and the diagnosis can only be established subjective to the clinician. Since these discolorations may be a result of several factors, it is usually challenging to arrive at an accurate diagnosis for the same.

2. Aetiology/causes

WSL usually has a multifactorial manifestation. It is vital to ascertain the causes, before planning and providing treatment options to the patient. This is because the results of the treatment will vary depending on the substructure available [8–12].

Causes of WSL include,

- high fluoride intake in childhood
- complications in pregnancy
- trauma
- poor oral hygiene

2.1 Fluorosis

During the phase of enamel mineralisation, if there is excessive fluoride exposure, and as a result the enamel would become hypomineralized, leading to a condition called fluorosis. Studies conducted by McKay and Black [11] conclude, that fluoride can be beneficial or harmful depending on certain factors, like the age, dosage, and health of the patient [13]. In preventive measures, many times a dentist uses fluoride to reinforce the enamel, hence a controlled dosage is required to make the use of fluoride extremely beneficial (**Figure 1**).

It is observed that fluorosis generally appears symmetrically and can present itself in 3 ways i.e., white spots, brown spots or pitting. In milder cases, it presents itself as narrow white lines, following the perikymata, cuspal snow capping or snowflaking whereas, in severe cases the brown discoloration is apparent due to the infiltration of chromophoric proteins [3] (**Table 1**). In any case, WSL and fluorosis are two different entities and can be differentiated as follows [14]:

WSL:

- Occurs due to the hypomineralization of enamel.
- Surfaces appear translucent when the tooth surface is moist and, opaque white when the surface is air-dried.
- The surface of WSL is softer and rougher with easy dental plaque formation.

Fluorosis:

- Occurs due to hypomineralization because of excessive incorporation of fluoride during the formation of enamel.
- In the early phase, the surfaces have convergent horizontal white lines leading to a "Parchment-like" appearance along with irregular chalky areas. Then the colour changes to brown, due to the infiltration of exogenous chromophoric proteins.
- Histopathologically, fluorosis occurs on the sub-surface of the external third of enamel.

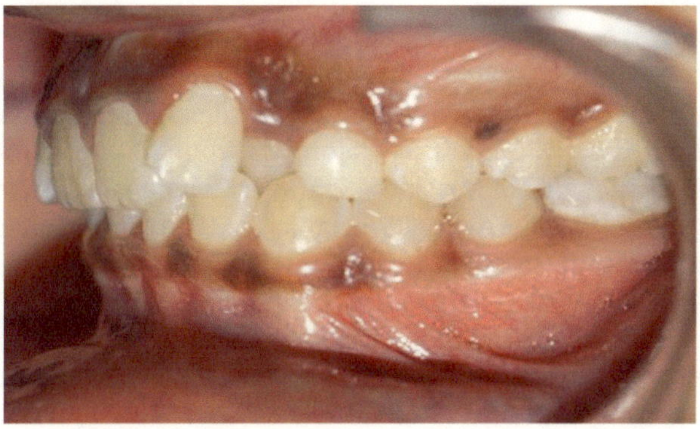

Figure 1.
Mild fluorosis.

Classification	Criteria—description of enamel (teeth not air-dried)
Normal	No evidence of fluorosis
Questionable	Enamel discloses slight aberrations from the translucency of normal enamel, ranging from a few white flecks to occasional white spots. This classification is utilised in those instances where a definite diagnosis is not warranted and a classification of 'normal' not justified
Very mild	Small, opaque, paper-white areas scattered irregularly over the tooth involving up to 25% of the tooth surface. Frequently included in this classification are teeth showing up to 1–2 mm of white opacity at the cusp tips of the premolars or second molars
Mild	More extensive white opaque areas in the enamel of the teeth involving up to 50% of the tooth surface (**Figure 1**)
Moderate	All enamel surfaces of the teeth are affected and are at risk of attrition. Brown stain is frequently a disfiguring feature
Severe	All enamel surfaces are affected and the hypoplasia affects the general form of the tooth. The major diagnostic sign of this classification is discrete or confluent pitting. Brown stains are widespread and teeth often present with a corroded-like appearance

Table 1.
Dean's fluorosis index [12].

2.2 Traumatic hypomineralization

It is not unusual to find white spot lesions due to trauma in the primary dentition stage. An incidence rate of 74.1% is seen [15] following which the succeeding tooth may be hypoplastic, or display discoloration (**Figure 2**).

Traumatic hypomineralization is usually asymmetric in presentation and involves a single tooth with unusual patches.

Physical trauma such as a break or fracture of the tooth or chemical trauma such as a periapical infection of the primary tooth can cause a severe periapical inflammation which disturbs and influences the underlying mineralisation of the tooth, resulting in accelerated deposition of minerals. These are commonly seen as punctiform lesions of the dental crowns or the incisal one thirds [16].

2.3 Demineralization

Enamel demineralization is a complication associated with poor hygiene during orthodontic treatment. When there is prolonged and excessive plaque accumulation, in the course of treatment, WSLs are seen along the appliance margins at various sites. 46–73% is the prevalence rate of demineralization following orthodontic treatment and this poses a grave challenge to the clinicians [17]. The subsurface demineralization is a predisposing factor to caries formation and is commonly seen around the bracket attachments and underneath the molar bands.

These areas are mostly noticed in orthodontic patients who are unable to adequately clean the tooth surface with the toothbrush which later appears as white spots. They are white chalky in appearance and unusually located (**Figure 3**).

2.4 Molar incisor hypomineralization (MIH)

Weerheijm et al. introduced the term molar-incisor hypomineralization (MIH) [18], wherein they defined it as a hypomineralization of systemic origin, which presented itself as a demarcated, qualitative defect of the enamel of 1–4 first permanent molars, frequently associated with enamel opacities. In these cases, due to the qualitative defects, the teeth exhibit post-eruptive breakdown of the enamel. This causes rapidly progressive caries and severe sensitivity of the teeth.

The causes of MIH are still not clear, it is thought that there is a systemic disruption of amelogenesis which includes, malnutrition, hypoxia, common childhood illness and use of antibiotics before the age of 3 years that causes this effect [16].

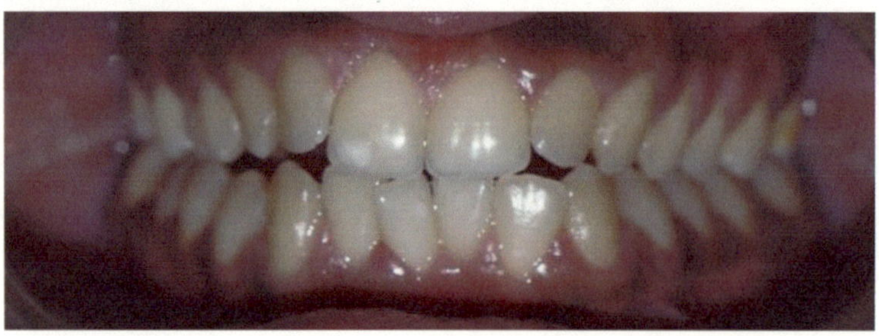

Figure 2.
Traumatic hypomineralization.

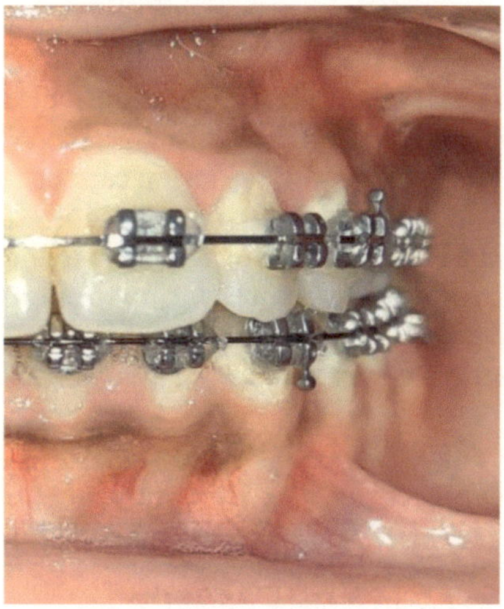

Figure 3.
Demineralization with braces.

Clinically they are seen as white-creamy or yellow-brown opacities, usually larger than 1 mm and post-eruptive breakdown of at least one first permanent molar.

A history of illness in the first three years, difficulty during birthing, or prenatal illness helps with the diagnosis.

3. Diagnosis

3.1 Importance

The clinical manifestation of WSL starts as early as 4 weeks in case of orthodontic treatment. Unnoticed WSL can lead to the disintegration of enamel surface followed by carious lesion which may require aesthetic restorations or in more advanced cases a prosthodontic intervention. This is more commonly seen in high caries risk individuals. In people with low caries activity, the repair mechanisms help in the potential healing of the lesion.

Hence, it is important to plan the treatment according to the caries activity in individuals after a proper diagnosis. The emphasis given to new technologies has made it possible to detect initial lesions before they turn into irreversible cavitation [19].

3.2 Methods

The ideal method for the detection of WSLs should have a high level of sensitivity (the ability to detect disease when present) and specificity (the ability to confirm that disease is absent).

3.2.1 Conventional methods

The conventional methods of diagnosing WSLs are visual examination, tactile examination with probing and digital photographic examination. These methods are simple to use, inexpensive, and clinically valid.

3.2.1.1 Visual examination

For visual examination, the tooth surface must be air-dried for at least 5 s after cleaning with pumice under adequate light to visualise the WSLs. The opacities on the enamel surface will not be visible and the lesion cannot be distinguished the enamel gets wet. Because the micro pores in the surface are filled with water and the refractive index of enamel becomes 1.33, which is close to that of healthy enamel. On the other hand, after the air drying, the pores within the lesion will be filled with air, which has a refractive index of 1.0. Hence, the opaque enamel lesions become evident and distinct from the healthy enamel surface [20].

3.2.1.2 Photographic examination

The recommended specifications for taking intraoral images are 100 mm macro lens with a small aperture of 25. While taking a photograph the teeth should be inaccurate axial position i.e. the occlusal plane should be parallel to the horizontal plane. Although, these methods are useful in the detection, they do not quantify the depth of the lesions [21].

3.2.2 Contemporary methods

They are more consistent and enhanced sensitivity towards lesion diagnosis when compared to the conventional methods. This can be classified as:

3.2.2.1 Electric resistance (electronic conductance and impedance)

An intact enamel surface is a good electrical insulator due to its high inorganic content. Demineralization causes loss of minerals, resulting in increased porosities filled with saliva, this acts as a conductive pathway for electric current. The electric conductivity is directly proportional to the amount of demineralization [22].

E.g., Electrical Caries Monitor, Caries Meter L, CarieScan Pro.

3.2.2.2 Fluorescence

The autofluorescence of tooth tissue decreases as the demineralization activity increases .This could be attributed to protoporphyrin, a photosensitive pigment present in demineralized dental tissues that are generated due to bacterial metabolic activity [23].

E.g., Fibre-Optic Transillumination (FOTI), Digital imaging Fibre-Optic Transillumination (DIFOTI), Near-infrared digital imaging transillumination (NIDIT), Laser fluorescence (LF), Quantitative light-induced fluorescence (QLF), and Multiphoton imaging

3.2.2.2.1 Fibre-Optic Transillumination (FOTI)

The concept of transillumination for the detection of WSL is based on the refractive index of different tooth structures [23]. The refractive index will vary when light is passed through different tissues. The demineralized enamel appears as a grey hue whereas dentin gives an orange-brown or a bluish hue. Due to the intra and inter-observer disparity, Digital imaging FOTI (DIFOTI) was developed in the 1990s. In DIFOTI the images are captured and stored by a CCD camera. Another advanced method is near-infrared digital imaging transil-lumination (NIDIT). In this technique two near-infrared laser diodes are used, which allows superior light to spread into the dental tissues and get better picture quality than visible light [23].

3.2.2.2.2 Laser fluorescence (LF)

LF uses a red wavelength of 655 nm for caries detection [23]. It is based on the principle when light is applied to the tooth surface, the caries-related changes in the tooth tissues lead to an increase in fluorescence. This can be translated into numeric values, which can vary from 0 to 99.

For example, in DIAGNOdent pen scores from 0 to 10 are interpreted as healthy, while scores above 30 indicate a lesion that requires restorative treatment [23].

3.2.2.2.3 Quantitative light-induced fluorescence (QLF)

It measures the percentage of fluorescence change in demineralized enamel. This technique allows us to detect the lesion activity as well as to predict the lesion progression. Since demineralized tissue has limited penetration of light, it gives a dark image in QLF [24].

3.2.2.2.4 Multiphoton imaging

Unlike conventional fluorescence imaging, it uses two infrared photons simul¬taneously to excite a fluorescent compound in the tooth. Caries will appear as a dark form within a bright fluorescing tooth. It also helps to collect information from carious lesions up to 500 μm of depth [25].

3.2.2.3 Thermography

The concept of thermography for the detection of early enamel caries has been discovered by Kaneko in 1999. It measures the lesion activity rather than its presence or absence. This is based on the principle of change in thermal radiation energy that occurs when fluid is lost from a lesion by evaporation just as in WSLs [25].

E.g., Infrared thermography, Frequency-domain infrared photothermal radiometry and modulated luminescence (PTR/LUM).

3.2.2.4 Terahertz imaging

Terahertz parametric imaging (TPI) has great potential in the diagnosis of WSL [25]. Terahertz radiation is located between the high-frequency microwave and long-wavelength infrared region of the spectrum. This helps identification of infected tissue inside the tooth followed by 3D plotting which can be applied to obtain the depth of the demineralized tissue. It can also be used to measure the remineralization of enamel [25].

3.2.2.5 Based on the optical behaviour

3.2.2.5.1 Midwest caries ID probe

It works on the principle of difference in the optical behaviour inside the tooth. The probe when placed on the tooth surface emits 635–880 nm wavelength and the light reflected from the surface of the tooth converts it to electrical signals [25].

3.2.2.5.2 Optical coherence tomography (OCT)

It is a novel, non-irradiative, non-invasive imaging technique. The concept of OCT is based on the differences in the optical absorption and scattering properties of the dental tissue. It uses infrared light to produce a real-time cross-sectional image of dental tissue. Demineralized tissue can be distinguished from sound tissue based on the following principles:

- Increased light scattering in porous demineralized tissue and
- Depolarization of incident light by demineralized tissue.

Enamel caries appear brighter on grayscale OCT images whereas dentin caries gives the image a continuous bright area throughout the enamel into the dentin [26].

3.3 Evaluation

Conventional methods: [21]

1. Visual examination: on visual examination, if the lesion is active or inactive can also be determined. If the tooth surfaces are chalky and rough, it indicates active lesions. If the tooth surfaces are smooth and shiny, it indicates inactive lesions. Different methods are used for evaluation on clinical examination. They include:

- Ekstrand assessment scale (1995)
- The Nyvad system (1999)
- The Dundee Selectable Threshold Method for Caries Diagnosis (DSTM in 2000)
- The International Caries Detection and Assessment System (ICDAS in 2004) [26].

The scores are given in **Table 2**.

2. Photographic examination: for the evaluation on photographic examination, frontal and lateral photos are taken and it's done using the Gorelick index. The scoring is done on the labial surfaces of incisors, cuspids and buccal surfaces of premolars. The inference is given in **Table 3**.

Contemporary methods [21]

1. Electrical conductance measurement (Caries meter L):

The tooth surface is inserted with conducting gel and is gently air-dried. Every tooth surface is dampened between the measurements to establish proper contact between the electrode and tooth surface. The device has colour codes to indicate the extent of caries as given in **Table 4**.

Ekstrand system	Nyvad system	DSTM system	ICDAS system
0—no/slight changes in enamel translucency after prolonged air dry (5 s)	0—healthy tooth	G—healthy tooth	0—sound
1—opacity/discoloration distinctly visible after air drying, hardly on wet surfaces	1—active (intact)	W—white spot lesion	1—first visual change in enamel
2—opacity/discoloration distinctly visible without air drying	2—active (surface discontinuity)	B—brown spot lesion	2—distinct visual change in enamel
3—localised enamel breakdown in opaque or discoloured enamel and/or greyish discoloration from the underlying dentine	3—active (cavitated)	E—enamel cavitation	3—localised enamel breakdown
4—cavitation in enamel exposing the dentine	4—inactive (intact)	D—dentine lesion (non-cavitated)	4—underlying dark shadow from dentine
	5—inactive (surface discontinuity)	C—dentine cavity	5—distinct cavity with visible dentine
	6—inactive (cavity)	P—pulp involvement	6—extensive distinct cavity with visible dentine
	7, 8, 9—presence or absence of caries which might be active or inactive in the filling or restorations	A—arrested dentinal decay F—filled surfaces contiguous with the upper types of lesions	

Table 2.
Different systems for evaluation on clinical examination.

Score	Inference
0	No lesion
1	Thin rims of white spot lesion
2	Thick bands of white spot lesion
3	Cavitation due to white spot lesion

Table 3.
Gorelick index scoring.

2. Quantitative light fluorescence (QLF):

According to Rodrigues et al. in 2011, there are two devices used in QLF. They are DIAGNOdent device and DIAGNOdent pen. The device consists of a laser diode, photo diode and a long pass filter [27]. A tip is placed on the tooth surface at a certain angle and fluorescence values are calculated as in **Table 5**.

3. Light-emitting diode fluorescence:

LED fluorescence is based on the principle of difference in optical property. There are two available systems: Midwest caries (MID) and Vista Proof (VP). MID probe is a small battery-operated device with a portable handpiece and a probe [27]. When the probe touches the demineralized tooth surface there is an audible signal with a colour change from green to red as given in **Table 6**.

4. Frequency-domain infrared photothermal radiometry and modulated luminescence (PTR/LUM) [21]:

A recent technology called the Canary system has been introduced in the year 2011. This system consists of a laser tip along with an intra-oral camera. The laser tip is placed on the tooth surface that has to be examined and the WSL is recorded based on the scoring from 0 to 100 on the digital display. The scores and inferences are given in **Table 7**.

Colour	Inference
Green	No caries
Yellow	Caries in enamel
Orange	Caries in dentine
Red	Caries reaching pulp

Table 4.
Colour codes and inference of caries meter L.

Readings	Inference
0–14	Absence of caries
15–20	Caries present in enamel
21–99	Caries present in dentine

Table 5.
Scoring of DIAGNOdent device.

Score	Inference
0	Green light without any signal indicates healthy tooth
1	Red light with medium signal indicates enamel caries
2	Red light with rapid signal indicates dentinal caries

Table 6.
Scoring of Midwest caries device (LED fluorescence).

Score	Inference
0–20	Healthy tooth
21–70	Demineralization and caries
71–100	Advanced caries

Table 7.
Scores and inference of PTR/LUM.

4. Remineralization and white spot lesions

The pathophysiology of dental caries is a continuous process of demineralization and remineralization wherein a net mineral gain is required to prevent lesion progression. To achieve this, the balance between the pathological factors such as fermentable carbohydrate ingestion, salivary function inhibition, acidogenic bacteria and protective factors like antibacterial agents, composition and rate of flow of saliva, fluoride and diet needs to be maintained [28]. Fermentation of carbohydrates leads to formation of organic acid by acidogenic bacteria that cause diffusion of calcium and phosphate ions out of the tooth leading to the formation of white spot lesions at an early stage, which further progresses to cavitation if the process continues [5]. This can be prevented by remineralization or mineral gain which is defined as the process whereby calcium and phosphate ions are supplied from a source external to the tooth to promote ion deposition into crystal voids in demineralized enamel [29].

Saliva is the major source of these minerals consists of calcium (Ca), phosphate (P), fluoride (Fl) ions in addition to salivary proteins such as proline-rich proteins, statherin, histatins which increases the concentration of calcium ions and salivary enzymes such as lysozymes and peroxidases. Normally the saliva is supersaturated with calcium and phosphate ions but when the pH decreases (<5.5) due to the fermentation of carbohydrates, as mentioned above, this equilibrium is lost and demineralization starts. To prevent this, saliva acts as a remineralizing agent by providing Fl ions to regain homeostasis and thereby acts by preventing demineralization, promoting remineralization and having an antibacterial effect. Therefore, a variety of treatment modalities are available to treat initial carious lesions also known as white spot lesions based on the above theory, which will be discussed in the upcoming treatment modalities [30].

5. Treatment

5.1 Various methods of treatment

There are various treatment options available to treat WSLs depending on their extent and severity [31] (**Table 8**).

5.1.1 Micro-abrasion

Micro-abrasion is the application of an acidic and abrasive compound to the surface of the enamel. The micro abrasion process removes small amounts of surface enamel but also leaves a highly polished enamel surface. The micro-abraded enamel surface does not have the ideal enamel surface appearance as interprismatic spaces would be absent.

White spot lesion	Presentation	Treatment options
Fluorosis	Can vary from symmetrical lesions, presence of white lines, 'snowflake appearance', to pitting and mottling in severe cases	• Whitening • Micro-abrasion • Resin infiltration • Restorations
Traumatic hypomineralisation	Presents as a punctiform lesion on the incisal 3rd of the crown, usually asymmetrical	• Whitening • Resin infiltration • Restorations
MIH	Condition where there is hypomineralised permanent first molars along with or without the incisors, presenting yellowing of the teeth, mottling and post eruptive breakdown of molars	• Chemical remineralisation • Micro-abrasion • Whitening with/without CPP-ACP • Restorations • Extraction
Demineralisation	Presents as faint white lesions around the orthodontic brackets	• Chemical remineralisation • Whitening • Resin infiltration • Micro-abrasion
WSL (natural)	Presents itself as isolated white spots with a diameter less than 0.5 mm on the incisors	• Whitening

Table 8.
Various WSLs and their treatment options.

The micro-abrasion process abrades surface enamel while compacting calcium and phosphate into the interprismatic spaces. This polished surface reflects light differently than natural enamel. Therefore, a portion of the whitened enamel is removed and a portion is camouflaged by the highly polished surface.

Following this procedure, a 4-min 2% sodium fluoride treatment is recommended. If the micro-abrasion technique does not produce optimal aesthetic results, and if the whitened enamel is still prominent, vital tooth bleaching should be considered [32].

5.1.2 Whitening

Also known as vital tooth bleaching or bleaching. It is the process of lightening the colour of enamel. To date, there are two techniques of tooth whitening that have been prescribed:

a. Ambulatory—that requires an intraoral device/tray to apply a gel of peroxide, which can be done at home and is more cost-effective. It must be kept in mind that major changes are not observed before the 7th day.

b. In-office method, which requires a professional to perform the procedure, uses photoactivation, where the changes of colour in the enamel can be witnessed from the first session [33].

5.1.3 Resin infiltration

Also known as an ICON (infiltration concept) was designed as a minimally invasive resin infiltration system for treating incipient caries in patients of all ages. The low viscosity unfilled resin, developed by the company DMG (Germany) camouflages white spots using optical manipulation, and no tooth tissue removal is strictly necessary (**Figure 4**).

The clear resin flows into the demineralized enamel, and has similar optical properties (similar refractive index) to the enamel, therefore reflecting light to match the tooth's natural shade [34, 35].

5.1.4 Chemical remineralization

CPP-ACP (Casein Phosphopeptide-Amorphous Calcium Phosphate) also known as the stabilised ACP, was developed based on the idea that CPP being saliva biomimetic solubilises the nano complexes readily, and creates a diffusion gradient that allows them to localise in supragingival plaque [36].

Low pH conditions that arise during a cariogenic attack, facilitate the release of Ca and P ions, inhibiting demineralization and favours the remineralization of the incipient lesions by precipitation of the released ions. This subsurface remineralization pattern produced by CPP-ACP has shown significant improvement in the aesthetics, and strength of the remineralized white spot lesion [29]. Some of the commercially available products are GC tooth mousse, flouride varnish, nanohydroxyapatite system and bioactive glass.

5.1.5 Restorations

Dental restorations also known as dental fillings are treatments used to restore the function, integrity and morphology of the missing tooth structure. Dental restorations include glass ionomer cement, composites (light-cured, chemically cured or dual-cure), giomers, compomers and veneers.

Restorations are done in cases where aesthetics is of major concern and when there are lesser chances of reversing the damage. Restorations are also considered as a permanent solution [37].

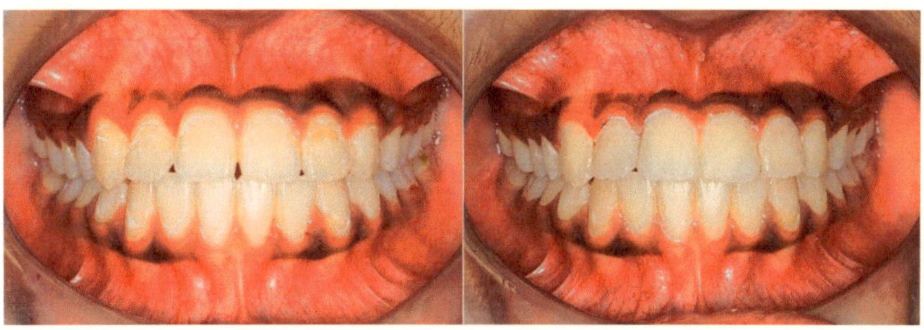

Figure 4.
ICON treatment: pre and post treatment.

6. Prevention

Without a doubt, enamel decalcification/demineralization is a major clinical problem. Once the lesions are established, it is hard to achieve complete remineralization. Fluoride is a major ingredient that is cariostatic and is capable of arresting the lesion. Hence judicious use of fluoridated toothpastes and mouthwashes are advocated. Newer agents like CPP-ACP, hydroxyapatite systems, bioactive glasses are also being experimented [2]. Optimal oral hygiene is necessary to evade white spot lesions. Regular dental visits and the use of oral prophylactic aids are not negotiable. Patients undergoing fixed orthodontic treatment are required to maintain their oral hygiene and use oral hygiene products that would help in remineralizing the demineralized enamel.

7. Conclusion

Prevention of enamel demineralization is of utmost importance. Should enamel demineralization occur (white spot lesions), early diagnosis and intervention are appropriate. Improved brushing with fluoridated dentifrice and over-the-counter fluoride rinses would be the first recommended intervention.

Patients may also develop demineralized enamel during orthodontic treatment, which exhibits itself as white spot lesions adjacent to brackets and the free gingival margin area. As previously discussed, topical fluoride therapy is appropriate to be sure remineralization of enamel has occurred. Mild whitened enamel can often be camouflaged by bleaching with standard tray-based whitening systems used overnight or with the hydrogen peroxide-impregnated polyethylene strips. If 2 to 4-week bleaching with these regimens is ineffective at camouflaging this whitened enamel, microabrasion followed by bleaching is recommended.

Author details

Monisha Khatri[1*], Shreya Kishore[2], S. Nagarathinam[1], Suvetha Siva[2] and Vanita Barai[3]

1 Department of Conservative Dentistry and Endodontics, SRM Dental College, SRM Institute of Science and Technology, Chennai, India

2 Department of Orthodontics, SRM Dental College, SRM Institute of Science and Technology, Chennai, India

3 Private Practitioner, India

*Address all correspondence to: drkhatrimonisha@gmail.com

References

[1] Bergstrand F, Twetman S. A review on prevention and treatment of post-orthodontic white spot lesions—Evidence-based methods and emerging technologies. The Open Dentistry Journal. 2011;**5**:158

[2] Paula AB, Fernandes AR, Coelho AS, et al. Therapies for white spot lesions—A systematic review. The Journal of Evidence-Based Dental Practice. 2017;**17**(1):23-38

[3] Denis M, Atlan A, Vennat E, Tirlet G, Attal JP. White defects on enamel: Diagnosis and anatomopathology: two essential factors for proper treatment (part 1). International Orthodontics. 2013;**11**(2):139-165

[4] AlShehri A, Kwon SR. Etiology and management of white spot lesions. Prosthetics Restorative. Journal of Multidisciplinary Care Decisions in Dentistry. 2016:10-19

[5] Kudiyirickal MG, Ivancaková R. Early enamel lesion part I. Classification and detection. Acta Medica (Hradec Kralove). 2008;**51**(3):145-149

[6] Guzmán-Armstrong S, Chalmers J, Warren JJ, Ask us. White spot lesions: Prevention and treatment. American Journal of Orthodontics and Dentofacial Orthopedics. 2010;**138**(6):690-696

[7] Axelsson P. Diagnosis and Risk Prediction of Dental Caries. Chicago: Quintessence Pub. Co; 2000. p. 307

[8] Gorelick L, Geiger AM, Gwinnet AJ. Incidence of whitespot formation after bonding and banding. American Journal of Orthodontics. 1982;**81**:93-98

[9] Ekstrand KR, Kuzmina I, Bjørndal L, Thylstrup A. Relationship between external and histologic features of progressive stages of caries in the occlusal fossa. Caries Research. 1995;**29**(4):243-250. [Crossref]

[10] Pitts N. "ICDAS"—An international system for caries detection and assessment being developed to facilitate caries epidemiology, research and appropriate clinical management. Community Dental Health. 2004;**21**(3): 193-198

[11] Black GV. Mottled teeth: an endemic developmental imperfection of the enamel of the teeth heretofore unknown in the literature of dentistry. Dental Cosmos. 1916;**58**:129-156

[12] Dean HT. Classification of mottled enamel diagnosis. Journal of the American Dental Association (Chicago, IL). 1934;**21**:1421-1426

[13] Watts A, Addy M. Tooth discolouration and staining: A review of the literature. British Dental Journal. 2001;**190**:309-316

[14] Deveci C, Çınar Ç, Tirali RE. Management of white spot lesions. In: Dental Caries—Diagnosis, Prevention and Management. Zühre Akarslan: IntechOpen; 2018. DOI: 10.5772/intechopen.75312. Available from: https://www.intechopen.com/chapters/60376

[15] De Amorim LFG, Estrela C, da Costa LRRS. Effects of traumatic dental injuries to primary teeth on permanent teeth—A clinical follow up study. Dental Traumatology. 2011;**27**:117-121

[16] Deveci C, Çınar C, Tirali RE. Management of white spot lesions. In: Akarslan Z, editor. Dental Caries: Diagnosis, Prevention and Management.

London: IntechOpen; 2018. Available from: https://www.intechopen.com/books/dental-caries-diagnosis-prevention-and-management/management-of-white-spot-lesions [Accessed: August 2020]

[17] Mizrahi E. Enamel demineralization following orthodontic treatment. American Journal of Orthodontics. 1982;**82**:62-67

[18] Weerheijm KL, Jälevik B, Alaluusua S. Molar-Incisor hypomineralisation. Caries Research. 2001;**35**:390-391

[19] https://clinicaltrials.gov/ct2/show/NCT04827966

[20] Sadikoglu IS. White spot lesions: Recent detection and treatment methods. Cyprus Journal of Medical Sciences. 2020;**5**(3):260-267

[21] Izhar D, Batra D, Miglani D. Diagnostic tools for early diagnosis of white spot lesions. European Journal of Molecular & Clinical Medicine. 2021;**8**(2):680-695

[22] Vimal k Sikri Textbook of Operative Dentistry. 4th ed. Diagnosis and Treatment Planning. pp. 97-98

[23] Mital P, Mehta N, Saini A, Raisingani D, Sharma M. Recent advances in detection and diagnosis of dental caries. Journal of Evolution of Medical and Dental Sciences. 2014;**3**(1): 177-192

[24] Pretty IA. Caries detection and diagnosis: Novel technologies. Journal of Dentistry. 2006;**34**(10):727-739

[25] Yadav NP, Hu G, Yao Z, Kumar A. Diagnosis of dental problem by using terahertz technology. Journal of Electronic Science and Technology. 2021;**19**:100082

[26] Abogazalah N, Ando M. Alternative methods to visual and radiographic examinations for approximal caries detection. Journal of Oral Science. 2017;**59**(3):315-322

[27] Rodrigues J, Hug I, Neuhaus KW, Lussi A. Light-emitting diode and laser fluorescence-based devices in detecting occlusal caries. Journal of Biomedical Optics. 2011;**16**(10):107003

[28] Philip N. State of the art enamel remineralization systems: The next frontier in caries management. Caries Research. 2019;**53**(3):284-295

[29] Cochrane NJ, Cai F, Huq NL, Burrow MF, Reynolds EC. New approaches to enhanced remineralization of tooth enamel. Journal of Dental Research. 2010;**89**(11):1187-1197

[30] Farooq I, Bugshan A. The role of salivary contents and modern technologies in the remineralization of dental enamel: A narrative review. F1000Research. 2020;**9**:171

[31] Sampson V, Sampson A. Diagnosis and treatment options for anterior white spot lesions. British Dental Journal. 2020;**229**(6):348-352

[32] Donly KJ, Sasa IS. Potentioal remineralization of post orthodontic demineralized enamel and the use of enamel microabrasion and bleaching for esthetics. Seminars in Orthodontics. 2008;**14**:3, 220-225

[33] Feliz-Maltos L, Hernandez LM, Abreu N. Dental bleaching techniques; hydrogen-carbamide peroxides and light sources for activation, an update—Mini review article. The Open Dentistry Journal. 2014;**8**:264-268

[34] Manoharan V, Arun Kumar S, Arumugam SB, Anand V,

Krishnamoorthy S, Methippara JJ. Is resin infiltration a microinvasive approach to white lesions of calcified tooth structures? A systemic review. International Journal of Clinical Pediatric Dentistry. 2019;**12**:53-58

[35] Omar S. Using resin infiltration to treat developmental defects of enamel. Three case reports. Journal of Restorative Dentistry. 2013;**1**:31-35

[36] Reynolds EC, Cai F, Cochrane NJ, Shen P, Walker GD, Morgan MV, et al. Fluoride and casein phosphopeptide-amorphous calcium phosphate. Journal of Dental Research. 2008;**87**:344-348

[37] Bishara SE, Ostby AW. White spot lesions: Formation, prevention, and treatment. Seminars in orthodontics. 2008;**14**(3):174-182

Chapter 6

Oral Cancer around Dental Implants: Are the Clinical Manifestations and the Oncogenic Mechanisms Unique?

Gabriela Lopes dos Santos, Kaique Preto Alberto, Silas Antonio Juvêncio de Freitas Filho, Kellen Cristine Tjioe and Denise Tostes Oliveira

Abstract

Osseointegrated implants have been an optimal treatment option for dental rehabilitation of fully or partially edentulous patients. Although peri-implantitis remains as the most common local risk factor for dental implant failure, the development of oral cancer involving the soft tissue around the titanium may lead to early implants loss and impact the quality of life of the patient negatively. Oral squamous cell carcinoma (OSCC) is the most common malignancy among head and neck tumors. It has higher prevalence in men over 50 years old, and in tobacco and/or alcohol users. Unfortunately, oral cancer is often detected in advanced stages, when the treatment options are limited. Thus, OSCC typically has poor prognosis. Despite the recent advances in oral carcinogenesis understanding, the relationship between dental implants and the development of malignant lesions around them is not completely understood. It has been suggested that the titanium corrosion occurring at the top of dental implants causes the release of metal ions. These ions might lead to oral epithelial genetic damage and higher susceptibility of normal mucosa to malignant transformation. The aim of this chapter was to review the clinical characteristics, diagnosis, and the possible carcinogenic mechanisms involved in oral cancer around dental implants.

Keywords: oral cancer, carcinogenesis, dental implants, titanium corrosion, delayed diagnosis

1. Introduction

Oral cancer remains as a significant cause of mortality worldwide as most of these the tumors are detected and treated in late stages. The etiology of oral cancer is multifactorial. Tobacco and alcohol are still considered the main risk factors as about 80% of the patients who develop oral tumors are tobacco and/or alcohol users [1].

Additional etiologic factors have also been suggested such as infection by human papillomavirus (HPV) and other oncogenic viruses, immunosuppression states, genetic alterations, and deficient nutrition.

Dental implants are one of the top choices for the oral rehabilitation of partially or totally edentulous patients. The stability and comfort provided by the implants-anchored crowns are among their clinical advantages. Moreover, the success rate of dental implants surpasses 94.6% [2]. However, the soft tissue and supporting structures around the dental implants remain exposed to the oral cavity and may undergo pathological changes. The most frequent lesions are those of inflammatory nature triggered by the accumulation of bacterial biofilm. When the inflammatory lesion is confined to the soft tissue, it is named as peri-implant mucositis. On the other hand, when there is loss of supporting bone, the lesion is known as peri-implantitis. Due to the high incidence of peri-implant inflammatory diseases, some dental professionals treat the lesion but do not send the specimens to the microscopical analysis. About 3.6% of the lesions are malignant tumors (mainly squamous cell carcinomas, the most common malignancy of the oral cavity) [3]. In 2001, the first cases of malignant lesions developing around dental implants were published [4–22]. Since then, the potential relationship of titanium implants with malignant tumor development has been discussed [1, 5, 13].

The aim of this chapter was to offer the readership the most recent information regarding the clinical features of oral cancer around dental implants, its differential diagnosis, and potential oncogenic mechanisms.

2. Clinical features of oral cancer around dental implants

A review of literature available until September 2021 was conducted in the PubMed/Medline database using the term "Oral squamous cell carcinoma around dental implants." Only cases with definitive microscopic diagnosis of OSCC arising in the soft tissue around one or more dental implants were included. The literature review revealed 43 cases of patients with OSCC around dental implants in the 19 published manuscripts [4–22]. All clinical and epidemiological information about the sample is summarized in the **Table 1**.

The age of patients with oral cancer around dental implants ranged from 61 to 75 years old. There was a predominance of females (24 cases - 57.14%) when compared to males (18 cases - 42.86%). The typical clinical appearance of oral cancer around dental implants was an exophytic mass (20 tumors—47.62%) with few cases presenting as ulcer (4 tumors—9.52%). The bone osteolysis was frequently observed in the area of tumor causing the implant loss in some patients. The tumors affected mainly mandible (38 cases—90.47%) of the patients with multiples osseointegrated implants. Of note, oral cancer around dental implants is frequently clinically mistaken as peri-implantitis (**Table 1**).

Although peri-implantitis is the most common local risk factor for dental implant failure, the development of oral cancer involving the soft tissue around the titanium also impact the quality of life of the patient negatively. The oral cancer can manifest as hypertrophy, erythema, and/or ulcerative lesion of the soft tissue, and these features are similar to inflammatory peri-implant diseases such as peri-implantitis and/or peri-implant mucositis, as described by others [7, 10, 11]. Furthermore, these inflammatory peri-implant diseases frequently present the same epidemiological pattern and risk factors for oral cancer, that is, patients older than 60 years old and

Author	Gender/age	Cancer site	Lesion	Risk factors*	Prev. Rep. CA	Primary diagnosis
Block et al. 2001 [4]	M/72	Mandible	Mimicked PI	Yes	Yes	PI
Shaw et al. 2004 [5]	M/67	Mandible	Exophytic mass	NA	Yes	PI
	F/69	Mandible	Mimicked PI	NA	Yes	NA
Czerninski et al. [15]	F/52	Mandible	Mimicked PI	Yes	No	PI
	M/80	Mandible	Mimicked PI	No	Yes	PI
Abu El Naaj [16]	F/70	Mandible	Exophytic white	No	Yes	NA
Schache el al. [17]	F/77	Mandible	Exophytic mass	No	No	NA
Gallego et al. [18]	F/81	Mandible	PI mass	No	Yes	OL
Kwok et al. [19]	M/71	Mandible	"Inflammatory process"	Yes	No	PI
	F/67	Mandible	Exophytic mass	Yes	Yes	NA
	M/62	Mandible	Non-healing ulcer	Yes	No	Na
De Ceulaer et al. [20]	F/77	Mandible	Mimicked PI	Yes	Yes	PI
	M/71	Mandible	Swelling	Yes	Yes	PI
	F/62	Mandible	Mimicked PI	Yes	Yes	PI
Meijer et al. [21]	F/69	Mandible	Exophytic mass	No	Yes	PI
Orhan et al. [22]	F/69	Mandible	Numb chin syndrome, with mixed RO-RL lesion	NA	Yes	NA
Pfammatter et al. [6]	F/55	Mandible	mimicked PI, numbness	Na	Yes	Metastasis
Moergel et al. [7]	F/63	Mandible	Exophytic mass	No	Yes	NA
	F/70	Mandible	Exophytic mass	Yes	Yes	NA
	M/72	Mandible	Exophytic mass	No	Yes	NA
	M/57	Mandible	mimicked PI	Yes	Yes	PI
	M/72	Mandible	Exophytic mass	NA	No	NA
	F/54	Mandible	Exophytic mass	No	NA	NA
	M/47	Mandible	Ulcer	Yes	No	NA
	M/88	Mandible	Ulcer	No	No	NA
	F/42	Mandible	Ulcer	NA	Yes	NA
	F/59	Mandible	Ulcer	NA	Yes	NA
	M/73	Maxilla	Exophytic mass	Yes	Yes	NA
	M/77	Mandible	Exophytic mass	Yes	No	NA
	F/68	Mandible	Exophytic mass	Yes	Yes	NA
	F/69	Mandible	Exophytic mass	No	Yes	NA
Marini et al. [8]	F/51	Mandible	Exophytic mass	No	No	PI
Bhandari et al. [9]	F/71	Maxilla	Erythematous	No	No	PI
Chainani-Wu et al. [10]	F/60	Maxilla	Fistula	No	No	PI

Author	Gender/age	Cancer site	Lesion	Risk factors*	Prev. Rep. CA	Primary diagnosis
Vadim Raiser et al. [11]	F/55	Maxilla	White Exophytic mass	NA	NA	OL
	F/70	Mandible	Erythematous mass	NA	NA	NA
Noguchi et al. [12]	F/65	Mandible	gingival swelling	Yes	NA	Neoplasia
Malthiéry et al. [13]	M/77	Mandible	Mimicked PI	NA	No	PI
Granados et al. [14]	M/83	Mandible	Ulcerous lesion	NA	Yes	NA
	M/60	Mandible	Verrucous lesion	NA	NA	NA
	F/54	Mandible	"Gum lesion"	NA	NA	NA
	M/64	Mandible	Excrescent lesion	NA	NA	NA

*M = Male; F = Female; Pre.Rep.CA = Previously reported cancer; PI = Peri-implantitis; OL = Oral lichen planus; NA = Not available. * Patients who smokers and/or drinkers were considered.*

Table 1.
Demographic and clinical features of patients diagnosed with oral squamous cell carcinoma around dental implants.

chronic tobacco and/or alcohol consumers [1]. Although there are protocols for peri-implantitis treatment, frequently, the peri-implant tissue removed during this surgical treatment is not submitted for histopathological analysis [23, 24]. Then, the number of reported cases of peri-implant malignancy seems to be low in mouth but it may be being underreported by health professionals [24]. Recently, in a study of 111 biopsies of peri-implant lesions, 3.6% of those had histopathological diagnosis of oral squamous cell carcinomas [3]. Another investigation demonstrated that 2.9% of 68 dental implant-related lesions were oral squamous cells carcinomas [25].

Figure 1 illustrates a case report of an edentulous 64-year-old woman. She had an exophytic mass associated with ulcerated area and covered by a yellowish membrane in the anterior region of the mandible. The lesion was surrounded multiple osseointegrated implants (**Figure 1A**). She did not report adverse habits, for example, tobacco or alcohol consumption. Periapical radiographic exhibited an ill-defined bone destruction underneath the area of the lesion (**Figure 1B**). The histopathological analysis exhibited keratinizing well-differentiated epithelial neoplastic cells, some undergoing atypical mitosis, and invading the subjacent fibrous connective tissue (**Figure 1C**). The diagnosis of oral cancer was confirmed.

The early diagnosis of malignant tumors around dental implants is challenging because incipient lesions may resemble inflammatory peri-implant lesions [1, 2, 4–7, 10, 12, 15–18, 21]. In the **Table 1**, 14 out of 43 cases of oral cancer surrounding dental implants (33.33%) had the primary diagnosis of peri-implant lesions. Therefore, this clinical misinterpretation might delay the diagnosis of oral cancer facilitating its dissemination and resulting in a worst prognosis of the disease. These facts underscore how critical is the histological exam of every lesion around dental implants surgically removed. Furthermore, the peri-implant lesion that does not present the classical features of an inflammatory condition and that does not respond to conventional treatment, particularly if the patient has risk factor for oral cancer, should be submitted to the biopsy and histopathological analysis [23–25].

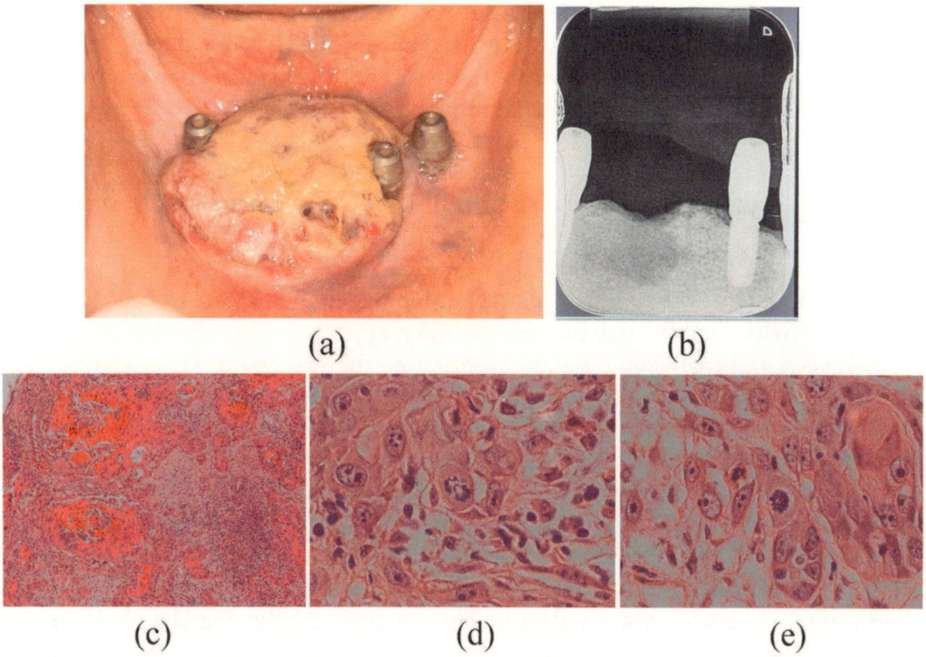

Figure 1.
Clinical and microscopic findings of oral squamous cell carcinoma around dental implants. a) Exophytic ulcer covered by necrotic tissue at the anterior-inferior alveolar ridge.b) Periapical radiograph showing an ill-defined bone loss in the peri-implant region. c) Neoplastic squamous epithelium-infiltrating subjacent submucosa with corneal pearls and discrete pleomorphism. d and e) epithelial cells with atypical mitotic figures infiltrating the tissue.

3. Risk factors for oral cancer around dental implants

The etiology of oral cancer is multifactorial. OSCC is the most prevalent oral malignant tumor and it is associated with lifestyle risk factors such as alcohol consumption and smoking [26]. Curiously, tobacco smoking is also the predictor of dental implants failure and more smokers have post-operative infections and peri-implant crestal bone loss than nonsmokers [27, 28]. Although the information about lifestyle-related factors that predispose to oral cancer was incomplete in most of cases included in the **Table 1**, 34.88% of patients diagnosed with squamous cell carcinoma around dental implants were smokers and/or drinkers. These overlapping risk factors may drive the clinician to attribute the onset of an atypical lesion involving dental implants to a deficient or anomalous immune response of a patient who consumes tobacco and/or alcohol. However, it is essential that the clinicians are aware that the classic signs of inflammation persist in such patients and that these features are useful to distinguish a benign from a malignant lesion. Additionally, the histopathological analysis remains as the gold standard for the diagnosis of lesions located in the oral cavity [23].

A well-defined concept is that patients with previous history of cancer have higher risk of developing other tumors. Twenty-three (54.76%) of all cases of squamous cell carcinoma around dental implants arose in patients with history of cancer. Interestingly, we observed that 19 (82.60%) patients had OSCC previously. Furthermore, other patients had lung [6, 15], intestine [15], thyroid [17], and breast [17, 22] cancer previously. As the development of OSCC has been also associated with genomic instability and genetic predisposition [1], one can hypothesize that a patient who had a malignant lesion are more susceptible to local aggressions such as the contact of the soft tissue with dental implant materials.

4. Carcinogenic mechanisms associated with osseointegrated dental implants

Titanium is one of the most common components in implants alloys used in dental and medical fields [1, 29]. High biocompatibility, appropriate mechanical properties, inertness, and corrosion resistance are among the main advantages of titanium [25, 29, 30]. When the titanium implant is installed in extra oral sites, where it is protected from the contact with the environment, it has inert behavior. On the other hand, dental implants are continuously exposed to the oral cavity hostile conditions [31]. The area between the implants and the abutment or the prosthetic crown is particularly susceptible to the bacterial biofilm accumulation, saliva, pH and temperature changes, and functional micromotion (**Figure 2**) [31].

When the dental implant surface is exposed to any source of oxygen or nitrogen, a chemical reaction takes place and a thin layer of titanium dioxide (TiO_2) is formed and deposited in the outer surface of the implants. This layer is extremely resistant to corrosion. However the chemical agents of the oral cavity can reduce the protection of the dioxide deposit and induce the corrosion development [31]. Saliva and other chemicals introduced into the oral cavity through feeding or in contact with bacterial biofilms influence the gradual biodegradation of metallic structures including the titanium used in dental implants [29]. Furthermore, acidic solution combined with mechanical friction strength potentiates the damages to the implants surfaces. Interestingly, some studies with cytology have demonstrated the presence of titanium

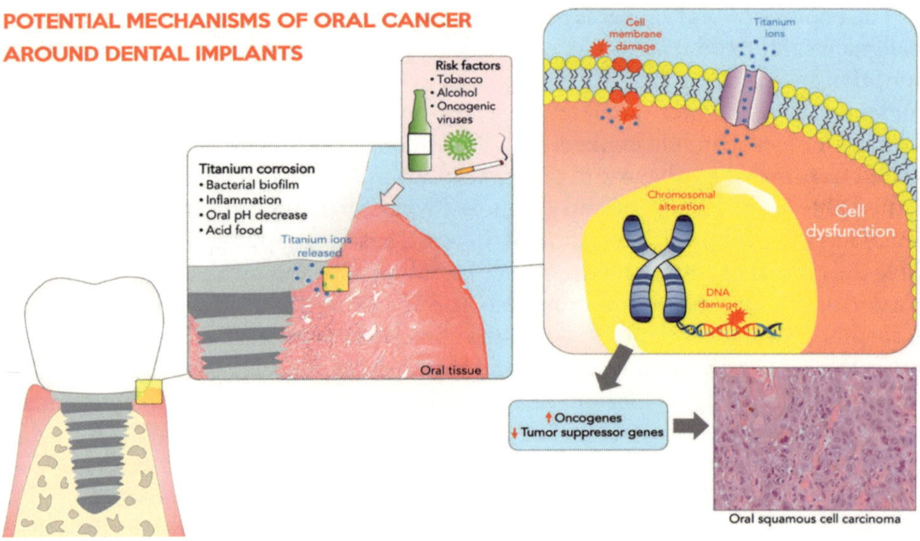

Figure 2.
Illustration of potential risk factors and mechanisms on the development of squamous cell carcinoma around dental implants.

particles in the peri-implant tissues [23, 25] regardless of the presence of peri-implantitis or peri-implant mucositis. It has been suggested that this material accumulation may be the result of the corrosive process of the dental implants [29, 30, 32], implant-abutment friction at the installation of the implants, and/or implantoplasty [29, 31, 33, 34]. The degree of titanium corrosion can be influenced by quality and quantity of saliva, diet, alloy polishing, genetics, oral hygiene, amount and distribution of the occlusal forces, and microbiota [29, 30, 32].

The above data show that titanium is not entirely bioinert as suggested years ago. Then, even with their good biological properties, titanium alloys are susceptible to corrosion attack with release of metal ions to the surrounding hard and soft oral tissues, lymph nodes, peripheral, and even distant organs [30]. Consequently, titanium ions have been implicated in the development of oral cancer around dental implants [1, 34].

As stated previously, the relationship between titanium dental implants and oral cancer has been suggested based on the increasing number of tumors arising in the peri-implant tissue. However, as far as we know, there is not any study dedicated to unveil the potential carcinogenic mechanisms triggered by titanium ions.

Titanium particles have been shown to induce the expression of breast cancer gene 1 (BRCA1) and checkpoint kinase 2 (CHK2) in epithelial cells *in vitro* [35]. These proteins are markers of DNA damage response. Additionally, titanium also triggered the generation of reactive oxygen species (ROS) [36, 37]. The chronic exposure of the epithelial cells to aggressive factors may increase the probability of mutations that might not be detected by the immune system. Indeed, the chronic inflammatory response seems to be also modulated by titanium, especially when there is accumulation of bacterial biofilm. Higher amounts of titanium ions in peri-implant soft tissue with inflammatory process are observed when compared to healthy tissues [25, 38]. Accordingly, titanium nanoparticles induced stronger pro-inflammatory response in macrophages regardless of the association with lipopolysaccharide from *Porphyromonas gingivalis* [39] and by increasing the secretion of interleukin (IL)-6, IL-1β, and tumor necrosis factor-alpha (TNF-α) by macrophages *in vitro* [38, 40]. Taken together, all these disturbances in the peri-implant microenvinoment may persist for years and, gradually, predispose the epithelial cells to sequential mutations until the malignant state is reached.

In 2006, the International Agency for Research on Cancer (IARC) classified the titanium dioxide as a possible carcinogen for humans [41]. However, in view of the few case reports of oral cancer around dental implants the authors were unable to exclude the existence of other confounding carcinogens as tobacco and/or alcohol [1, 7, 19].

5. Conclusion

The literature review showed that most cases of OSCC around dental implants had initial clinical features compatible with peri-implantitis. Therefore, this clinical misinterpretation of an inflammatory process in peri-implant mucosa may delay the diagnosis of oral cancer facilitating the local progression and dissemination of cancer cells, resulting in worst patient's prognosis. Thus, the peri-implant lesion not responding to conventional anti-inflammatory treatment, particularly if the patient has risk factor for oral cancer, should be submitted to the biopsy and histopathological analysis, avoiding delay in the diagnosis of the tumor.

Acknowledgements

This study was supported by the Coordenação de Aperfeiçoamento de Pessoal de Nível Superior—Brasil (CAPES)—Finance Code (#001). We also thank Dr. Marcelo Júnior Zanda for providing the clinical images.

Conflict of interest

The authors declare they do not have conflict of interest.

Author details

Gabriela Lopes dos Santos[1], Kaique Preto Alberto[1],
Silas Antonio Juvêncio de Freitas Filho[1], Kellen Cristine Tjioe[2]
and Denise Tostes Oliveira[1*]

1 Department of Surgery, Stomatology, Pathology and Radiology, Area of Pathology, Bauru School of Dentistry, University of São Paulo, Bauru, Brazil

2 Department of Surgery, Stomatology, Pathology and Radiology, Area of Stomatology, Bauru School of Dentistry, University of São Paulo, Bauru, Brazil

*Address all correspondence to: denisetostes@usp.br

References

[1] Ramos JC, dos Santos ES, Normando AGC, Alves FA, Kowalski LP, Santos-Silva AR, et al. Oral squamous cell carcinoma around dental implants: a systematic review. Oral Surgery, Oral Medicine, Oral Pathology, Oral Radiology. 2021;**131**(6):660-674. DOI: 10.1016/j.oooo.2021.01.019

[2] Moraschini V, Poubel LA da C, Ferreira VF, Barboza E dos SP. Evaluation of survival and success rates of dental implants reported in longitudinal studies with a follow-up period of at least 10 years: a systematic review. International Journal of Oral and Maxillofacial Surgery 2015;**44**:377-388. DOI:10.1016/J.IJOM.2014.10.023

[3] Sotorra-Figuerola D, Lafuente-Ibáñez de Mendoza I, Parra-Pérez C, Aguirre-Urizar JM. Histopathological analysis of biopsies of "peri-implant inflammatory lesions." Everything is not what it seems. Clinical Implant Dentistry and Related Research. 2020; **22**:366-372. DOI: 10.1111/cid.12905

[4] Block MS, Scheufler E. Squamous cell carcinoma appearing as peri-implant bone loss: A case report. Journal of Oral and Maxillofacial Surgery. 2001;**59**:1349-1352. DOI: 10.1053/JOMS.2001.27532

[5] Shaw R, Sutton D, Brown J, Cawood J. Further malignancy in field change adjacent to osseointegrated implants. International Journal of Oral and Maxillofacial Surgery. 2004;**33**:353-355. DOI: 10.1016/J.IJOM.2003.09.017

[6] Pfmmatter C, Lindermuller IH, Lugli A, Filippi A, Kuhl S. Metastases and primary tumors around dental implants: a literature review and case report of peri-implant pulmonary metastasis. Quintessence Int (Berl). 2012;**43**:563-670. DOI: 10.1016/J.STOMAX.2007.04.004

[7] Moergel M, Karbach J, Kunkel M, Wagner W. Oral squamous cell carcinoma in the vicinity of dental implants. Clinical Oral Investigations. 2014;**18**:277-284. DOI: 10.1007/s00784-013-0968-5

[8] Marini E, Spink MJ, Messina AM. Peri-implant primary squamous cell carcinoma: A case report with 5 years' follow-up. Journal of Oral and Maxillofacial Surgery. 2013;**71**:322-326. DOI: 10.1016/j.joms.2012.06.184

[9] Bhandari S, Rattan V, Panda N, Vaiphei K, Mittal BR. Oral cancer or periimplantitis: A clinical dilemma. The Journal of Prosthetic Dentistry. 2016; **115**:658-661. DOI: 10.1016/j.prosdent.2015.10.022

[10] Chainani-Wu N, Chang C, Sim C, Wu TC, Cox D, Sirjani D, et al. Oral Squamous Cell Carcinoma Mimicking Peri-Implantitis. Clin Adv Periodontics. 2016;**6**:83-88. DOI: 10.1902/cap.2015.150041

[11] Raiser V, Abu-El Naaj I, Shlomi B, Fliss DM, Kaplan I. Primary Oral Malignancy Imitating Peri-Implantitis. Journal of Oral and Maxillofacial Surgery. 2016;**74**:1383-1390. DOI: 10.1016/j.joms.2016.02.008

[12] Noguchi M, Tsuno H, Ishizaka R, Fujiwara K, Imaue S, Tomihara K, et al. Primary peri-implant oral intra-epithelial neoplasia/carcinoma in situ: a case report considering risk factors for carcinogenesis. Int. J Implant Dent. 2017;**3**:1-5. DOI: 10.1186/s40729-017-0109-z

[13] Malthiéry E, De Boutray M, Koren C, Albouy JP, Torres JH, Fauroux MA. Squamous cell carcinoma around a dental implant: A case report and literature review. Oral Oncology. 2019;**91**:134-136. DOI: 10.1016/j.oraloncology.2019.02.005

[14] Granados F, Santos-Ruiz L, Contreras M, Mellado J, Martin G, Bermudo L, et al. Squamous cell carcinoma related with dental implants. A clinical cases report. Journal of Clinical and Experimental Dentistry. 2020;**12**:e98-e102. DOI: 10.4317/jced.55964

[15] Czerninski R, Kaplan I, Almoznino G, Maly A, Regev E. Oral squamous cell carcinoma around dental implants. Quintessence Int (Berl). 2006;**37**:707-711. DOI: 10.3390/MEDICINA56020053

[16] Abu El-Naaj I, Trost O, Tagger-Green N, Trouilloud N, Robe N, Malka G, et al. Peri-implantitis or squamous cell carcinoma? Revue de Stomatologie et de Chirurgie Maxillo-Faciale. 2007;**108**: 458-460. DOI: 10.1016/J.STOMAX.2007.04.004

[17] Schache A, Thavaraj S, Kalavrezos N. Osseointegrated Implants: A Potential Route of Entry for Squamous Cell Carcinoma of the Mandible. The British Journal of Oral & Maxillofacial Surgery. 2008;**46**:397-399. DOI: 10.1016/j.bjoms.2007.09.009

[18] Gallego L, Junquera L, Baladrón J, Villarreal P. Oral Squamous Cell Carcinoma Associated With Symphyseal Dental Implants: An Unusual Case Report. Journal of the American Dental Association (1939). 2008;**139**:1061-1065. DOI: 10.14219/JADA.ARCHIVE.2008.0308

[19] Kwok J, Eyeson J, Thompson I, McGurk M. Dental implants and squamous cell carcinoma in the at risk patient – report of three cases. British Dental Journal. 2008;**205**:543-545. DOI: 10.1038/sj.bdj.2008.980

[20] De Ceulaer J, Magremanne M, Scheerlinck J. Squamous cell carcinoma recurrence around dental implants. Journal of Oral and Maxillofacial Surgery. 2010;**68**:2507-2512. DOI: 10.1016/J.JOMS.2010.01.023

[21] Meijer GJ, Dieleman FJ, Bergé SJ, Merkx MA. Removal of an oral squamous cell carcinoma including parts of osseointegrated implants in the marginal mandibulectomy. A case report. Oral Maxillofac Surg. 2010;**14**:253-256. DOI: 10.1007/S10006-010-0208-Y

[22] Orhan K, Bayndr H, Aksoy S, Seker BK, Berberoğlu A, Ozan O. Numb chin syndrome as a manifestation of possible breast cancer metastasis around dental implants. The Journal of Craniofacial Surgery. 2011;**22**:942-945. DOI: 10.1097/SCS.0B013E31820FE1AF

[23] Sotorra-Figuerola D, Lafuente-Ibáñez de Mendoza I, Parra-Pérez C, Aguirre-Urizar JM. Histopathological analysis of biopsies of "peri-implant inflammatory lesions." Everything is not what it seems. Clinical Implant Dentistry and Related Research. 2020; **22**:366-372. DOI: 10.1111/cid.12905

[24] Kaplan I, Zeevi I, Tal H, Rosenfeld E, Chaushu G. Clinicopathologic evaluation of malignancy adjacent to dental implants. Oral Surgery, Oral Medicine, Oral Pathology, Oral Radiology. 2017; **123**:103-112. DOI: 10.1016/j.oooo.2016.08.023

[25] Paparella ML, Domingo MG, Puia SA, Jacobi-Gresser E, Olmedo DG. Titanium dental implant-related pathologies: A retrospective histopathological study. Oral Diseases. 2021 [In press]. DOI: 10.1111/ODI.13794

[26] Capote-Moreno A, Brabyn P, Muñoz-Guerra MF, Sastre-Pérez J, Escorial-Hernandez V, Rodríguez-Campo FJ, et al. Oral squamous cell carcinoma: Epidemiological study and risk factor assessment based on a 39-year series. International Journal of Oral and Maxillofacial Surgery. 2020;**49**:1525-1534. DOI: 10.1016/j.ijom.2020.03.009

[27] Berglundh T, Armitage G, Araujo MG, Avila-Ortiz G, Blanco J, Camargo PM, et al. Peri-implant diseases and conditions: Consensus report of workgroup 4 of the 2017 World Workshop on the Classification of Periodontal and Peri-Implant Diseases and Conditions. Journal of Clinical Periodontology., vol. 45, Blackwell Munksgaard; 2018, pp. S286–S291. DOI:10.1111/jcpe.12957.

[28] Javed F, Rahman I, Romanos GE. Tobacco-product usage as a risk factor for dental implants. Periodontology 2000. 2000;**2019**(81):48-56. DOI: 10.1111/prd.12282

[29] Mombelli A, Hashim D, Cionca N. What is the impact of titanium particles and biocorrosion on implant survival and complications? A critical review. Clinical Oral Implants Research. 2018;**29**:37-53. DOI: 10.1111/clr.13305

[30] Noumbissi S, Scarano A, Gupta S. A literature review study on atomic ions dissolution of titanium and its alloys in implant dentistry. Materials (Basel). 2019;**12**:1-15. DOI: 10.3390/MA12030368

[31] Rucha Shah S, Deepika Shree Lakshmi P, Raison T, Dhoom SM. Titanium Corrosion: Implications For Dental Implants. The European Journal of Prosthodontics and Restorative Dentistry. 2016;**24**:171-180. DOI: 10.1922/EJPRD_1531SHAH10

[32] Dias Corpa Tardelli J, da Costa L, Valente M, Theodoro de Oliveira T, Cândido dos Reis A. Influence of chemical composition on cell viability on titanium surfaces: A systematic review. The Journal of Prosthetic Dentistry. 2021;**125**:421-425. DOI: 10.1016/J.PROSDENT.2020.02.001

[33] Oliveira M, Schunemann W, Mathew M, Henriques B, Magini R, Teughels W, et al. Can degradation products released from dental implants affect peri-implant tissues? Journal of Periodontal Research. 2018;**53**:1-11. DOI: 10.1111/JRE.12479

[34] del AFS-L, Garaicoa-Pazmiño C, Fretwurst T, Castilho RM, Squarize CH. Dental implants-associated release of titanium particles: A systematic review. Clinical Oral Implants Research. 2018;**29**: 1085-1100. DOI: 10.1111/CLR.13372

[35] Suárez-López del Amo F, Rudek I, Wagner V, Martins M, O'Valle F, Galindo-Moreno P, et al. Titanium activates the DNA damage response pathway in oral epithelial cells: A pilot study. The International Journal of Oral & Maxillofacial Implants. 2017;**32**:1413-1420. DOI: 10.11607/JOMI.6077

[36] Bressan E, Ferroni L, Gardin C, Bellin G, Sbricoli L, Sivolella S, et al. Metal nanoparticles released from dental implant surfaces: Potential contribution to chronic inflammation and peri-implant bone loss. Maternité. 2019;**12**:2036. DOI: 10.3390/MA12122036

[37] Yang F, Tang J, Dai K, Huang Y. Metallic wear debris collected from patients induces apoptosis in rat primary osteoblasts via reactive oxygen species-mediated mitochondrial dysfunction and endoplasmic reticulum stress. Molecular Medicine Reports. 2019;**19**:1629-1637. DOI: 10.3892/MMR.2019.9825

[38] Messous R, Henriques B, Bousbaa H, Silva FS, Teughels W, Souza JCM.

Cytotoxic effects of submicron- and nano-scale titanium debris released from dental implants: an integrative review. Clinical Oral Investigations. 2021;**25**:1627-1640. DOI: 10.1007/S00784-021-03785-Z

[39] Dodo CG, Meirelles L, Aviles-Reyes A, Ruiz KGS, Abranches J, Cury AADB. Pro-inflammatory Analysis of Macrophages in Contact with Titanium Particles and Porphyromonas gingivalis. Brazilian Dental Journal. 2017;**28**:428-434. DOI: 10.1590/0103-6440201701382

[40] Vallés G, González-Melendi P, Saldaña L, Rodriguez M, Munuera L, Vilaboa N. Rutile and titanium particles differentially affect the production of osteoblastic local factors. Journal of Biomedial Materials Research Part A. 2008;**84A**:324-336. DOI: 10.1002/JBM.A.31315

[41] International Agency for Research on Cancer. Carbon Black, Titanium Dioxide, and Talc. IARC Monographs on the Evaluation of Carcinogenic Risks to Humans; 2006:93.

Chapter 7

Variability of Saliva Viscosity - Potential Impact

Lara Eltze, Maren Eltze and Antonio Garcia

Abstract

As novel COVID-19 testing develops, saliva has become of increasing interest as an alternate biological sample for rapid testing. The appeal in saliva-based testing lies within the ease of which samples are collected, as well as patient comfort throughout the collection process. With this, it has become increasingly important to delineate the characteristics of saliva viscosity due to its effects on the movement and interactions of the substances and molecules found within it. The characteristics that affect saliva viscosity include the presence of aggregates, variations in temperature, and time elapsed between sample collection and testing. Understanding how physicochemical properties and temperature affect saliva's viscosity are important in generating guidelines for proper sample handling in saliva testing to ensure consistent and reliable results. In this study, passive sampling of saliva was analyzed. This type of collection ensures a more uniform saliva composition, suggesting that variations in viscosity can be attributed solely to modifications in saliva handling post-collection. The data suggested that saliva viscosity is greatest immediately following collection of the saliva sample, increases with higher quantities of aggregates in saliva, and decreases tremendously when the sample has been frozen and thawed to room temperature. These findings suggest that to ensure accuracy and uniformity in quantitative saliva-based test results, protocols should favor the testing of a sample immediately following its collection. The implications of these results in optimizing saliva testing are far reaching. The value of saliva based testing extends far beyond COVID-19 or other disease testing. It is also gaining utility in understanding daily fluctuations in hydration state and in other wellness applications.

Keywords: saliva, viscosity, point-of-care, diagnostics, Cannon-Fenske, viscometer

1. Introduction

As novel COVID-19 testing develops, saliva has become of increasing interest as an alternate biological sample for rapid testing [1]. The appeal in saliva-based testing lies within the ease of which samples are collected, as well as patient comfort throughout the collection process [2]. Yacoubian Jr., Wish, and Perez (2001) found that the benefits in the ease of saliva collection were multifaceted. These benefits include the uncomplicated nature of collection, which, coupled with a low risk of direct contact and contamination, makes salivary diagnostics an attractive alternative to biological sample collection where contamination may be more challenging to avoid, such as with blood or urine analyses. For these reasons, saliva-based testing has become an increasingly popular choice in the creation of novel forms of diagnostic testing. With this, it has become increasingly important to delineate the characteristics of saliva viscosity due to its effects on the movement and interactions of the substances and molecules found within it. In the context of this study, viscosity refers to internal friction of a fluid, which is marked by the resistance of a fluid to flow [3].

While viscosity can affect the interactions and molecules within saliva is important to note in developing diagnostic tests, salivary viscosity itself can also be seen as an important factor in maintaining oral and overall health. A study by Katsuhiro Kitada and Takahiko Oho (2011) found that an increase in saliva viscosity decreases the bacterial co-aggregation between *Streptococcus oralis* and *Actinomyces naeslundii* [4]. Under normal circumstances, co-aggregation can prevent bacterial infection in the oral cavity, as co-aggregated bacteria may be swallowed before forming attachments within the oral cavity. The study indicated that increasing saliva viscosity decreased formation of these co-aggregated bacteria, which may allow for further health problems, such as pneumonia or other infections that may be brought on by the aspiration of oral bacteria or microorganisms [4]. The demonstrated health implications surrounding salivary viscosity further suggests the importance of developing protocols to accurately measure salivary viscosity following saliva collection.

The characteristics of salivary viscosity, namely the presence of aggregates, variations in temperature, sample handling, and time elapsed between sample collection and testing, serve as points of interest in the creation of laboratory protocols for salivary-based rapid diagnostic testing. Understanding how external factors affect saliva viscosity are important in generating guidelines for proper sample handling in saliva testing to ensure consistent and reliable results.

Multiple studies demonstrated in the literature reflect the variability of saliva viscosity. The 1998 Rantonen and Meurman study concluded that salivary viscosity can be dependent on the method of its production. Particularly, whether secreted by the submandibular, sublingual, or palatal glands [5]. Although the study demonstrated that the quantity of mucin within each saliva sample of differing origin did not change, the species of mucin did. Particularly, it was demonstrated that the saliva stemming from the sublingual glands demonstrated more elasticity than those of the submandibular and palatal glands, which would affect the viscosity of the saliva. In addition, the 2016 study by Antoon Ligtenberg, Erwin Liem, Henk Brand, and Enno Veerman found that acute exercise correlated with a significant increase of saliva viscosity when collected shortly thereafter [6]. These findings were parallel with the Rodica Murineanu, Corina Stefanescu, Agripina Zaharia, Carolina Davidescu, and Sorin Popsor (2011) study that found medication, general illness, and acrylic dentures to all correlate with a change in saliva viscosity [7]. This study suggested medication and disease state may affect saliva viscosity. For example, complete acrylic dentures were specifically found to correlate with an increase in salivary viscosity. It is also interesting to note the apparent correlation between salivary viscosity and dental cavities. A 2014 study by Animireddy et al found that in a sample of 75 school children, the cavity-free children had on average higher salivary viscosity than their counterparts [8]. These findings delineate some of the known variability to saliva viscosity discussed in the literature, which further demonstrate the necessity of qualifying the properties and behavior of saliva viscosity.

Beyond the variability of salivary viscosity, the level of normal viscosity is very different from that of other commonly used human biofluids in diagnostic testing. This is an important factor to note in the development of such tests, especially when considering technologies previously developed for other biofluids. The viscosity of normal cerebrospinal fluid, for example, is remarkably close to that of water, which is 1.00 cSt at 20°C [9, 10] Similarly, the kinematic viscosity of urine is 1.07 cSt at the same temperature [11]. These examples are lower than the kinematic viscosity of normal blood, which is around 3.65 cSt at 21.2°C [12]. While there is variability within the viscosities of these human biofluids, they are far lower than what we expect of human saliva, an important challenge to overcome in developing diagnostic testing.

Due to the interest in point-of-care saliva-based diagnostic testing, and based on the current literature demonstrating potential variabilities in saliva viscosity and associated causes, it is rather surprising that the literature on salivary viscosity characterization for protocol creation is rather sparse. This study hopes to address some of the gaps in the literature pertaining to salivary properties by exploring how viscosity changes upon freezing and subsequent thawing, and how it changes over time with consecutive trials, using the Cannon-Fenske experimental protocol, with the goal of aiding in the development of laboratory protocols pertaining to salivary-based diagnostic testing.

Based on the previous literature at hand, the research questions of this study are as follows:

How does the viscosity of collected saliva change over time with subsequent trials? How does the viscosity of collected saliva change after freezing and subsequent thawing?

2. Application of research

In the absence of detailed information in the research literature, this study seeks to better understand the specific properties of saliva viscosity, and how saliva viscosity reacted to factors that are integral in the creation of lab protocols; specifically, how the samples are stored. It is not uncommon for biological samples to be frozen or cooled, and this makes sense with respect to slowing down bacterial contamination and maintaining biological molecules of interest. It is well understood that many human proteins, enzymes, vitamins, degrade over time [9] and that the degradation over time can be diminished by freezing or cooling samples beyond given temperature degradation thresholds, to allow for long-term storage.

Changes within the aggregates commonly found in human saliva, such as mucins, may also be affected by temperature and shear forces. Enzymes, such as salivary alpha-amylase, and hormones, such as cortisol, will degrade over time unless this process is inhibited, typically by freezing samples to −20 degrees Celsius, or below [10]. However, it is important to determine the effects of sub zero temperatures on viscosity itself, as the viscosity of the saliva may be impactful in how the aggregates are measured via point-of-care salivary biosensors. This was reflected in the 2013 Robles et al. study which found that the most consistent and reliable salivary alpha-amylase biosensor data was obtained from frozen and centrifuged passive saliva samples, rather than samples that were collected as fresh, passive, drool [11]. The authors hypothesize this discrepancy to be due to various factors of the saliva itself (such as mucin molecules), which may interfere with the device in question by preventing close binding to the sensor surface, as it attempts to detect quantities of salivary alpha-amylase. Also, this hypothesis reflects the prediction that salivary viscosity is an important factor in molecular measurements. While the aggregation effect was disadvantageous when in reference to the assessing quantities of the enzyme salivary alpha-amylase, it may actually be preferable when measuring quantities of different gases within saliva samples. This further delineates the importance of taking a closer look at physical salivary properties, in order to approach proposed handling methodologies appropriately, depending on the given purpose of the saliva sampling.

3. Protocols

As previously mentioned, we hoped to better understand the properties of saliva viscosity in regards to different methodologies in sample preservation or usage. For this reason, two cycles of laboratory trials were conducted, with the aim of determining how saliva viscosity was affected. The first study aim is to determine how time alone affects saliva samples. The second trial aims at determining whether freezing and subsequent thawing affect the viscosity of the sample, as well. Both phases of data collection were done at a Biomedical Engineering laboratory, at Arizona State University, Tempe, and human saliva samples were collected within this department.

Participants were instructed to not eat within an hour of sample collection, and were then asked to drink approximately 100 mL of water immediately prior to saliva collection. This was to prevent short-term dehydration effects from confounding our variables. In addition, this aided in the ease of saliva collection. Participants were then asked to collect approximately 15 mL of passive saliva over a span of 25 minutes, into a plastic vial. The goal for saliva collection included diminishing the amount of air bubbles trapped within the saliva, by collecting the saliva very carefully, slowly, and with as little movement as possible. Foam-like saliva that is saturated with small air bubbles was not included in the overall 15 mL amount of passive saliva collected.

The viscosity of the collected saliva sample was measured using a Size 350 Cannon-Fenske apparatus, with a capillary radius of 0.045 cm, a shear rate of 2.08 1/s at 10cSt, and a viscometer constant of 0.5 cSt/s, which was cleaned and dried prior to commencing the viscosity protocol. The saliva sample was then poured into the apparatus, and allowed to flow through, while efflux time was measured concomitantly, indicating the time required for the meniscus of the viscous fluid to flow between the designated markings. This viscometer procedure was replicated 10 times consecutively for each collected sample, after which each sample was frozen and subsequently thawed the following day, at which point the viscometer procedure was performed again. A series of viscosity measurements of a 50% glycerol/water control solution was tested in the same manner to act as a control variable.

The kinematic viscosity of each trial was calculated using the efflux time and viscosity constant in the following relationship:

$$Kinematic\ Viscosity = (viscometer\ constant)\ x\ (efflux\ time\ (s)) \quad (1)$$

This procedure reflected the first half of the research questions, as to how saliva viscosity changes with time [12]. By comparing the time elapsed for the viscosity of human saliva with the glycerol/water solution, we are able to visualize how viscosity properties may be affected by the presence of the aggregates in unprocessed human saliva, which are not present in the glycerol/water mixture.

4. Results

Data was collected for each measurement of salivary viscosity. The initial graph (**Figure 1**) represents the methodology behind the first research question; how does

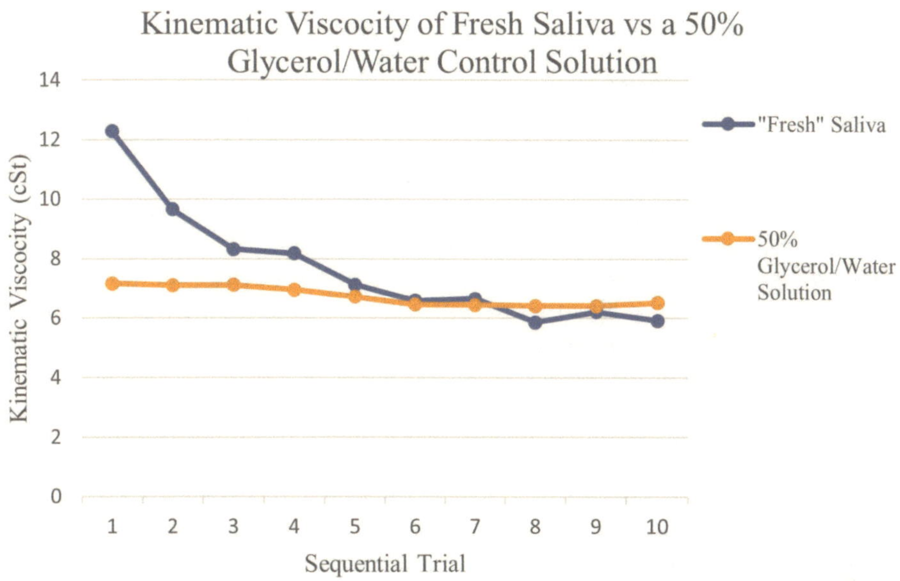

Figure 1.
This figure evaluates how salivary viscosity changes with time over subsequent trials following collection. This arbitrary time is demonstrated in sequential trials, as trials were completed one after the other following collection. This saliva kinematic viscosity is contrasted with that of a 50% glycerol water solution, acting as a control. In the passive saliva trials, we see a stark decrease in kinematic viscosity with each subsequent trial, however, the glycerol/water solution shows a slight variation within an expected range given the experimental apparatus and simple laboratory control of room temperature (22 C).

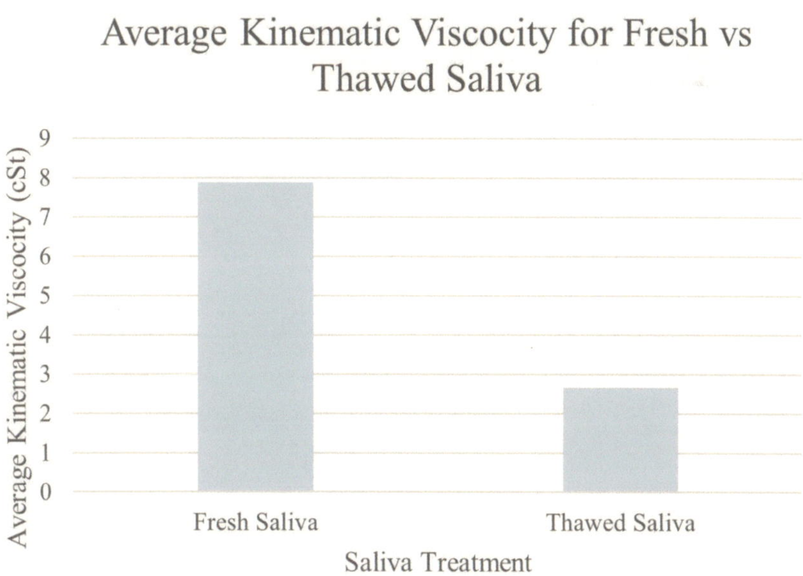

Figure 2.
This figure demonstrates the statistically significant discrepancy between fresh and thawed passive saliva samples at 22 C. each bar represents an average of 10 trials. One outlier was removed from the thawed trial group as it was handled outside the guidelines of the lab protocol.

salivary viscosity behave over time? **Figure 2** represents the viscosity of saliva (as average kinematic viscosity), with freshly collected samples of saliva, compared to with samples that were frozen, and subsequently, thawed for analysis.

5. Discussion

There are several points of interest with regards to the conclusions drawn from the experimental design that reflect the difference in how fresh saliva behaves, compared to fresh saliva, and compared to saliva that had been frozen and re-thawed. Such comparisons are reflected in the literature by the 2019 study by Johannsen et al. which found that salivary viscosity measurements varied depending on whether the saliva was untreated or subject to magnet-beating prior to viscosity measurements at low shear rates [13].

One aspect that is of interest is whether there is a methodology that can guide how fresh saliva can be processed in order to have a consistent flow property or ensure that the major aggregates, presumably due to entangled mucin chains, can be minimized quickly so that a rapid test can be performed (**Figure 3**).

Bansil et al. [14] provide a molecular interpretation on how the structure of mucin leads to entanglements among the biopolymers in solution and create a range of viscosity effects depending upon concentration and mucin type. They suggest that a dilute solution of mucin generally has viscoelastic behavior that depends upon shear rate. A more general approach to the viscosity behavior of biopolymer solutions is given by Picout and Ross-Murphy [15] who provide experimental verification of the Cross equation:

$$\eta = \eta_\infty + (\ \eta_o - \eta_\infty)/[1 + (\lambda^m \gamma^m)] \tag{2}$$

with lambda being a time constant and gamma the shear rate.

Comparing the Cross equation to the data shown in this study in **Figure 2** suggests that repeated shearing with a Cannon-Fenske viscometer is a cumulative effect, so one may conjecture the following modified forms of the Cross equation could explain the apparent viscosity change in saliva after repeated shearing due to the capillary flow within the viscometer.

$$\eta = \eta_\infty + (\ \eta_o - \eta_\infty)/\sum_{n=0}^{k}[1 + k\ (\lambda^m \gamma^m)] \tag{3}$$

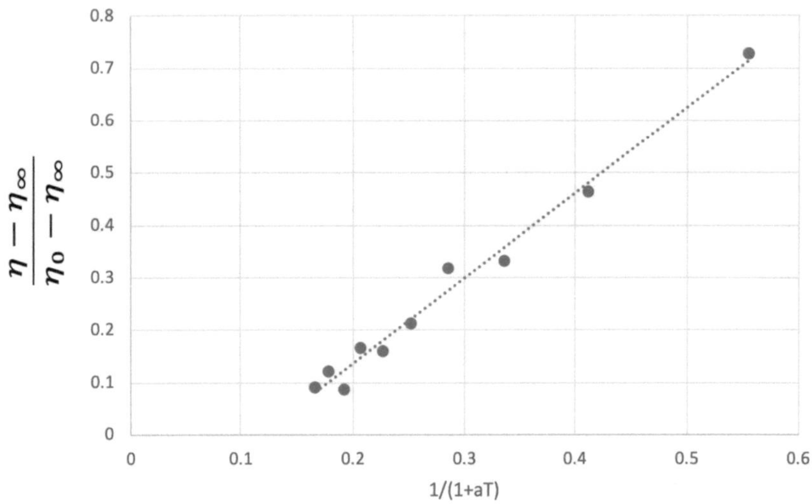

Figure 3.
This figure demonstrates the cross equation fit, using the limits of η_∞ and η_0. The independent variable is demonstrated to be $1/(1 + aT)$.

or

$$\eta = \eta_\infty + (\eta_o - \eta_\infty)/\{[1 + (\lambda^m \gamma^m)T]\} \quad (4)$$

where n is an integer and k is the number of repeat measurements in the first equation and T is the total elapsed time of shear for the combined repeat measurements. It is not as important to determine which equation may be better at predicting data than to understand how to use the concept to prepare saliva samples in a variety of ways rather than relying solely on freezing or centrifugation which can be cumbersome and time consuming.

The potential utility of these modified Cross equations is in determining a way to rapidly shear saliva samples using a simple microfluidic device or mixer, rather than subjecting the saliva to freezing or flowing the saliva through a longer tube to simulate the cumulative shear thinning shown in **Figure 2**. The shear rate experienced in the Cannon Fenske viscometer used for these experiments is on the order of 2 s^{-1}, so based on the **Figure 2** data of approximately a total time of 80 seconds of shearing is needed in order to reach a stable and minimum kinematic viscosity a device capable of deliver a shear rate of 200 s^{-1} which is well within the reach of portable and low cost homogenizers [16–19].

6. Conclusions

Salivary viscosity can be an important parameter to consider when designing diagnostic devices for rapid testing. Consideration should be given to the fact that not only is saliva viscoelastic, but its apparent viscosity can change by mild shearing over a period of time. Shearing at rates as low as 2 s^{-1} can decrease its kinematic viscosity by more than half, which could change some kinetics of enzyme action, sensor signal development, or diffusive transport. After approximately a total time of 80 seconds of shearing at 2 s^{-1} can lead to a stable and minimum kinematic viscosity. The concept of biopolymer viscosity behavior being modeled by the Cross equation suggests that a device capable of delivering shear rates of 200 s^{-1} and above may be able to modify the mucin superstructure sufficiently to provide saliva samples with consistent apparent viscosities. Microfluidic devices or low cost handheld homogenizers could very quickly deliver the needed shearing action in order to provide a more consistent saliva sample, in terms of its viscous properties.

Acknowledgements

The institutions involved in the findings for this paper are Arizona State University, Tempe, and New Mexico State University. The data was collected at a Arizona State University Biomedical Engineering laboratory in Tempe, Arizona. This project was done under the supervision of Professor Antonio A. Garcia, who is now Associate Dean of Engineering at New Mexico State University in Las Cruces, New Mexico.

Conflict of interest

The authors declare no conflict of interest.

Notes/Thanks/Other declarations

Special thanks to Professor Antonio A. Garcia, Associate Dean of Engineering at New Mexico State University. His mentorship is invaluable.

Author details

Lara Eltze[1*], Maren Eltze[1] and Antonio Garcia[2]

1 Arizona State University, Tempe, United States

2 New Mexico State University, Tempe, United States

*Address all correspondence to: leltze@asu.edu

IntechOpen

References

[1] Khurshid Z, Asiri FYI, Al Wadaani H. Human saliva: Non-invasive fluid for detecting novel coronavirus (2019-nCoV). International Journal of Environmental Research and Public Health. 2020;**17**(7):2225

[2] Speckl I, Hallbach J, Guder W, Meyer L, Zilker T. Opiate Detection in Saliva and Urine—A Prospective Comparison by Gas Chromatography–Mass Spectrometry. Journal of Toxicology – Clinical Toxicology [Internet]. 1999 Jun [cited 2020 Jul 14];37(4):441. Available from: https://search-ebscohost-com.ezproxy1.lib.asu.edu/login.aspx?direct=true&db=aph&AN=7430260&site=ehost-live

[3] Cleveland CJ. Morris C. Dictionary of Energy. 2nd ed. Elsevier Science & Technology; 2014

[4] Kitada K, Oho T. Effect of saliva viscosity on the co-aggregation between oral streptococci and Actinomyces naeslundii. Gerodontology. 2011 Nov 13; **29**(2):e981-e987

[5] Rantonen PJ, Meurman JH. Viscosity of whole saliva. Acta Odontologica Scandinavica. 1998;**56**(4): 210-214

[6] Ligtenberg AJM, Liem EHS, Brand HS, Veerman ECI. The Effect of Exercise on Salivary Viscosity [Internet]. MDPI. Multidisciplinary Digital Publishing Institute; 2016 [cited 2020Jul25]. Available from: https://www.mdpi.com/2075-4418/6/4/40/htm

[7] Romanian Journal of Oral Rehabilitation. [cited 2020Jul25]. Available from: http://www.rjor.ro/evaluation-of-total-unstimulated-saliva-viscosity-in-complete-edentulous-patients/?lang=ro

[8] Animireddy D, Reddy Bekkem VT, Vallala P, Kotha SB, Ankireddy S, Mohammad N. Evaluation of pH, buffering capacity, viscosity and flow rate levels of saliva in caries-free, minimal caries and nursing caries children: An in vivo study. Contemporary Clinical Dentistry. 2014;**5**(3):324-328. DOI: 10.4103/0976-237X.137931

[9] Irani, D.N., Cerebrospinal Fluid in Clinical Practice. Philadelphia, PA: Saunders/Elsevier; 2009. Chapter 10: Properties and Composition of Normal Cerebrospinal Fluid; pp. 69–89.

[10] Kestin J, Sokolov M, Wakeham WA. Viscosity of liquid water in the range −8 °C to 150 °C. Journal of Physical and Chemical Reference Data. 1978;**7**(3):941-948

[11] Inman BA, Etienne W, Rubin R, et al. The impact of temperature and urinary constituents on urine viscosity and its relevance to bladder hyperthermia treatment. International Journal of Hyperthermia. 2013;**29**(3): 206-210. DOI: 10.3109/02656736.2013.775355

[12] Haya L, Tavoularis S. Effects of bileaflet mechanical heart valve orientation on fluid stresses and coronary flow. Journal of Fluid Mechanics. Cambridge University Press. 2016;**806**:129-164

[13] Tworoger SS. Collection, processing, and storage of biological samples in epidemiologic studies: Sex hormones, carotenoids, inflammatory markers, and proteomics as examples. Cancer Epidemiology Biomarkers & Prevention. 2006;**15**(9):1578-1581. DOI: 10.1158/1055-9965.epi-06-0629

[14] Amadeu JK et al. Effect of storage time and temperature on salivary Total

antioxidant capacity, Total oxidant status, and oxidant stress index. Acta Stomatologica Croatica. 2019;**53**(2):119-124. DOI: 10.15644/asc53/2/3

[15] Robles TF et al. Saliva sampling method affects performance of a salivary α-amylase biosensor. American Journal of Human Biology. 2013;**25**(6):719-724. DOI: 10.1002/ajhb.22438

[16] Instructions for the use of The Cannon-Fenske Routine ... [Internet]. [cited 2020Jul25]. Available from: https://www.cannoninstrument.com/Image/GetDocument/437?language=en

[17] Johannsen B, Müller L, Baumgartner D, Karkossa L, Früh S, Bostanci N, et al. Automated Pre-Analytic Processing of Whole Saliva Using Magnet-Beating for Point-of-Care Protein Biomarker Analysis. Micromachines [Internet]. MDPI AG; 2019 Nov 30;10(12):833. Available from: http://dx.doi.org/10.3390/mi10120833

[18] Bansil R et al. Mucin biophysics. Annual Review of Physiology. 1995;**57**:635-657

[19] Picout DR, Ross-Murphy SB. Rheology of biopolymer solutions and gels. The Scientific World. 2004;**3**:105-121

Chapter 8

Metabolomics Distinction of Cigarette Smokers from Non-Smokers Using Non-Stationary Benchtop Nuclear Magnetic Resonance (NMR) Analysis of Human Saliva

Benita C. Percival, Angela Wann, Sophie Taylor, Mark Edgar, Miles Gibson and Martin Grootveld

Abstract

Implementations of high-field nuclear magnetic resonance (NMR) facilities into metabolomics studies are unfortunately restricted by their large dimensions, high costings, and specialist technical staff requirements. Therefore, here the application and practical advantages offered by low-field (60 MHz), compact NMR spectrometers for probing the metabolic profiles of human saliva was explored, as was their value in salivary metabolomics studies. Saliva samples were collected from cigarette smoking (n = 11) and non-smoking (n = 31) human participants. ^{1}H NMR spectra were acquired on both low-field (60 MHz) and medium-field (400 MHz) spectrometers. Metabolomics analyses were employed to evaluate the consistencies of salivary metabolite levels determined, and their abilities to distinguish between smokers and non-smokers. Low-field ^{1}H NMR analysis detected up to 15, albeit permitted the reliable quantification of 5, potentially key diagnostic biomolecules simultaneously (LLOQ values 250–400 μmol/L), although these were limited to those with the most prominent resonances. Such low-field profiles were also found to be suitable for salivary metabolomics investigations, which confirmed the successful discrimination between smoking and non-smoking participant sample donors. Differences observed between these groups were largely ascribable to upregulated salivary levels of methanol, and its metabolite formate, in the smoking group, but higher smoking-mediated concentrations of acetate, propionate and glycine may arise from a diminished salivary flow-rate in these participants. In conclusion, determination of salivary biomolecules using low-field, benchtop ^{1}H NMR analysis techniques were found to be valuable for bioanalytical and metabolomics investigations. Future perspectives for the applications of this non-stationary NMR technique, for example for the on-site 'point-of-care' testing of saliva samples for diagnostic oral disease screening purposes at dental surgeries and community pharmacies, are considered.

Keywords: compact low-field NMR analysis, NMR spectroscopy, NMR-linked metabolomics, bioanalytical chemistry, saliva, salivary biomarkers, oral diseases, tobacco smoking, salivary biomarkers for smoking, methanol

1. Introduction

'State-of-the-art' developments of novel devices and facilities for the metabolic screening of biofluids through 'omics' strategies provide an encouraging and thoroughly emerging outlook for future healthcare management prospects, including those focused on the diagnosis of diseases and/or their prognostic stratification [1]. Indeed, high-field (HF) nuclear magnetic resonance (NMR) facilities are routinely used for metabolomics investigations in order to rapidly recognize unusual metabolic patterns in patients suffering from a wide range of diseases. However, deployments in healthcare settings have been prohibitively impacted by the large sizes and costs of the instrumentation required for these purposes [2].

Imbalances in the human metabolome have long been associated with health-mediated disturbances, with ancient societies employing very crude methods to assess biofluids [3], including the smell and taste of urine samples to detect urinary ketone bodies and glucose, respectively, in cases of diabetes, for example. However, more recently there have been many notable developments in this research area, and these have given rise to the development of multicomponent metabolic profile analysis by many researchers since the early 1970s [4–7]. Whilst tandem liquid-chromatographic- and gas-chromatographic-mass spectrometric methods (LC-MS and GC-MS, respectively) can be employed for the reliable and sensitive determination of low concentrations of metabolites in biofluids, these approaches suffer from issues associated with matrix effects, and both are destructive techniques, which usually require a substantial knowledge of sample composition, and the likely identities of key biomarker analytes, prior to analysis [8]. Conversely, high-resolution NMR-based metabolomics analysis offers a highly selective means of simultaneously identifying a wide range of biomolecules present in complex biofluids at a minimal detectable concentration of $\leq$5 μM, providing an untargeted methodology ideal for the analysis of a very large number of biomolecules simultaneously [9] (up to 120 or so and *ca.* 80 in human urine and saliva, respectively at operating frequencies of $\geq$600 MHz). Therefore, the multicomponent ^{1}H NMR analysis of biofluids such as blood plasma, urine and saliva, and tissue biopsies, offers a high level of potential regarding the investigation of metabolic processes, and when coupled with conventional and/or newly-developed multivariate (MV) data analysis techniques, serves as an extremely powerful means of probing the biochemical basis of human disease aetiology [1–5]. Indeed, this form of combined multianalyte-MV analysis is generally classified as metabolomics, and has been extensively applied in a very wide range of biomedical and clinical investigations, including the identification of diagnostic or prognostic biomarkers for a very wide range of diseases.

Although previous applications of low-field (LF) rather than HF NMR spectroscopy to the multicomponent analysis of intact or near-intact biofluids, or other biological media, have been severely limited, our laboratory has paved the way forward for the performance of such studies. Indeed, one of our recent investigations explored the ability of a LF (60 MHz) NMR spectrometer to provide valuable urinary metabolite data for the monitoring of type 2 diabetes (T2D) in humans [10]. Indeed, this application displayed a high level of chemopathological classification success, although this is perhaps not completely unexpected, since uncontrolled or poorly controlled T2D samples all contain quite high levels of glucose (both ^{1}H NMR-distinguishable α- and β-anomers), along with the ketone bodies acetoacetate, acetone and 3-D-hydroxybutyrate, whereas little or none of these biomolecules are normally detectable in healthy control samples. However, one of the major advantages of the ^{1}H NMR technique is that it can simultaneously detect and monitor abnormal levels of a range of further metabolites involved in human disease pathology and associated co-morbidities, for example excessive urinary creatinine concentrations arising from kidney dysfunction and damage in T2D, together with hypoglycaemic drugs such as metformin [11].

Saliva serves as a multifunctional biofluid which plays important roles in facilitating the chewing, swallowing and tasting of foods, and also the regulation of oral flora; hence, it is of much importance for the maintenance of overall health in humans. Indeed, human saliva comprises an agglomerate hypertonic 'solution' which contains oral mucosal exudates, salivary acini and gingival crevicular fluid (GCF) [12]. Since this biofluid is readily accessible, it offers much potential as a medium for the identification and monitoring of established or potential biomarkers for human diseases, particularly oral health conditions, but not exclusively so. Indeed, it's collection can be self-performed by participants with minimal training and without clinical supervision. Therefore, here we have employed optimized LF NMR-based metabolic profiling strategies for the global analysis of human saliva in order to assess the viabilities of these compact instruments for biomedical applications in metabolic profiling, metabolomics, oral health assessments, and potentially future screenings of the efficacies of oral healthcare products. Coupling of this LF salivary analysis technique to MV analysis strategies may indeed serve to facilitate the development of favourable outcome strategies for such investigations, and therefore here we also demonstrate, for the first time, the applications of LF NMR-based metabolomics protocols to the distinction of saliva samples collected from non-smoking and tobacco cigarette-smoking subjects. The future clinical monitoring applications of this novel technique are discussed.

2. Materials and methods

2.1 Saliva sample collection from human participants

Whole mouth saliva samples (n = 61) were collected from healthy human participants (n = 42, age range 21–65 years, 14 male/28 female), of whom 31 were non-smokers, and 11 were regular 'mild-to-heavy' smokers of tobacco cigarettes (an average of 3 to ≥20 cigarettes per day, with 44% of these smoking ≥20 per day). These non-smoking and tobacco-smoking participant groups were age-matched, with their mean ± SEM ages being 42.52 ± 2.25 and 41.91 ± 2.70 years respectively. All ethical considerations were in accord with those of the Declaration of Helsinki 1975 (7th amendment made in 2013). All samples were collected with informed consent and approved by the Faculty of Health and Life Sciences Research Ethics Committee, De Montfort University, Leicester, UK (reference no. 1082). Participants were fasted for a 12-h period prior to providing saliva specimens. All participants were requested to refrain from all oral activities, including eating, drinking, tooth-brushing and smoking, etc. throughout this period, including the short, *ca*. 5 min. duration between awakening and sample donation. They were also requested not to consume any alcoholic beverages 24 h prior to the sample collection time-point. A range of 1–3 samples were collected from each participant, and those donating >1 sample provided these on separate daily a.m. 'wake-up' episodes. All samples were collected in sterile plastic universal containers and were transferred to the laboratory on ice. These were then immediately centrifuged at 3500 rpm at 4°C for a period of 15 min, and following sample preparation as outlined below, the clear human salivary supernatants (HSSs) arising therefrom were then stored at −80°C for a maximal duration of 72 h until ready for NMR analysis.

2.2 Sample preparation and ^{1}H NMR analysis

All reagents and chemicals were purchased from Sigma-Aldrich (Gillingham, UK) unless otherwise stated. Aliquots (500 μL) of HSS samples were treated with 60 μL of pH 7.00 phosphate buffer (1.00 mol/L) containing 0.04% (w/v) sodium azide, and 50 μL of ^2H_2O containing 0.05% (w/v) sodium 3-(trimethylsilyl)propionate-2,2,3,3-d4 (TSP) (final added HSS concentration 238 μmol/L). TSP served as an internal chemical shift reference and quantitative calibration standard; sodium azide acted as a microbicidal preservative in order to protect against the artefactual generation and/or consumption of microbial catabolites during the sample transport and preparation stages; phosphate buffer served to control sample pH values; and ^2H_2O acted as a field frequency lock. Admixtures were then homogenized and transferred to 5-mm diameter NMR tubes (Norell, Morganton, NC, USA). LF ^{1}H NMR spectra were acquired on a 60 MHz Magritek Spinsolve Ultra Benchtop spectrometer (Magritek GmbH, Philipsstr. 852068, Aachen, Nordrhein-Westfalen, Germany) with 64 and/or 384 scans, acquisition and repetition times of 6.4, and 10 or 15 s respectively, and a pulse angle of 90°; the H_2O/HOD presaturation frequency was optimized at δ = 4.80 ppm using the programmed 1D PRESAT function. For the calibration and metabolomics studies described here, scan number and repetition time were standardized at 64 and 10 s respectively. Notwithstanding, total analysis times of <15 min per sample were possible. These samples also underwent medium-field (MF) ^{1}H NMR analysis at an operating frequency of 400 MHz (Bruker Avance-I 400 spectrometer (Bruker AXS, GmbH, Östliche Rheinbrückenstr. 49 76187, Karlsruhe, Germany, Leicester School of Pharmacy facility, De Montfort University, Leicester, UK), operating at a frequency of 400.13 MHz, and using the noesygppr1d pulse sequence for water suppression (H_2O, δ = 4.80 ppm); 32 k data points were acquired in 128 scans, with 2 dummy scans, a sweep width of 4844 Hz, and an automatically-adjusted receiver gain.

^{1}H NMR resonances present in each HSS spectrum acquired were routinely assigned by a consideration of chemical shift values, coupling patterns and coupling constants with reference to literature sources, and where required, two-dimensional ^{1}H-^{1}H correlation and total correlation (COSY and TOCSY respectively) spectra were acquired to confirm these assignments. Median ^{1}H NMR signal-to-noise (STN) ratios were determined from the formula STN = 2.50A/Npp, where A represents resonance height, and Npp the highest peak-to-peak noise difference determined at each chemical shift region selected. Lower limits of detection and quantification (LLOD and LLOQ respectively) values were computed as 3- and 10-times these median STN values. HSS spectral resonances were manually-bucketed, and their intensities determined using *ACD/Spectrus Processor 2019* software; that of residual H_2O/HOD was removed prior to performing univariate (UV) or MV statistical analysis. Salivary biomolecule levels were determined from calibration plots of ratios of their pre-selected resonance intensities to that of internal TSP against their known concentrations in a series of analytical calibration standard solutions.

Calibration and Bland-Altman dominance plots of the ^{1}H NMR-determined concentrations of acetate, propionate, formate, glycine and methanol featured matched analysis sample datasets, with determinations made on these salivary metabolites at both 60 and 400 MHz operating frequencies. All determinations which were found to have none detectable (nd, specifically those with values <LLOD) at both operating frequencies utilized, were removed from the datasets. As recommended [13], corresponding ^{1}H NMR profiles of blank samples, which were prepared as outlined above, but with HPLC-grade water in place of HSSs, were acquired, and their 'noise' intensities at the appropriate δ values were included in these calibration plots. Spectra were acquired on replicate (n = 3) preparations of such blank samples for these purposes.

2.3 UV and MV statistical and metabolomics analyses

2.3.1 UV analysis

A paired sample t-test was applied to test for any differences between LF 60 MHz spectra acquired with relaxation delays of 10 or 15 s, and an *XLSTAT2020* software module was employed for this purpose.

An analysis-of-covariance (ANCOVA) experimental design was employed to test the statistical significance of the 'between-smoking status' source of variation, along with the potential effects of essential demographic variables recorded on participant sample donors, on salivary acetate, formate, propionate, glycine and methanol concentrations (Eq. (1)). Overall, this model evaluated the influences of the 'between-participant' (random) effect $P_{(k)l}$, and the 'between-participant ages' (A_i), 'between-participant-genders' (G_j), and'between-smoking status' (S_k) sources of variation (all fixed) on these five sets of ^{1}H NMR-determined levels. Moreover, the statistical significance of the age × gender, age × smoking status, and gender × smoking status first-order interaction effects (AG_{ij}, AS_{ik} and GS_{jk} respectively) were also assessed. ANCOVA was performed using *XLSTAT2014* and *2020* software modules.

$$y_{ijklm} = \mu + A_i + G_j + S_k + P_{(k)l} + AG_{ij} + AS_{ik} + GS_{jk} + e_{ijklm} \quad (1)$$

An additional ANCOVA model explored the significance of any differences between the two operating frequencies in the non-smoking group only, and in this experimental design, the 'between-ages', 'between-genders' and 'between-participants' sources of variation were also evaluated, as was the age × gender first-order interaction effect (Eq. (2)). In this design, O_k represents the 'between-spectrometer operating frequencies' effect (fixed).

$$y_{ijklm} = \mu + A_i + G_j + O_k + P_{(k)l} + AG_{ij} + e_{ijklm} \quad (2)$$

2.3.2 MV metabolomics analysis

Principal component analysis (PCA) was primarily employed to identify any possible outlier samples present in the 60 MHz operating frequency ^{1}H NMR dataset, and in total 8 of these were found and classified as such, and then subsequently removed prior to the performance of further MV analysis. PCA was then employed to determine the reproducibility of replicate salivary metabolite determinations made on the LF benchtop spectrometer, and this check was performed with n = 9 duplicated salivary samples randomly selected from the smoking group of participants, with all the above five metabolite variables included, and not non-smokers in view of the restricted availability of data on salivary methanol and, to a lesser extent, formate concentrations above their LLOQ indices. For this PCA analysis, salivary metabolite concentrations were not constant sum-normalized (CSN), nor transformed, and nor auto- or Pareto-scaled.

For the major objective of this study, a LF benchtop ^{1}H NMR-based metabolomics investigation featured a comparison of saliva specimens collected from the non-smoking and tobacco-smoking participants, and for this purpose all the above 5 potential predictor variables, determined via TSP-normalization as described above, were incorporated. For these purposes, the dataset was product quotient normalized (PQN), generalised $\log_{10}$ (glog)-transformed, and Pareto-scaled prior to MV analysis, which involved PCA, partial least squares-discriminatory analysis (PLS-DA), orthogonal partial least squares-discriminatory analysis (OPLS-DA), random forest (RF) and agglomerative hierarchical clustering (AHC) techniques (*MetaboAnalyst 5.0*, University of Alberta and National Research Council, National Institute for Nanotechnolgy, (NINT), Edmonton, AB, Canada). Distinctions found between the two groups with the above PLS-DA and OPLS-DA strategies were cross-validated with determination of Q^2 statistics, and also permutation tests with 2000 permutations. A Q^2 value of $\geq$0.50 was considered as a significant discriminatory cut-off threshold [14].

PQN converts ^{1}H NMR metabolomics profiles according to an overall estimate of the most probable 'dilution' influence [15], and for saliva this includes reductions in salivary flow-rate (SFR), which has been reported to be significantly reduced in cigarette smokers [16]. This strategy usually involves the subtraction of a mean or median column-bucketed reference spectral profile from those of either all or a subset of study samples, and for this investigation the non-smoking control group was employed for this purpose.

At an operating frequency of 60 MHz, some missing data in the MV datasets were unavoidable in view of resonance overlap complications. Therefore, for this metabolomics model, these randomly missing values, *ca.* 9% of the total available ^{1}H NMR-determined concentrations, were estimated and imputed using the non-linear iterative partial least squares (NIPALS) approach (*XLSTAT2020*) [17], since this method is considered appropriate for MV metabolomics datasets such as that analyzed in the current study. For UV data analysis, these imputations were accompanied by a corresponding decrease in degrees of freedom available for the parametric statistical evaluations conducted. Metabolite concentration values below the detection limit (i.e., zero analyte values or '*less-thans*') were replaced using the simple multiplicative replacement approach described in Ref. [18], specifically as 65% of their metabolite LLOD values.

Multivariate ANOVA (MANOVA) was performed using *XLSTAT2014* software. The non-parametric RF analysis featured 1000 trees and 2 predictor variables selected at each node following tuning. The dataset was randomly split into training and test sets comprising *ca.* two-thirds and one-third of the samples respectively. The training set was used to construct the RFs model and determine an out-of-the-bag (OOB) error value in order to assess classification performance.

3. Results

3.1 Outline of ^{1}H NMR analysis results: detection and quantitative determination of salivary biomolecules at 60 MHz operating frequency

Figure 1 shows the 60 MHz ^{1}H NMR profile of a typical human salivary supernatant (HSS) sample obtained with 384 scans, a process which took 60 min to acquire. This spectrum contains clear ^{1}H resonances assignable to acetate (signal 7) and methanol (signal 14), which are both ascribable to their —$C\underline{H}_3$ groups. Further prominent resonances in the spectra acquired were those of propionate (both —$C\underline{H}_3$ and —$C\underline{H}_2$ functions, signals 1 and 8 respectively) and glycine (α-$C\underline{H}_2$ protons, signal 15), together with that of the single ^{1}H NMR-detectable proton ($\underline{H}$-CO_2^-) of formate (signal 20). Further, albeit weak signals were those assignable to dimethyl- and trimethylamine, the terminal-CH_2 groups of amine species such as lysine and 5-aminovalerate, and the >N—$C\underline{H}_3$ group of creatinine/creatine, together with two aromatic resonances (one a composite phenylalanine/tyrosine one), although all these biomolecules predominantly had salivary concentrations below their LLOQ values. A full list of all resonances identified in the 60 MHz 1H (superscript 1) NMR profiles of HSS samples analysed is provided in **Table 1**.

Acceptable benchtop 60 MHz spectra were also obtained with only 64 scans, which involved a 10 min acquisition time, although all ^{1}H NMR resonances therein were, however, notably affected by significantly lower signal-to-noise (STN) parameters, as expected. All carboxylic acid anions detectable represent oral microbial catabolites, and the simultaneous ^{1}H NMR measurement of their salivary concentrations in this manner may offer significant potential regarding the provision of valuable diagnostic and prognostic screening information for dental surgeons and oral healthcare specialists alike, especially those regarding conditions such as dental caries and periodontal diseases, as previously noted in studies performed with conventional specialist NMR laboratory-based medium- and high-resolution 400 and 600 MHz operating frequency spectrometers respectively [19, 20]. Moreover, amino acids detectable such as glycine are potentially derived from the actions of proteolytic bacteria on salivary proteins, although there are, of course, also host sources of this metabolite [21], as indeed there are for some of the organic acid anions, such as acetate.

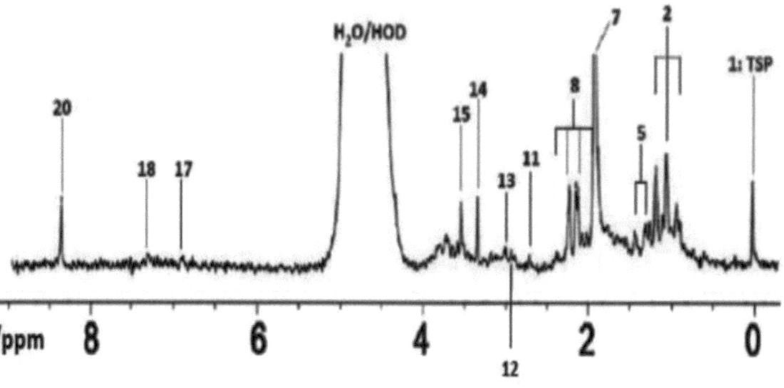

Figure 1.
*Experimental 60 MHz ^{1}H NMR profile of a HSS sample acquired with 384 scans. Numerical assignment codes correspond to those in **Table 1**. TSP represents the 3-(trimethylsilyl)propionate-2,2,3,3-d4 chemical shift reference and internal quantitative ^{1}H NMR standard, and H_2O/HOD the residual water signal.*

Resonance code	Chemical shift (*multiplicity*)	Assignment
1	0.00 (*s*)	3-Trimethylsilyl-(2,2,3,3-$^2H_4$)-1-propionate (TSP)-Si($C\underline{H}_3$)$_3$: internal chemical shift reference and quantitative integration intensity calibration standard
2	1.06 (*t*)	Propionate-$C\underline{H}_3$
3	1.13 (*d*)	Propane-1,2-diol-$C\underline{H}_3$*
4	1.18 (*t*)	Ethanol-$C\underline{H}_3$*
5	1.33 (*d*)	Lactate-$C\underline{H}_3$
6	1.48 (*d*)	Alanine-$C\underline{H}_3$
7	1.92 (*s*)	Acetate-$C\underline{H}_3$
8	2.18 (*q*)	Propionate-$C\underline{H}_2$
9	2.23 (*t*)	5-AV-α-$C\underline{H}_2$
10	2.41 (*s*)	Succinate-$C\underline{H}_2$
11	2.75 (*s*)	Dimethylamine-N($C\underline{H}_3$)$_2$
12	2.90 (*s*)	Trimethylamine-N($C\underline{H}_3$)$_3$
13	3.04 (*m*)	Creatinine-N($C\underline{H}_3$)/Creatine-N($C\underline{H}_3$)/Lysine-ε-CH_2/5-AV-δ-$C\underline{H}_2$
14	3.37 (*s*)	Methanol-$C\underline{H}_3$*
15	3.57 (*s*)	Glycine-α-CH_2
16	3.67 (*m*)	Ethanol-$C\underline{H}_2$*
17	6.91 (*d*)	Tyrosine aromatic ring protons-C$\underline{H}$
18	7.22 (*d*)/7.30–7.45 (all *m*)	Tyrosine/phenylalanine aromatic ring protons-C$\underline{H}$
19	7.91 (*s*)	Histidine imidazole ring-C$\underline{H}$
20	8.45 (*s*)	Formate-C$\underline{H}$

Abbreviation: 5-AV, 5-aminovalerate.
**Indicates resonances of molecules which may also arise from exogenous sources, e.g., propane-1,2-diol and methanol from tobacco smoking [23], and ethanol from alcoholic beverage ingestion [19].*

Table 1.
*Assignments for resonances present in the 60 MHz ^{1}H NMR spectra shown in **Figure 1** (coupling patterns for these are also provided). Resonances highlighted in red are visible in both LF (60 MHz) and HF (400 MHz) ^{1}H NMR profiles, whereas those in blue are observable but not readily quantifiable at the lower operating frequency in view of overlap with or close localization to other biomolecule signals, or being below the lower limits of quantification (LLOQ) values for their assigned metabolites. The identities of selected signals were confirmed via reference to [22].*

Although the 60 MHz spectral profiles of HSS specimens investigated are largely dominated by the highest intensity resonances therein (i.e. those assigned to biomolecules of the highest salivary concentrations such as acetate and propionate), this technique also lent itself to the assignment of lower intensity signals, and the quantification of salivary metabolites present at significantly lower concentrations. Indeed, the singlet resonances of formate, methanol and glycine were clearly resolved from potential overlapping signals, and therefore appeared suitable for quantification purposes. As previously documented [23], one major source of salivary methanol in humans is the ingestion of cigarette smoke. However, in some HSS specimens, the lactate-CH_3 function doublet resonance at δ = 1.33 ppm was also clearly visible in 60 MHz spectra, most especially those with quite high millimolar salivary levels. Although highly variable, reported mean levels for salivary lactate in adults are 0.1–20.3 mmol/L [24]. However, our previously reported overall mean lactate concentration in saliva samples collected from a pre-fasting healthy control population was found to be 13.3 mmol/L, although those of replicate samples from n = 20 participants also varied substantially, i.e. from 0.08 to 100.9 mmol/L [18].

TSP was present in HSS analyte solutions at an added level of only 238 μmol/L (i.e. a 238/9 = 26.44 μmol/L single ^{1}H nucleus equivalent value), and because this was also one of the most intense signals present in the spectra acquired (*s*, δ = 0.00 ppm), concentrations of <60 μmol/L were also readily visible in spectra of chemical model systems containing this internal standard. However, since this intense resonance arises from a total of 9 protons (i.e. 3 equivalent Si-C$\underline{H}_3$ units), it is conceivable that many salivary and perhaps other biofluid metabolites containing only single, or one or more magnetically-distinguishable —CH_3 functions with singlet resonances (for example, acetate) are clearly detectable and potentially also quantifiable at concentrations of ≤150 μmol/L in this complex, multicomponent biofluid matrix, although further investigations are required to explore this. Moreover, for such —CH_3 function-containing analytes, a LLOD value of *ca.* 100 μmol/L was estimated for HSS samples (i.e. 3 × the mean spectral noise intensities at their specified chemical shift values in water blank solution spectra acquired under the same experimental conditions, or a SNR value of 3). Such LLOD values will also be influenced by further factors, such as T_2-dependent resonance line-widths (the potential influence of which will be much greater at LFs), the dependence of noise on chemical shift values, saturation effects, digital resolution and baseline slants, etc. Notwithstanding, further key experiments are required to determine these LLOQ values (with SNR = 10) for key biomolecules present within LF salivary spectra, particularly oral disease-linked biomarkers of interest.

The relaxation delay employed for acquisition of LF 60 MHz ^{1}H NMR spectra, i.e. 10 or 15 s, did not give rise to any differences in the estimated salivary concentrations of acetate, propionate, formate, glycine and methanol (paired sample t-tests performed on untransformed datasets, n ≥ 10 matched spectra for each biomolecule). These data demonstrated that a relaxation delay of 10 s was sufficient for full T_1 relaxation of the ^{1}H environments involved.

3.2 Comparative evaluations of the ^{1}H NMR profiles of human salivary supernatants at 60 and 400 MHz operating frequencies

All resonances detectable in the above 60 MHz 1H NMR profiles were, of course, also readily detectable in corresponding 400 MHz spectra, and as expected, median resonance STN values were much greater, and hence corresponding LLOQ and LLOD parameters were substantially lower with this MF spectrometer. Indeed, signals arising from metabolites with detectable but not quantifiable signals in the 60 MHz profiles acquired, for example the malodorous amines DMA and TMA, and the amino acids phenylalanine and tyrosine, were readily quantifiable at the 400 MHz operating frequency. Additionally, in view of the much improved spectral resolution and quality, metabolites which were only detectable but unquantifiable, or completely undetectable at 60 MHz, were also detectable and predominantly quantifiable at MF, and these included leucine (—C$\underline{H}_3$ (*t*), δ = 0.96 ppm); valine (—CH_3s (both *d*), δ = 0.98 and 1.03 ppm); alanine (—CH_3 (*d*), δ = 1.48 ppm); glutamate (γ-CH_2 (*m*), δ = 2.34 ppm); glutamine (γ-CH_2 (*m*), δ = 2.44 ppm); taurine (—$C\underline{H}_2NH_3^+$ and —$C\underline{H}_2SO_3^-$ (both *t*), δ = 3.23 and 3.47 ppm respectively); *n*-butyrate (—$C\underline{H}_3$, —$C\underline{H}_2$- and $C\underline{H}_2CO_2^-$ (*t*, *m* and *t*), δ = 0.94, 1.55 and 2.15 ppm respectively); 2,2-dimethylsuccinate (—$C\underline{H}_3$s (*s*), δ = 1.22); 3-D-hydroxybutyrate (—$C\underline{H}_3$ (*d*), δ = 1.24 ppm); lactate (—$C\underline{H}_3$ and —$C\underline{H}$ (*d* and *q*), δ = 1.33 and 4.13 ppm respectively); 5-aminovalerate (β/γ-, α- and δ-$C\underline{H}_2$s (*m*, *t* and *t*), δ = 1.63, 2.23 and 3.05 ppm respectively); pyruvate (—CH_3 (*s*), δ = 2.39 ppm); succinate (—CH_2s (*s*), δ = 2.405 ppm); choline (—$N(C\underline{H}_3)_3^+$ head group (*s*), δ = 3.21 ppm); ethanol (—$C\underline{H}_3$ and —$C\underline{H}_2OH$ (*t* and *q*), δ = 1.18 and 3.66 ppm respectively); carbohydrates such as glucose and sucrose (C1$\underline{H}$ anomeric protons located at 4.66/5.25 for the former (both *d*s), and 5.41 ppm (*d*) for the glycosidic proton of the latter, respectively), where detectable; dihydroxyacetone (—$C\underline{H}_2OH$ (s), δ = 4.46 ppm), and N-acetylsugars and N-acetylamino acids, both high- and low-molecular mass (broad and narrow —$NHCOC\underline{H}_3$ signals respectively (*s*), δ = 2.01–2.08 ppm); aromatic amino acids (aromatic ring resonances of tyrosine (2 × *d*, δ = 6.88 and 7.25 ppm), phenylalanine (3 × *m*, δ = 7.32, 7.38 and 7.43 ppm) and histidine (2 × s, δ = 7.07 and 7.81 ppm); and those assignable to a number of pyrimidine, or nicotinate and nicotinamide pathway metabolite(s).

Plots of salivary acetate, glycine and methanol concentrations determined on the LF 60 MHz NMR facility *versus* those obtained on the HF 400 MHz instrument were all linear (r = 0.990, 0.987 and 0.995 respectively), and these results confirmed good-to-excellent correlations and agreements between these two methods of ^{1}H NMR analysis for these biomolecules. However, this correlation was found to be less strong for formate (r = 0.927). Moreover, for propionate, despite a strong linear correlation between these two forms of NMR analyses (r = 0.973), 95% confidence intervals (CIs) for its regression coefficient were found to be significantly greater than the 1.00 value expected for good agreement between these values (i.e. 1.22–1.41). This observation is explicable by potential interferences arising from further ^{1}H NMR resonances located within the δ = 0.92–1.18 ppm chemical shift range spanned by the propionate-CH_3 signal at 60 MHz (15.3 Hz in total: J = 7.67 Hz for this signal). These potential interfering signals are those assignable to the terminal-CH_3 functions of both long- and alternative short-chain fatty acids (including that of *n*-butyrate at δ = 0.94 ppm and those of branched-chain amino acids such as valine). Therefore, the apparent propionate concentration determined at 60 MHz was significantly inflated by a mean value of approximately 1.32-fold over those determined at the more conventional 400 MHz operating frequency.

In order to explore the significant LF spectral overestimations of propionate further, the complete chemical shift span of its -CH_3 function triplet at 60 MHz (0.92–1.18 ppm) was integrated in the corresponding 400 MHz spectra acquired, and apparent propionate concentrations obtained in this manner were then plotted against those determined at 60 MHz (**Figure 2**). As expected, this plot was found to display a much-improved agreement between the two estimated concentration values, with 95% CI values for the regression coefficient and y-intercept both covering unity and 0.00 respectively (r = 0.985). However, a comparison of these bioanalytical calibration plots indicated only a relatively marginal interference from the above potentially overlapping, albeit minor signals for the direct determinations of propionate at 60 MHz when its salivary level was *ca.* ≤1.0 mmol/L. Therefore, for the LF NMR determination of salivary propionate, one possible solution is that samples with concentrations greater than this value are first diluted to levels close to or below this limit in order to facilitate its quantification.

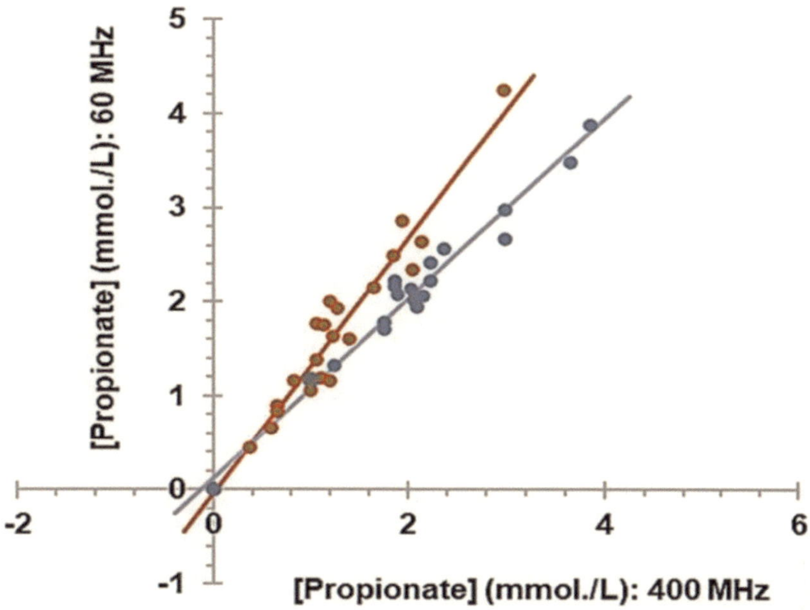

Figure 2.
Comparison of a plot of the estimated salivary concentrations of propionate determined at 60 MHz with that from spectra acquired at 400 MHz for its —$\underline{CH}_3$ *function resonance encompassing its chemical shift span i.e. 2 × 7.67 = 15.34 Hz at both operating frequencies, and equivalent to 0.256 and 0.038 ppm at 60 and 400 MHz respectively (red data-points and regression line), with that obtained from employment of the corresponding 60 MHz 0.256 ppm bucket span for integration purposes at 400 MHz, i.e. 0.92–1.18 ppm (blue data-points and regression line).*

Nevertheless, a novel statistical approach was employed for determining the maximal concentration determinable at this operating frequency. Firstly. an alternative ANCOVA model (model 2) was designed and employed for statistical analysis of the non-smoking participant group only (Eq. (2)), and this included a consideration of variance contributions from differential ages, genders, participants and spectrometer operating frequencies, plus the age × gender first-order interaction effect. Secondly, p values for the statistical significance of the fixed 'between-operating frequencies' (O_k) effects were isolated for a series of these ANCOVA models arising from sequential removal of the highest or highest remaining estimated salivary propionate concentration, i.e. $[\text{propionate}]_{max}$ (at 60 MHz), starting from a prior sample size of n = 30 observations (i.e. with coupled 60 and 400 MHz ^{1}H NMR determinations for each of n = 15 participants), down to only n = 6 (with coupled measurements made for only n = 3 participants); as expected, these p values increased with decreasing sample size, i.e. the degree of statistical significance between the two operating frequencies tested decreased. Thirdly, $-\log_{10}$ transformations of these p values were then plotted as a function of $[\text{propionate}]_{max}$ value (**Figure 3**), and the ordinate axis value of this curve set at $p = 0.05$ served to provide an estimate for the latter value's limit for bioanalytical purposes, i.e. that at which the difference observed between salivary concentrations determined at 60 and 400 MHz operating frequencies became statistically insignificant at the 5% level. This limit was therefore estimated as 1.2 mmol/L for salivary propionate concentrations determined at 60 MHz, a value similar to the 1.00 mmol/L limit proposed above.

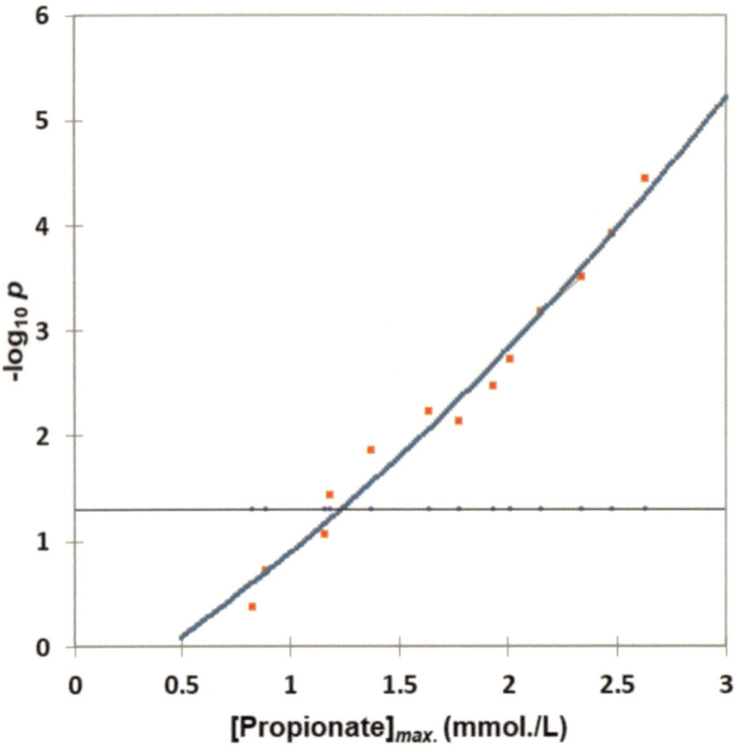

Figure 3.
(a) Polynomial plot of -$\log_{10}$ p value obtained for the significance of the 'between-operating frequencies' mean square of the ANCOVA model of Eq. (2) as a function of decreasing maximal salivary propionate concentration ([propionate]$_{max}$) with sample size, the latter diminishing via the sequential removal of the [propionate]$_{max}$, value (from n = 15 to n = 3 matched duplicate samples, one determination made at 60 MHz, one at 400 MHz ^{1}H NMR operating frequencies). The horizontal black line represents the $-\log_{10}$ p index arising from a p value of 0.05, i.e. the minimal level required for statistical significance; its crossing with blue polynomial plot yields a [propionate]$_{max}$ value of 1.2 mmol/L. The quadratic equation fitted to the experimental data was $-\log_{10}$ p = 0.603 + 1.261[Propionate]$_{max}$ + 0.226[Propionate]$_{max}^2$ (R^2 = 0.9795), which was an improved fit over that obtained with a standard linear relationship.

3.3 PCA and MANOVA assessments of the bioanalytical precision of metabolite determinations at 60 MHz operating frequency

Subsequently, principal component analysis (PCA) was utilized to monitor the precision of duplicate, 'between-assay'sample analyses with this facility in a model containing 5 LF NMR-detectable salivary metabolites with quantifiable concentrations (acetate, propionate, formate, glycine and methanol). For this purpose, n = 9 duplicate sets of samples were randomly drawn from the tobacco-smoking group, and analyzed in different assay batches conducted with LF 60 MHz spectral acquisitions made on separate work-days. With the exception of two sets of matched analyses, there was a good agreement of both PC1 and PC2 scores obtained for all duplicate samples analyzed (**Figure 4**). Moreover, MV analysis-of-variance (MANOVA) of these experimental data found that the 'between-replicates' and the participant × replicate interaction effects were both statistically insignificant (p = 0.80 and 0.97 respectively), although there was a very highly significant difference observed 'between-participants' ($p = 5.50 \times 10^{-4}$), as expected.

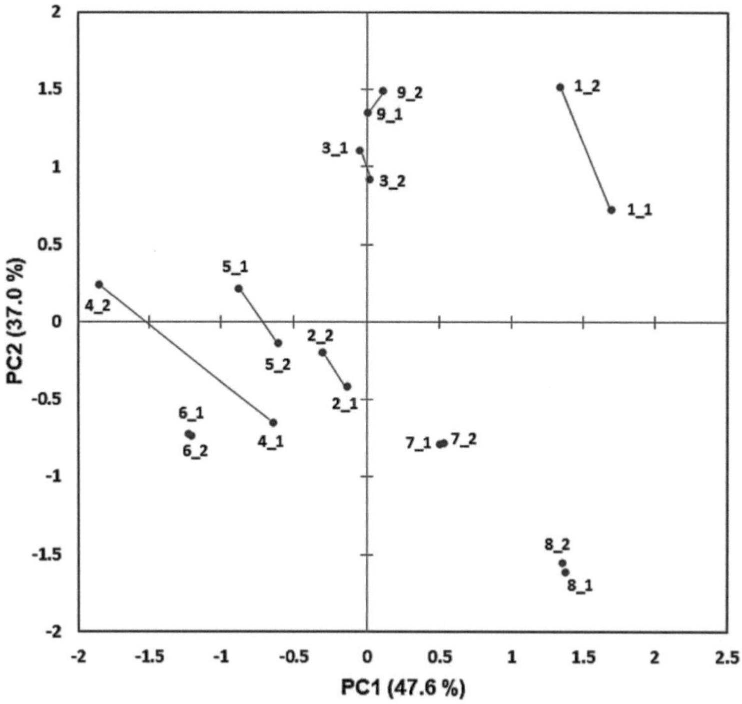

Figure 4.
PCA scores plot of PC2 versus PC1 for duplicate LF NMR determinations of 5 metabolites in saliva specimens collected from n = 9 tobacco smoking participants at an operating frequency of 60 MHz. This plot demonstrates that, with the exception of samples 1 and 4, there was a satisfactory agreement between the repeated determinations. Abbreviations: n_1 and n_2 refer to the first and second duplicate determinations made on sample n, and so on.

3.4 UV evaluations of metabolic differences between smoking and non-smoking participants

Mean ± SEM salivary levels of acetate, propionate, formate, glycine and methanol determined using the LF 60 MHz benchtop spectrometer for both the non-smoking and smoking groups are provided in **Table 2**. Univariate statistical analyses of these data revealed that the salivary concentrations of methanol, glycine and acetate were all significantly higher in smokers, the substantial upregulation in methanol observed being concordant with results previously acquired by Percival et al. [23].

The above model 1 experimental design featured the 'between-age (A_i), -gender (G_j) and -smoking status (S_k)' main factors (fixed effects), the 'between-participants' random effect ($P_{(k)l}$), and the AG_{ij}, AS_{ik} and GS_{jk} first-order interactions effects. Results from this factorial analysis are shown in **Table 3**. Overall, the participant age factor was not significant for any metabolite; the gender predictor variable was only close to statistical significance for glycine, with males having higher concentrations than females; cigarette smoking exerted highly significant effects on acetate, glycine and, of course, methanol. For the first-order interactions investigated, only the GS_{jk} effect was statistically significant, but only for acetate and glycine, i.e., non-additive responses to the four differential gender-smoking status combinations were observed. The random s_P^2 effect confirmed very highly significant differences 'between-participants' for all metabolites investigated.

Metabolite	Non-smokers (mmol/L)	Smokers (mmol/L)
Acetate	5.54 ± 0.95 (range 0–30.92)	11.20 ± 2.00 (range 0–30.20)*
Propionate†	1.89 ± 0.18 (range 0–5.59)	2.43 ± 0.35 (range 0–4.95)
Formate	0.14 ± 0.04 (range 0–0.95)	0.37 ± 0.09 (range 0–1.27)
Glycine	0.34 ± 0.04 (range 0–1.04)	0.80 ± 0.17 (0–2.49)*
Methanol††	0.00 ± 0.00 (range 0–0.20)	0.48 ± 0.11 (0–1.58)**

†Propionate levels were determined at an operating frequency of 400 MHz in view of resonance overlap complications observed at 60 MHz.
††At an operating frequency of 60 MHz, this agent was ^{1}H NMR-quantifiable in n = 3 samples only in the non-smoking participant cohort.
**p < 0.05 for differences between the mean values of non-smokers and smokers; **p < 10^{-3} (test performed for determining the significance of the 'between-smoking status' mean square in the model 1 ANCOVA model design delineated in (Eq. (1))).*

Table 2.
Mean ± SEM concentrations of salivary biomolecules determined by LF 60 MHz ^{1}H NMR analysis of HSS samples in non-smoking and smoking sampling groups (sample sizes were n = 33 and 19 for these groups respectively; ranges are provided in brackets).

		Metabolite				
Effect	Status	Acetate	Propionate	Formate	Glycine	Methanol
Age	Fixed	ns	0.114	ns	ns	ns
Smoking Status	Fixed	0.044	0.127	0.086	0.041	0.00093
Gender	Fixed	ns	ns	ns	0.057	0.094
Age × gender	Fixed	ns	ns	ns	ns	ns
Age × Smoking Status	Fixed	ns	ns	ns	ns	ns
Gender × Smoking Status	Fixed	<0.05	ns	ns	<0.01	ns
s_p^2	Random	0.00032	0.00014	0.00072	0.00010	0.0000039*

Abbreviations: s_p^2, 'between-participant' component of variance; ns, not significant.
**As expected, this difference was statistically significant for only the smoking participants and not the non-smoking group, and this p value corresponds to that cohort only.*

Table 3.
Statistical significance (p values) of all main sources of variation (both fixed and random), and first-order interaction effects, from ANCOVA analysis of the model 1 salivary metabolite dataset.

3.5 Distinction between non-smoking and smoking participants using LF NMR-based MV metabolomics analysis

^{1}H NMR-based metabolomics analysis was, for the first time, utilized to determine the value of LF benchtop NMR analysis to discriminate between the salivary ^{1}H NMR profiles of the cigarette smoking *versus* non-smoking sampling groups. Therefore, the above ^{1}H NMR-detectable and validated 5 biomolecule variables, i.e. acetate, propionate, formate, methanol and glycine concentrations, as determined on the LF 60 MHz spectrometer, were employed to explore any MV differences between these. PCA, partial-least squares discriminatory analysis (PLS-DA), orthogonal partial least squares-discriminatory analysis (OPLS-DA), and agglomerative hierarchal clustering (AHC) techniques were used for this purpose, as was analysis using a RF model.

Figure 5(a) and **(b)** show three-dimensional (3D) PLS-DA, and a two-dimensional (2D) OPLS-DA scores plots, arising from these forms of MV analysis, and both revealed that it was possible to achieve a satisfactory level of distinction between these two groups. Cross-validating $Q^2(R^2Y)$ values for these analyses were found to be high (0.721(0.803) and 0.709(0.786) respectively), and permutation tests performed for these models with 2000 permutations were very highly significant indeed ($p < 5.0 \times 10^{-4}$ in both cases). These analyses revealed that only methanol and its potential *in vivo* metabolite formate were important discriminatory variables for this comparison, which were both significantly upregulated in the smoking group (PLS-DA variable importance parameter (VIP) values of 1.88 and 0.81 respectively), with corresponding values for acetate, propionate and glycine being only 0.06, 0.64 and 0.63 respectively, i.e. acetate offered no discriminatory potential whatsoever. These values were reflected by the PCA strategy applied, which had very strong PC1 positive loadings for methanol and formate (0.52 and 0.79 respectively), whereas those for acetate, propionate and glycine were negative, but only weakly so (−0.02, −0.08 and −0.32 respectively). These loadings vectors are fully consistent with PC1 being derived from a cigarette tobacco smoking source only: in addition to being an oral microbiome catabolite, formate is an important *in vivo* metabolite of cigarette smoke-containing methanol, the route proceeding through a toxic formaldehyde intermediate [33]. However, it also appears that 2 or more of the non-smoking group of participants are classifying or clustering as cigarette smokers. In view of this observation, it remains a possibility that self-reporting bias may be involved in such cases, as further discussed in Section 4 below.

Similarly, AHC analysis confirmed an at least partial distinction between these two HSS sample classifications (**Figure 5(c)**). However, despite a reasonable-to-good level of discrimination, 2 of the samples donated by non-smoking participants appeared within the smoking group cluster, and 5 of the smoking ones are clustered with the non-smoking cohort. This is possibly explicable by self-reporting bias in the former case, but for the latter, it is possible that the participants concerned smoked their last cigarette some considerable period of time prior to sample collection.

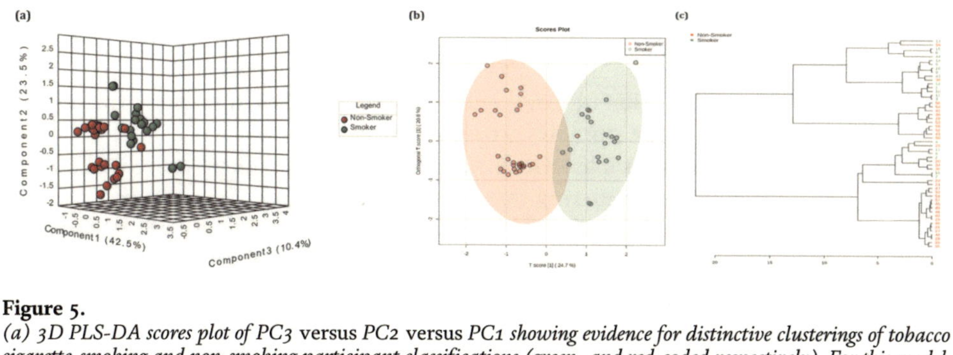

Figure 5.
(a) 3D PLS-DA scores plot of PC3 versus *PC2* versus *PC1 showing evidence for distinctive clusterings of tobacco cigarette-smoking and non-smoking participant classifications (green- and red-coded respectively). For this model, PC1, PC2 and PC3 accounted for 42.5, 23.5 and 10.4% of the total model variance respectively. (b) OPLS-DA plot of orthogonal T score {1}* versus *T score {1} also revealing a high level of distinction between the tobacco-smoking and non-smoking groups. (c) AHC analysis dendogram of this dataset, revealing an at least moderate level of differentiation between the smoking and non-smoking groups, with notable sub-clusterings within each classification. Two misclassified non-smoking participant sample donors may arise from a self-reporting smoking bias, whereas the five misclassified smoking participants may result from prolonged durations between sample collection and their last smoking episode. Eight potential outlier samples detected in a provisional PCA were removed from the dataset prior to analysis.*

Finally, an RF model demonstrated that 88 and 95% of the non-smoking and smoking participant donor samples were correctly classified (91% classification success rate overall). Hence, these MV comparisons demonstrate, for the first time, an important ^{1}H NMR-based metabolomics application which employs a non-stationary LF benchtop spectrometer. Four of the non-smoking participants were misclassified as smokers, whereas only one of the smokers was classified as a non-smoker with this analysis strategy.

3.6 Potential clinical and diagnostic significance of salivary metabolite tracking with LF benchtop NMR devices

In this study we have demonstrated the rapid, virtually non-invasive analysis of human saliva using a compact, LF 60 MHz benchtop NMR spectrometer. The major aim of the pilot investigations described here was to establish the abilities of LF NMR spectrometers to effectively perform the simultaneous quantitative analysis of a series of biomolecules in human saliva, and to consider their potential future value as trackable agents for the monitoring of selected oral diseases. We also critically examined limitations of the applications of this technique and their potential outcomes. Moreover, for the first time we have also applied 'state-of-the art' NMR-linked metabolomics techniques to distinguish between saliva samples donated by both non-smokers and tobacco cigarette-smoking participants in a case study.

Overall, we have shown that 60 MHz ^{1}H NMR measurements can be employed to reliably determine selected salivary metabolite concentrations, with potentially much scope for future diagnostic and prognostic applications to oral health conditions. The authors are fully aware of issues related to resonance overlap at low magnetic fields in view of the dependence of resonance frequencies on static magnetic field strength, in which ^{1}H NMR signals appear to be broader, and with a spectrally-wider chemical shift range for all multiplets, with decreasing spectrometer operating frequencies. Such studies are therefore highly challenging in view of these inherent analyte selectivity considerations, along with potential sensitivity issues expected at such lower magnetic field strengths. However, we found that complications arising from overlapping resonances in complex biofluid samples such as saliva were minimal, or were circumventable, for the most common prominent resonances, and also for those located within relatively interference-free spectral regions. The ability of this LF NMR technique to detect exogenous agents present in this biofluid should also be considered, for example the detection of drugs and other xenobiotics in saliva within specified time zones following their oral ingestion by humans.

Intriguingly, human saliva may afford a transference-dependent '*diluted picture*' of chemopathological changes occurring throughout the human body, in addition to more concentrated, localized metabolic features within the oral environment itself, since a large number of biomolecules, and disease biomarkers (of a range of specificities) have the ability to transfer to this biofluid from blood via intra-, extra-, trans- and pericellular pathways, which highlight active transport or passive diffusion within the gingival sulcus and salivary glands [25]. Indeed, researchers are now increasingly promoting the employment of saliva as a clinical diagnostic medium [26], and such applications have significant widespread potential. Correspondingly, salivary (particularly parotid salivary) metabolomic and proteomic modifications appear to mirror those observed in human blood [27–29].

In 2002, the study reported by Silwood et al. [19], was described in Ref. [9] as the very first untargeted metabolomics investigation of human saliva. This unique investigation successfully identified a total of 63 biomolecules therein using 600 MHz ^{1}H NMR analysis, and quantified 11 key microbial-derived catabolites, 9 of which displayed very highly significant 'between-participant' components of variance. These markers included acetate and lactate, with excessive levels of their corresponding acids being viewed as primary end-point biomarkers involved in the aetiology of dental caries [30]. However, formic and pyruvic acids (both present at millimolar or near-millimolar concentrations in human saliva, the former being higher in smokers as found here) are stronger acids than lactic acid, and therefore may also exert pro-cariogenic activities. Hence, the LF 60 MHz NMR detection and quantification of salivary formate demonstrated in the current study may indeed offer some diagnostic and/or prognostic monitoring potential. However, propionate, along with *n*- and *iso*-butyrates, are considered to be primary microbial catabolites involved in periodontal disease progression [31, 32]. Correspondingly, salivary short-chain organic acids/anions serve as biomarkers for the growth, preponderance and catabolic activities of micro-organisms, and hence species-dependent patterns of these agents may serve as biomarkers of pathologically-mediated alterations to the salivary microbiome [19, 33].

Furthermore, whilst modifications in salivary formate concentrations have been previously linked to between-gender differences (i.e. elevated concentrations in males) [28], which we did not find here, our data provides evidence that one potential source for it is the oxidative metabolism of methanol as an ingested and/or inhaled environmental toxin. Indeed, salivary methanol levels are markedly upregulated via tobacco smoke inhalation [23], and/or alternative exogenous sources such as dietary ones. In our study, although salivary formate levels were *ca.* 2-fold greater in males, which may arise from the impaction of an increased smoking frequency for this gender in our smoking cohort, this difference was found not to be statistically significant (**Table 3**).

Interestingly, the study reported in [28] found that salivary citrate, lactate, pyruvate and sucrose levels were significantly upregulated in saliva samples collected from smokers over those of non-smokers, and formate was downregulated therein. Moreover, although salivary methanol concentrations were *ca.* 3-fold greater in smokers than in non-smokers in this study, as might be expected from the current one, this difference was found not to be statistically significant. Similarly, cigarette humectant-derived propane-1,2-diol levels were higher in samples collected from smoking participants in Ref. [28], although again this difference was found not to be significant. Additionally, that investigation detected and determined glucose and sucrose in saliva samples. However, in those collected following the rigorous overnight fasting protocol involved in the current and our other studies, little or none of these carbohydrates are ^{1}H NMR-detectable in HSS samples collected from participant cohorts. Therefore, it appears that the quite limited pre-collection participant restrictions instigated in the study described in [28] was unsuccessful in completely precluding dietary-derived agents from the saliva samples analyzed. Indeed, participants were only required to not consume alcohol on the day of sample collection (and not also the evening before), and these samples were only collected at least 1 h following the last meal, which in our view is insufficient to remove interferences arising from dietary agents, along with those from alcoholic beverages consumed the previous day. Even with a protocol requesting that all participants refrain from the consumption of alcoholic drinks 24 h prior to the sample collection time-point (Section 2.1), traces of ethanol remain ^{1}H NMR-detectable in our saliva specimens when detected at operating frequencies of $\geq$400 MHz. Notwithstanding, generally ethanol consumed at time-points $\geq$ 24 h was not found in 60 MHz salivary ^{1}H NMR profiles in view of the lowered sensitivity of this approach. However, our pilot studies have also shown that if participants drank alcoholic beverages such as a beer, their salivary ethanol levels were indeed detectable and quantifiable using a 60 MHz benchtop NMR facility at least several hours or more thereafter. This observation clearly offers a high level of potential regarding future forensic investigations.

Likewise, citrate is only very rarely ^{1}H NMR-detectable in our HSS samples collected according to our rigorous overnight fasting protocol, and therefore its direct derivation from human diets (which serve as rich sources of this metabolite), and insufficient periods of fasting in Ref. [34], remains a strong possibility.

4. Limitations of the study

One major limitation of the application of LF salivary ^{1}H NMR analysis is inherent resonance overlap problems experienced at this operating frequency, which is much lower than those of more traditional MF or HF spectrometers coupled with restrictively-sized superconducting magnets (for example, those of 400–750 MHz operating frequencies). Hence, these resonance superimposition problems clearly give rise to major analytical limitations, notably in complex multianalyte biofluid spectra. Therefore, for future prospective studies involving the quantification of salivary biomolecules and/or xenobiotics, at least some level of caution should be applied when employing such devices. Unfortunately, these complications increase substantially when integrating resonances of higher first-order and more complex coupling patterns, which may markedly hinder such intensity determinations. Nevertheless, with the exception of the propionate-CH_3 resonance, these interference problems may be considered minimal for the determination of major, high concentration salivary metabolites, specifically those with prominent resonances in LF spectra obtained. Indeed, these signals have only low or negligible levels of superimposition with lower intensity signals, or appear in relatively 'spectroscopically clean' regions of the spectra acquired, for example formate. Therefore, although the LF 60 MHz ^{1}H NMR profiles of HSSs are largely commanded by resonances of the highest intensity and with simple coupling patterns and orders, and/or those arising from metabolites of high concentrations, in principle this novel NMR strategy potentially offers valuable quantitative information for those detectable at lower levels, most notably with the advent of higher-field compact benchtop instruments which operate at frequencies of 80 or 100 MHz.

As observed and further explored in Ref. [10], an additional limitation of ^{1}H NMR-based metabolomics studies featuring LF NMR spectrometers is the intensity-diminishing effects of the H_2O/HOD signal presaturation protocol, notably for signals located close to its chemical shift value (δ = 4.8 ppm). However, although such effects substantially influence the C1-$\underline{H}$ resonances of both the α- and β-glucose anomers (δ = 5.25 and 4.63 ppm respectively), such hurdles may be surmounted by the use of rigorous calibration processes with biomolecule standard solutions, and by the possible integration of alternative resonances derived from the agents affected, namely those with δ values sufficiently distant from the H_2O/HOD secondary irradiation one. An additional limitation arises from some significant differences between intramolecular ^{1}H relaxation times for a number of salivary metabolites, and also some long-range coupling phenomena, results which will be reported in detail elsewhere.

Finally, for the *prima facie* metabolomics investigation conducted here, data available in **Figure 5** indicates that this study may involve a small but significant level of self-reporting bias, since two, or perhaps more, of the non-smoking participant samples appeared to co-cluster with the tobacco-smoking cohort in PCA, PLS-DA and OPLS-DA scores plots, and AHC dendograms, as did those of five of the smoking cohort with the non-smoking group. These apparent erroneously-clustered non-smoking participants may represent those with only a limited or very limited smoking preference, but who preferred to report themselves as 'non-smokers' in this investigation in view of their low smoking incidences and/or smoking irregularities, for example those known as 'closet smokers'. Further investigations to explore this are currently in progress in our laboratories.

5. Conclusions

In this study, we have evaluated the viability of low-field (LF) benchtop ^{1}H NMR analysis technologies for metabolomics investigations of human saliva. This novel, convenient and near-portable technique was used to detect and/or potentially quantify and hence monitor up to 15 potentially healthcare-impacting oral metabolites in healthy human saliva, a strategy prospectively offering much potential for the direct 'on-site' testing of biofluids from patients affected by oral health or related conditions at clinical locations.

We report the detection of typical salivary metabolites, including propionate, acetate, succinate, glycine, dimethylamine, trimethylamine, methanol, formate and aromatic amino acids all at an operating frequency of only 60 MHz. However, quantification of the salivary levels of biomolecules was limited to only five of those with the most prominent ^{1}H NMR signals, although succinate (singlet signal, δ = 2.405 ppm) could also be considered if not significantly quantitatively impacted by salivary pyruvate (*s*, δ = 2.388 ppm) and/or glutamine (*m*, δ = 2.42 ppm) resonances. Indeed, since the singlet resonances of formate, methanol and glycine did not suffer from significant resonance overlap issues, and were therefore quite clearly resolved, the direct LF NMR determination of these biomolecules was possible. Excessive salivary levels of organic acid anion catabolites may serve as key biomarkers of the pathogenesis and development of dental caries [19, 20, 30] and periodontal diseases [19, 32], and herein it was found that both salivary acetate and propionate, which represent biomarkers of dental caries and periodontal diseases respectively, could be readily quantitated in this biofluid, despite some bioanalytical concentration limit/interference problems encountered with the latter.

This study also demonstrated for the first time that LF ^{1}H NMR-linked metabolomics analysis could be employed to discriminate between the salivary biomolecular profiles of tobacco-smoking and non-smoking participants. When detectable at sufficient salivary concentrations, these analyses may be transferable to the detection and perhaps quantification of exogenous agents such as ingested drugs in this biofluid. Moreover, the approach outlined here may indeed offer some forensic applications involving the identification of illicit drugs in human saliva samples collected at crime scenes, provided that such analytes have resonances present in spectrally-clear regions unaffected by overlapping signal interferences arising from endogenous species.

Notwithstanding, currently the authors recommend that future LF NMR investigations of human saliva and oral diseases should focus on the more prominent resonances present in spectra acquired, most notably those with relatively simple first-order coupling patterns (i.e., singlets, doublets, triplets, etc.) for quantification purposes, with the exception of those in which the targeted analyte has resonances(s) located in 'spectroscopically-clear' regions. However, future developments in LF benchtop NMR technologies operating at higher frequencies may serve to provide effective solutions to these issues.

The authors also suggest that this technique may also serve valuable diagnostic and/or prognostic tracking purposes in a clinical context for a range of human diseases. In principle, this non-stationary multi-analytical technique may be employed as a sensitive means of monitoring the salivary metabolic status of patients suffering from oral diseases, and potentially also physiologically-remote conditions, directly at dental surgery and primary healthcare sites, hospitals and hospital laboratories, and perhaps also community pharmacies. In this manner, such patient-contact sites may offer significant diagnostic and monitoring potential for oral health practitioners.

Acknowledgements

The authors wish to express the highest level of thanks to all project participants for the kind donation of their saliva samples for ^{1}H NMR analysis. We are also very grateful to Magritek GmbH, Aachen, Germany for the academic loan of a 60 MHz Magritek Spinsolve Ultra Benchtop NMR Spectrometer for research purposes.

Conflict of interest

The authors declare no conflict of interest.

Author details

Benita C. Percival, Angela Wann, Sophie Taylor, Mark Edgar, Miles Gibson and Martin Grootveld*
Leicester School of Pharmacy, De Montfort University, Leicester, United Kingdom

*Address all correspondence to: mgrootveld@dmu.ac.uk

References

[1] Grootveld M, Percival B, Gibson M, Osman Y, Edgar M, Molinari M, et al. Progress in low-field benchtop NMR spectroscopy in chemical and biochemical analysis. Analytica Chimica Acta. 2019;**1067**:11-30. DOI: 10.1016/j.aca.2019.02.026

[2] Teng Q. NMR-based metabolomics. In: Structural Biology. Boston, MA, US: Springer; 2013. pp. 311-392. DOI: 10.1007/978-1-4614-3964-6_9

[3] Trivedi DK, Hollywood KA, Goodacre R. Metabolomics for the masses: The future of metabolomics in a personalized world. European Journal of Molecular Clinical Medicine. 2017;**3**: 294-305

[4] Pauling L, Robinson AB, Teranishi R, Cary P. Quantitative analysis of urine vapor and breath by gas-liquid partition chromatography. Proceedings of the National Academy of Sciences. 1971;**68**: 2374-2376

[5] Nicholson JK, Buckingham MJ, Sadler PJ. High resolution ^{1}H NMR studies of vertebrate blood and plasma. Biochemical Journal. 1983;**211**:605-615

[6] Nicholson JK, O'Flynn MP, Sadler PJ, MacLeod AF, Juul SM, Sonksen PH. Proton-nuclear-magnetic resonance studies of serum, plasma and urine from fasting normal and diabetic subjects. Biochemical Journal. 1984;**217**:365-375

[7] Wishart DS. Emerging applications of metabolomics in drug discovery and precision medicine. Nature Reviews Drug Discovery. 2016;**15**:473-484

[8] Meiss E, Werner P, John C, Scheja N, Herbach N, Heeren J, et al. Metabolite targeting: Development of a comprehensive targeted metabolomics platform for the assessment of diabetes and its complications. Metabolomics. 2016;**12**:1-15

[9] Dame ZT, Aziat F, Mandal R, Krishnamurthy R, Bouatra S, Borzouie S. The human saliva metabolome. Metabolomics. 2015;**11**:1864-1883. DOI: 10.1007/s11306-015-0840-5

[10] Percival BC, Grootveld M, Gibson M, Molinari M, Jafari F, Sahota T, et al. Low-field, benchtop NMR spectroscopy as a potential tool for point-of-care diagnostics of conditions: Validation, protocols and computational models. High-Throughput. 2018;**8**(1):2. DOI: 10.3390/ht8010002

[11] Edgar M, Percival BC, Gibson M, Jafari F, Grootveld M. Low-field benchtop NMR spectroscopy as a potential non-stationary tool for point-of-care urinary metabolite tracking in diabetic conditions. Diabetes Research and Clinical Practice. 2021;**171**:108554. ISSN 0168-8227. DOI: 10.1016/j.diabres.2020.108554

[12] Gardner A, Carpenter G, So PW. Salivary metabolomics: From diagnostic biomarker discovery to investigating biological function. Metabolites. 2020; **10**(2):47 10.3390/metabo10020047

[13] Miller JN, Miller JC. Statistics and Chemometrics for Analytical Chemistry. London, UK: Pearson Higher Education; 2018. ISBN-13: 9781292186719

[14] Grootveld M. Metabolic Profiling: Disease and Xenobiotics. Cambridge, UK: Royal Society of Chemistry (Issues in Toxicology Series); 2014. ISBN: 1849731632 (395 p)

[15] Ruhl S. The scientific exploration of saliva in the post-proteomic era: From

database back to basic function. Expert Reviews in Proteomics. 2012;**9**:85-96. DOI: 10.1586/epr.11.80

[16] Rad M, Kakoie S, Niliye Brojeni F, Pourdamghan N. Effect of long-term smoking on whole-mouth salivary flow rate and oral health. Journal of Dental Research, Dentistry and Clinical Dental Prospects. 2010;**4**(4):110-114. DOI: 0.5681/joddd.2010.028. Epub 2010 Dec 21

[17] Andrecut MP, GPU. Implementation of iterative PCA algorithms. Journal of Computational Biology. 2009;**16**(11): 1593-1599. DOI: 10.1089/cmb.2008.0221

[18] Palarea-Albaladejo J, Martín-Fernández JA. Values below detection limit in compositional chemical data. Analytica Chimica Acta. 2013;**764**:32-43. ISSN 0003-2670. DOI: 10.1016/j.aca.2012.12.029

[19] Silwood CJL, Lynch E, Claxson AWD, Grootveld MC. ^{1}H and ^{13}C NMR spectroscopic analysis of human saliva. Journal of Dental Research. 2002;**81**:422-427

[20] Silwood CJL, Lynch E, Seddon S, Sheerin A, Claxson AWD, Grootveld MC. ^{1}H-NMR analysis of microbial-derived organic acids in primary root carious lesions and saliva. NMR in Biomedicine. 1999;**12**:345-356

[21] Gardner A, Parkes HG, So P-W, Carpenter GH. Determining bacterial and host contributions to the human salivary metabolome. Journal of Oral Microbiology. 2019;**11**(1):1617014. DOI: 10.1080/20002297.2019.1617014

[22] Pang Z, Chong J, Zhou G, de Lima A, Morais D, Chang L, et al. MetaboAnalyst 5.0: Narrowing the gap between raw spectra and functional insights. Nucleic Acids Research. 2021; **49**:W388-W396

[23] Percival BC, Wann A, Masania J, Sinclair J, Sullo N, Grootveld M. Detection and determination of methanol and further potential toxins in human saliva collected from cigarette smokers: A ^{1}H NMR investigation. JSM Biotechnology Bioengineering. 2018; **5**(1):1081-1088

[24] Park YD, Jang JH, Oh YJ, Kwon HJ. Analyses of organic acids and inorganic anions and their relationship in human saliva before and after glucose intake. Archives of Oral Biology. 2014;**59**(1):1-11. DOI: 10.1016/j.archoralbio.2013.10.006. Epub 2013 Oct 24

[25] Spielmann N, Wong D. Saliva: Diagnostics and therapeutic perspectives. Oral Diseases. 2011;**17**: 345-354

[26] Wong DT. Salivary diagnostics powered by nanotechnologies, proteomics and genomics. Journal of the American Dental Association. 2006;**137**: 313-321

[27] Sugimoto M, Wong DT, Hirayama A, Soga T, Tomita M. Capillary electrophoresis mass spectrometry-based saliva metabolomics identified oral, breast and pancreatic cancer-specific profiles. Metabolomics. 2010;**6**:78-95

[28] Takeda I, Stretchay C, Barnabya P, Bhatnagera K, Rankinb K, Fub H, et al. Understanding the human salivary metabolome. NMR in Biomedicine. 2009;**22**:577-584

[29] Chiappin S, Antonelli G, Gatti R, De Palo EF. Saliva specimen: A new laboratory tool for diagnostic and basic investigation. Clinica Chimimica Acta. 2007;**383**:30-40

[30] Hoppenbrouwers PMM, Driessens FCM. The effect of lactic and acetic acid on the formation of artificial caries lesions. Journal of Dental Research. 1988;**67**:1466-1467

[31] Niederman R, Zhang J, Kashket S. Short-chain carboxylic-acid stimulated, PMN-mediated gingival inflammation. Critical Reviews in Oral Biology and Medicine. 1997;**8**:269-290

[32] Niederman R, Buyle-Bodin Y, Lu BY, Naleway C, Robinson P, Kent R. The relationship of gingival crevicular fluid short chain carboxylic acid concentration to gingival inflammation. Journal of Clinical Periodontology. 1996; **23**:743-749

[33] Guerrant GO, Lambert MA, Moss CW. Analysis of short-chain acids from anaerobic bacteria by high-performance liquid chromatography. Journal of Clinical Microbiology. 1982;**16**:355-360

[34] Gardner A, Parkes HG, Carpenter GH, So P-W. Developing and standardising a protocol for quantitative proton nuclear magnetic resonance (1h nmr) spectroscopy of saliva. Journal of Proteome Research. 2018;**17**:1521-1531

Chapter 9

Molecular Docking of Phytochemicals against *Streptococcus mutans* Virulence Targets: A Proteomic Insight into Drug Planning

Diego Romário da Silva, Tahyná Duda Deps,
Otavio Akira Souza Sakaguchi,
Edja Maria Melo de Brito Costa,
Carlus Alberto Oliveira dos Santos,
Joanilda Paolla Raimundo e Silva,
Bruna Dantas da Silva, Frederico Favaro Ribeiro,
Francisco Jaime Bezerra Mendonça-Júnior
and Andréa Cristina Barbosa da Silva

Abstract

Streptococcus mutans (*S. mutans*) is the most prevalent and most associated with dental caries. Here we aim to identify, through an *in silico* study, potential bioactive molecules against *S. mutans*. Twenty-four bioactive molecules with proven action against S. mutans were selected: 1-methoxyficifolinol; 5,7,2′,4′-tetrahydroxy-8-lavandulylflavanone (sophoraflavanone G); 6,8-diprenylgenistein; apigenin; artocarpesin; artocarpin; darbergioidin; dihydrobiochanin A; dihydrocajanin (5,2′,4′-trihydroxy-7-methoxyisoflavanone); erycristagallin; Erystagallin; ferreirin; fisetin; kaempferol; licoricidin; licorisoflavan A; licorisoflavan C; licorisoflavan E; luteolin (3′,4′,5,7-tetrahydroxyflavone); malvidin-3,5-diglucoside; myricetin; orientanol B; quercetin; and quercitrin. Moreover, we selected nine important target proteins for the virulence of this microorganism to perform as drug targets: antigen I/II (region V) (PDB: 1JMM); Antigen I/II (carbox-terminal region) (PDB: 3QE5); Spap (PDB: 3OPU); UA159sp signaling peptide (PDB: 2I2J); TCP3 signaling peptide (PDB: 2I2H); ATP-binding protein ComA (PDB: 3VX4); glucanosucrase (PDB: 3AIC); dextranase (PDB: 3VMO), and Hemolysin (PDB: 2RK5). Five molecules were revealed to be the best ligands for at least three target proteins, highlighting the following compounds: 11 (erystagallin),

IntechOpen

10 (erycristagallin), 1 (methoxyficifonilol), 20 (malvidin-3,5-diglucoside), and 2 (sophoraflavanone G), which indicates a possible multi-target action of these compounds. Therefore, based on these findings, *in vitro* and *in vivo* tests should be performed to validate the effectiveness of these compounds in inhibiting *S. mutans* virulence factors. Furthermore, the promising results of these assays will allow the incorporation of these phytoconstituents in products for oral use for the control of tooth decay.

Keywords: dental caries, docking molecular, drug planning, phytochemicals, virulence

1. Introduction

The planning and development of new drugs require high-risk and high-cost investments [1]. This process can involve, for example, studying about 5000–10,000 compounds, a period of 7–12 years, and spending about $800 million for a single drug to be marketed [2]. Thus, alternatives that optimize the process and reduce these costs are considered promising [3].

Nevertheless, there are other issues to the success or failure of drugs that must be considered. The main factors responsible for the lack of success in the production of possible drugs during clinical trials are pharmacokinetic factors, such as absorption, distribution, metabolism, excretion, and toxicities [4].

With the evolution of biotechnology and bioinformatics, promising new approaches for drug planning and optimization have become possible [5]. To reduce costs, risks and have greater efficiency in the production process, the pharmaceutical industry has increasingly used *in silico* analysis, which enables the performance of various analytical tasks, such as the quantitative structure-activity relationship of a drug, definition of pharmacophores (region of a ligand molecule that is strongly bound to its receptors), and other forms of modeling [6].

The *in silico* approach to drug development assesses the properties and interactions of a given molecule using computational algorithms [7]. Research in the areas of "omics" (proteomics, genomics, and transcriptomics) has increased due to the use of computational analysis through spectrometry, crystallography, and magnetic resonance techniques, which allows detailed access to the structure of the molecule, thus enabling the planning of medications and also predict their effects [8]. Molecular docking, an *in silico* approach, has been widely used for the planning and development of new drugs [3].

In 1984, the Lock-Key model, proposed by Fisher, explained the theory of ligand-receptor interaction. The model suggested that the interaction between two corresponding structures (ligand and receptor) was due to geometric and energy affinity. In this model, both ligand and receptor were considered rigid structures. The Lock-Key model contributed to the understanding of the mechanism of action of drugs. Nonetheless, it does not explain the interactions in the environment or changes in the spatial conformation of the molecules. Considering these modifications is extremely important, as the conformation of structures can change before and after bonding. Consequently, modern molecular docking tools consider these factors.

Molecular docking assesses the interaction and recognition between macromolecules, in general proteins and ligands [9]. Besides, the algorithm can predict what would happen if these structures interacted in a microenvironment [10].

Prediction of these interactions allows for the creation of structure-based drug design, an advance in drug development as it allows screening of specific molecules for specific targets [11].

Therefore, computer-aided drug design (CADD) uses high-performance computational algorithms to design and optimize molecules to become new drugs. The use of CADD in drug development optimizes the development process, increasing success rate, decreasing laboratory and personnel costs, in addition to producing quick results [3].

Several drugs, currently available for use, have been discovered and improved with the aid of *in silico* tools, such as molecular dockings, zanamivir [12], imatinib [13], nelfinavir [14], and erdafitinib [15]. With the evolution of bioinformatics, biotechnology, and molecular biology, including the determination of protein structures by using X-ray crystallography or nuclear magnetic resonance (NMR) spectroscopy, it has become increasingly easier to use *in silico* tools to predict functioning drugs. Thus, in the last 20 years, more than 60 different molecular docking software were developed by universities and companies [16].

Molecular docking programs have different approaches and their characterization is according to incremental construction approaches, including shape-based algorithms, genetic algorithms, the Monte Carlo method, and systematic search techniques [17–20].

Despite the evidence of the effectiveness and advantage of using molecular docking for drug discovery, studies in this area are still incipient for oral diseases [5], which justifies the performance of new studies. Streptococcus mutans (*S. mutans*), a gram-positive, aciduric, and acidogenic bacterium, is the most prevalent in the dental biofilm [21] and the most studied [22]. This microorganism has relevant virulence factors that enable colonization of the tooth surface, including its high capacity to form biofilms, causing the development of carious lesions [23]. The dominant defense systems of S. mutans for biofilm formation and caries development are its ability to adhere to the surface of teeth and produce acids, associated with its resistance to this environment without suffering damage [24]. Thus, preventing the formation of this microbial complex is one of the most targeted strategies for caries control [23].

Additionally, natural products have been a promising source of positive molecules for drug development over the years [25]. Therefore, plants are a promising source of new chemical compounds (phytochemicals) with high biological potential. Phytochemicals are a class of organic compounds synthesized in small amounts from secondary plant metabolism and are related to plant defense, growth, reproduction, and adaptation, among others. Its main classes of compounds are terpenes, alkaloids, and phenolic compounds [26, 27].

In consequence, in this chapter, we performed, by molecular docking, a screening of molecules from plants that showed results of *in vitro* antimicrobial activity against *S. mutans*, to verify the possibility of interaction and inactivation of virulence factors of this bacteria.

2. Molecular docking between phytochemicals and S. mutans targets

2.1 Selection of the ligands

Ligands were selected from a literature search on phytoconstituents or plants with antimicrobial activity, *in vitro*, against *S. mutans*. The search was performed in the

Pubmed database (http://www.ncbi.nlm.nih.gov/pubmed), using the following terms as keywords: S. mutans, natural products, and anti-cariogenic effects, without language specification or deadline. All articles that addressed the antimicrobial activity of phytoconstituents (isolated molecules) with action on S. mutans, or with activity related to the reduction of cariogenic dental biofilm, were considered relevant. After these filters, 24 articles remained that had defined chemical structures of molecules with an inhibitory effect against S. mutans. The molecules identified and selected for the study in these articles are shown in **Figure 1**.

2.2 Selection of protein targets in *S. mutans*

The first inclusion criterion was the selection of S. mutans target proteins with high relevance for the virulence of this microorganism [28]. The availability of the crystallographic structures resolved and available in the Protein Data Bank (PDB) was the second inclusion criterion. The protein targets (receptors), their functions, PDB identifiers, and grid box coordinates are presented in **Table 1**.

2.3 Molecular docking analysis

Molecular modeling was performed as described by Rodrigues et al. [29]. Using Hyperchem v. 8.0.3, the chemical structures of all compounds of interest (ligands) were drawn and their geometric structures were optimized using the MM+ force field. Subsequently, a new geometry optimization was performed based on the AM1 semi-empirical method (Austin Model 1). The optimized structures were subjected to conformational analysis using Spartan software for Windows 10.0. The Monte Carlo computational method with 1000 interactions, 100 optimization cycles, and 10 conformations with the lowest energy level was selected. The dihedral angles were evaluated by rotation according to the standard conditions (default) of the program, in which the number of simultaneous variations was 1–8, acyclic chains were subjected to rotations from 60 to 180°, and the torsion rings, to rotations from 30 to 120°. The conformations with the lowest minimum energies were selected and saved in .sdf format. Receivers (protein target) were obtained from the PDB. Receiver, PDB id, and selected three-dimensional coordinates for docking are described in **Table 1**. Docking simulations were performed in AutoDock 4.2 software. The preparation of receptors and ligands was performed using VEGA ZZ 3.0.1 and MOLEGRO Molecular Viewer 2.5 software. Initially, ligand and receptor structures were saved in .pqbqt format to be used in docking calculations. Then, PyRx 0.9 software was used to assist in the docking steps and the analysis of the results. The "grid maps", which represent the boxes with three-dimensional coordinates determined for each receiver, were calculated with AutoGrid. Each ligand was docked inside its "grid" with the Lamarckian algorithm implemented in the AutoDock software. The genetics-based algorithm ran 12 simulations per ligand with 2,500,000 energy ratings and a maximum number of 54,000 generations. The crossover rate was increased to 0.8, the gene mutation rate was 0.02, and the number of individuals in each population was 200. All other parameters were left with the default AutoDock settings. The results for each calculation were analyzed to obtain the affinity energy of docking score (Edock) in kcal/mol values for each ligand conformation in its respective complex; structure inaccuracies were ignored in the calculations. To verify the number and positions of hydrogen bonds and non-covalent interactions between each ligand conformation and the catalytic residues of the receptors, the software PyMOL 1.4 and Molegro Molecular Viewer 2.5 were used.

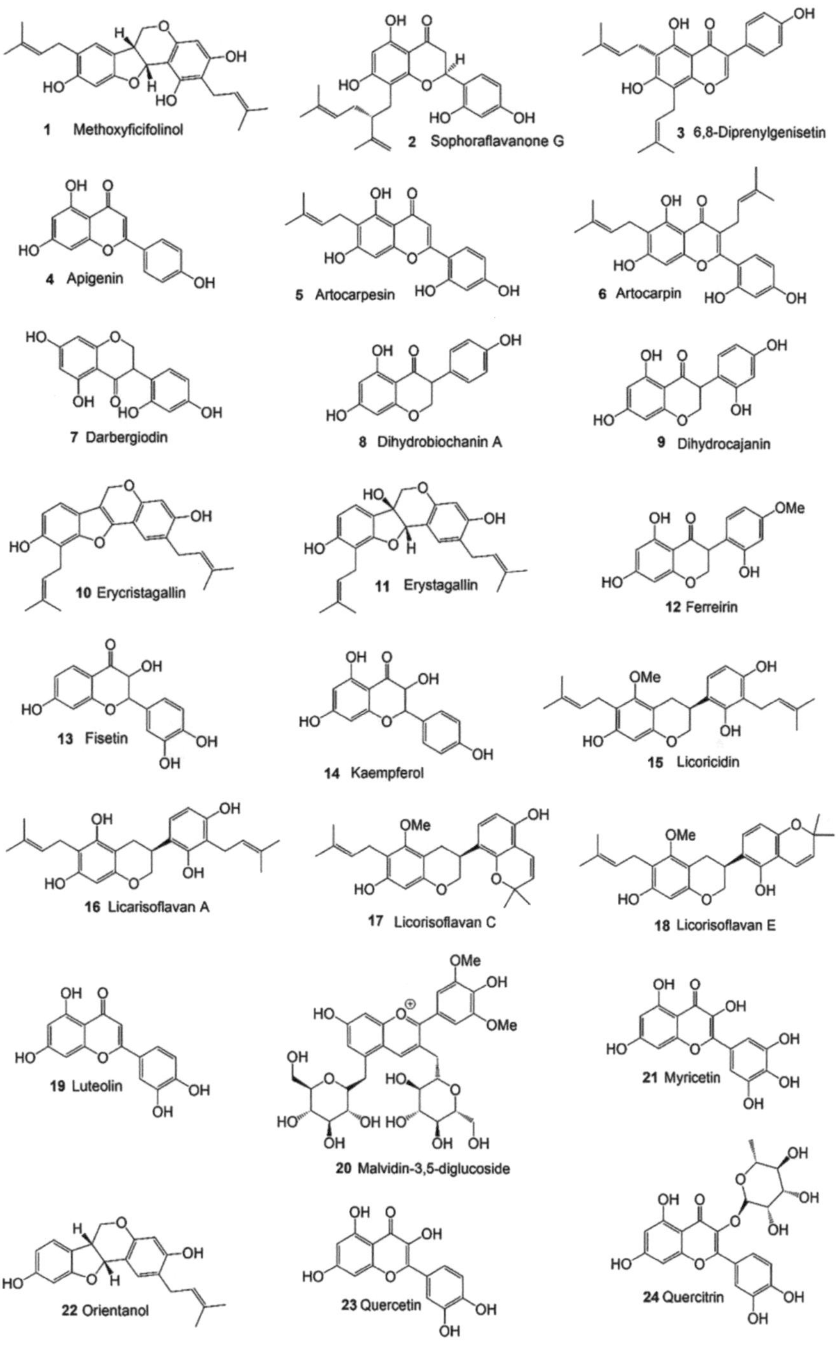

Figure 1.
Selected compounds for molecular docking in S. mutans *target proteins.*

Classification	Macromolecule (receiver)	PDB id	Coordinates			Ray (Å)
Function			X	Y	Z	
Adhesin	Antigen I/II (V-region)	1JMM	34.77	20.04	−7.82	20
Adhesin	Antigen I/II (carboxy-terminal)	3QE5	74.38	44.62	141.82	25
Adhesin	Spap	3OPU	−20.85	53.58	6.16	15
Signaling proteins *(quorum sensing)*	Signaling peptide UA159sp	2I2J	16.12	−1.42	3.73	15
Signaling proteins *(quorum sensing)*	Signaling peptideTCP3	2I2H	11.9	−3.45	0.99	15
Signaling proteins *(quorum sensing)*	ATP binding protein ComA	3VX4	35.31	35.17	13.77	15
Exoenzyme	Glucanosucrase	3AIC	192.19	44.63	197.26	15
Exoenzyme	Dextranase	3VMO	8.71	−13.02	−0.67	15
Exoenzyme	Hemolysin	2RK5	13.57	36.99	17.83	30

Table 1.
Names of macromolecules (receivers), identifier in the Protein Data Bank (PDB id), and selected three-dimensional coordinates for docking.

3. Molecular docking screening results

Molecular docking is an *in silico* methodology that makes it possible to simulate the orientation and conformations (poses) of a ligand near the active site of a target macromolecule, evaluating intermolecular forces, such as hydrophobicity, Van der Waals forces, hydrogen bonds, interactions electrostatic, and ionic bonds. Moreover, this methodology provides the energy of interaction (docking scores), the types of interaction, and the amino acid residues involved in the formation of the ligand-receptor complex [30].

The scores are used as a reference to rank the most stable poses of the ligand. Therefore, the lower the score value, the stronger and more stable the interaction with the selected target. The role and functioning of each of the nine selected S. mutans target proteins are briefly presented below, along with the presentation of the three best ligands for each of the proteins.

3.1 Adhesins

3.1.1 Region V of antigen I/II (PDB id: 1JMM)

The protein-antigen AgI/II is an adhesin present in the cell wall of S. mutans, which recognizes and binds to salivary glycoproteins on the tooth surface, enabling the formation of dental biofilm [31, 32]. Anti-AgI/II antibodies block the adhesion and colonization of S. mutans in the oral cavity [33, 34], justifying the interest in this adhesin in studies aimed at the development of an anticaries therapy [35].

AgI/II adhesin exhibits a functional supramolecular architecture on the cell surface [36], as well as an unusual tertiary structure, where a central variable domain (V-domain) appears like the tip of a formed stem by intertwined and flanked regions rich in alanine and proline [37]. The carboxy-terminal domain (C-domain), connected to a small N-terminal domain that attaches to the cell wall through an anchoring region [38]. AgI/II binding sites for DMBT1 agglutinin are located in the V-domain and C-domain [39].

Docking identified as the best ligands for antigen I/II (V-region) PDB id: 1JMM were the compounds: maldivin-3,5-diglucoside (20) (Edock = −160.78 kJ/mol), licorisoflavan C (17) (Edock = −151.50 kJ/mol), and erystagallin (11) (Edock = −139.85 kJ/mol). Common steric interactions in the complexes formed between Ser818 and Ser697 residues and compounds 17 and 20 were observed. As well as between residue Trp818 and compounds 11 and 17 (**Figure 2**).

3.1.2 Antigen I/II (carboxy-terminal) (PDB id: 3QE5)

The carboxy-terminal domain of antigen I/II, as well as other proteins in this family, can bind salivary glycoproteins, extracellular matrix molecules, and ligands from other bacteria. This category of proteins is not exclusive to **S. mutans**. Homologous proteins subsist in other *Streptococci* [40].

The I/II antigen is highly conserved and may be associated with M protein in other streptococcal species. The carboxy-terminal region (with 800–1540 amino acid residues) includes proline-rich (P) repeats, conferring hydrophobicity, a transmembrane domain (with 1537–1556 amino acid residues), and an LPXTG motif required for anchorage to the cell wall catalyzed by sortase [32, 41].

The phytochemicals with the most promising linkages with the antigen I/II (carboxy-terminus) PDB id: 3QE5 were: erycristagallin (10) (Edock = −128.98 kJ/mol), sophoraflavanone G (2) (Edock = −105.77 kJ/mol), and erystagallin (11) (Edock = −105.16 kJ/mol). All compounds had in common hydrogen bonds with the Lys1120 residue and steric interactions with the Thr1118 residue, thus indicating that these amino acids are important for minimizing the binding energies and stabilizing the complexes (**Figure 3**).

3.1.3 Spap (PDB id: 3OPU)

The Spap protein, also called P1, is a multifunctional adhesin that mediates the sucrose-independent adhesion of bacteria to salivary film glycoproteins on the tooth

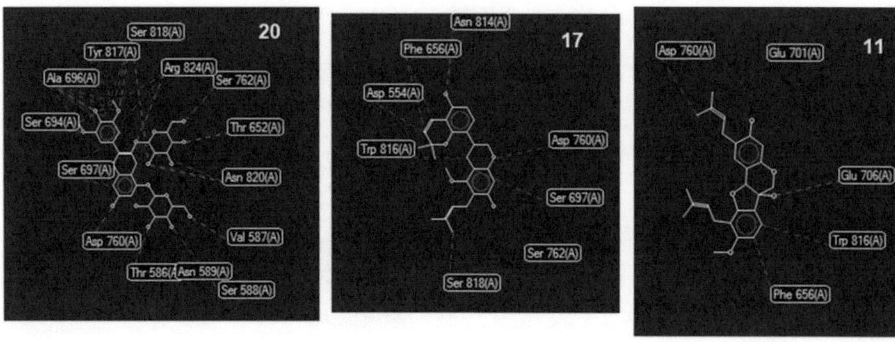

Figure 2.
Representations of the interactions between the three best ligands (compounds 20, 17, and 11) and the amino acid residues of the antigen I/II (V-region) PDB id: 1JMM. Blue dashed lines represent hydrogen bonds and red dashed lines represent steric interactions.

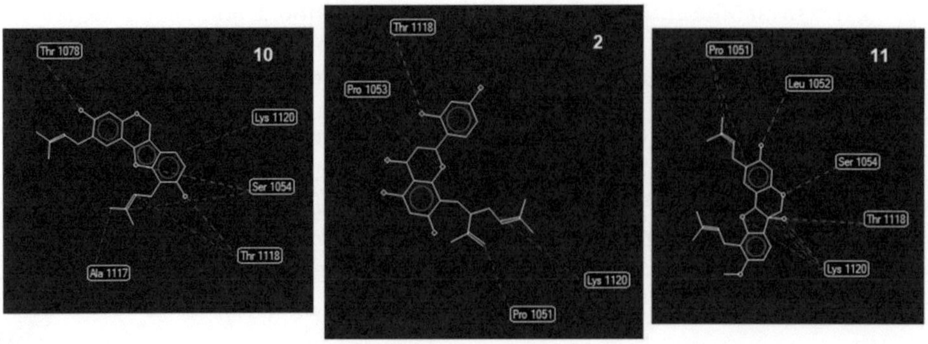

Figure 3.
Representations of the interactions between the three best ligands (compounds 10, 2, and 11) and the amino acid residues of antigen I/II (carboxy-terminal) PDB id: 3QE5. Blue dashed lines represent hydrogen bonds and red dashed lines represent steric interactions.

surface. Like other extracellular proteins, this adhesin can produce amyloid, which, in turn, is present in dental biofilms. Thus, this protein directly interferes with the facilitation and adhesion of cariogenic bacteria [21, 42].

The best interactions with Spap PDB id: 3OPU occurred with the compounds: sophoraflavanone G (2) (Edock = −136.98 kJ/mol), erystagallin (11) (Edock = −134.89 kJ/mol), and licorisoflavan (18) (Edock = −129.64 kJ/mol). The common interactions between these ligands and the active site of the protein, which contributed to the low values of the scores of these molecules, are the steric interactions with residues Lys1261 and Pro1210, and hydrogen bonds with residue Asp1208 (**Figure 4**).

3.2 Quorum sensing-associated signaling proteins

3.2.1 Signaling peptide UA159sp (PDB id: 2I2J)

The peptide-mediated quorum sensing in *S. mutans* is well conserved and regulates its genetic competence [28, 43, 44]. This signaling circuit plays regulatory roles in biofilm formation [43, 45, 46], stress response [47], and bacteriocin production, which are important virulence factors of this bacterium [43, 48].

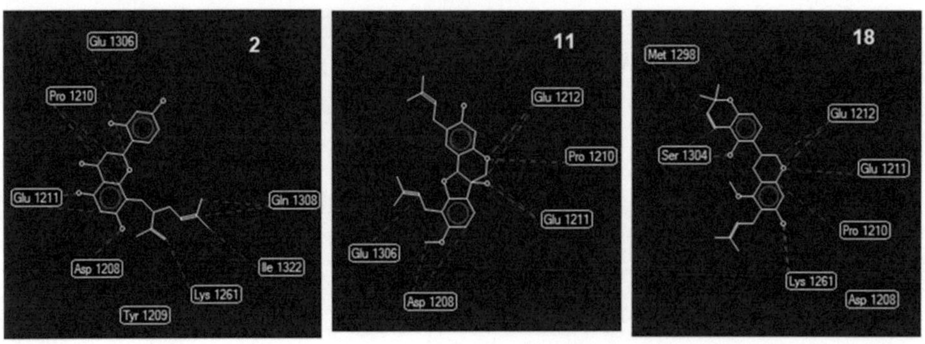

Figure 4.
Representations of the interactions between the three best ligands (compounds 2, 11, and 18) and the amino acid residues of Spap PDB id: 3OPU. Blue dashed lines represent hydrogen bonds and red dashed lines represent steric interactions.

Quorum-sensing allows bacterial communication, providing benefits during host colonization, defense against competitors, and adaptation to the environment [43, 49]. The chemical details of the signaling molecules of this system in **S. mutans** are known and only UA159sp has been identified as a signal peptide in wild-type **S. mutans** strain [44].

In a study, conducted by Syvitski et al. [50], peptides in which three or more residues were deleted from the C-terminal region of the signaling peptide UA159sp did not induce genetic competence and inhibited, by competition, the quorum sensing activated by UA159sp. Disruption of the amphipathic α-helix by replacing Phe-7, Phe-11, or Phe-15 residues with a hydrophilic residue resulted in a significant reduction or complete loss of peptide activity. In contrast to peptides truncated at the C-terminal region, these peptides with amino acid substitutions did not compete with UA159sp to activate quorum sensing, suggesting that disruption of the hydrophobic face of the α-helix structure results in a peptide that is not capable of binding to the receptor. Therefore, residues of the C-terminal region of the signaling peptide in the quorum-sensing system of streptococci are extremely important.

Quorum-sensing inhibitor drug design enables the development of more specific treatments for biofilm-dependent infectious diseases [51]. A benefit of using quorum sensing inhibitor drugs is that they are less susceptible to antimicrobial resistance than other antimicrobials, as they exert a lower selective pressure and do not directly kill bacterial cells [52].

Docking with the signaling peptide UA159sp PDB id: 2I2J identified as the best ligands the compounds: erystagallin (11) (Edock = −84.98 kJ/mol), erycristagallin (10) (Edock = −83.99 kJ/mol), and methoxyficifolinol (1) (Edock = −79.76 kJ/mol). In all ligands, the presence of hydrogen bonds with the Ser14 residue and steric interactions with the Ala18 residue is indicative of their importance for the stability of the interaction of these compounds with the active site (**Figure 5**).

3.2.2 Signaling peptide TPC3 (PDB id: 2I2H)

TPC3 peptide is a signal peptide synthesized by the mutant strain of **S. mutans** JH1005 that also can activate the quorum-sensing system.

For the signaling peptide TCP3 PDB id: 2I2H the best ligands were: erycristagallin (10) (Edock = −-99.74 kJ/mol), sophoraflavanone G (2) (Edock = −93.23 kJ/mol), and methoxyficifolinol (1) (Edock = −88.16 kJ/mol). As can be seen in **Figure 6**, hydrogen

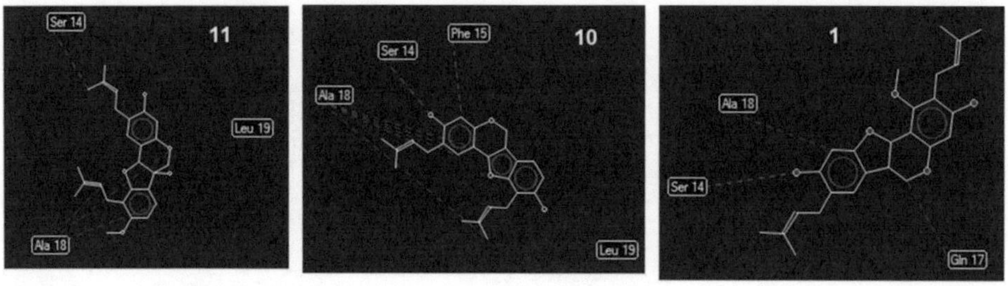

Figure 5.
Representations of the interactions between the three best ligands (compounds 11, 10, and 1) and the amino acid residues of the signal peptide UA159sp PDB id: 2I2J. Blue dashed lines represent hydrogen bonds and red dashed lines represent steric interactions.

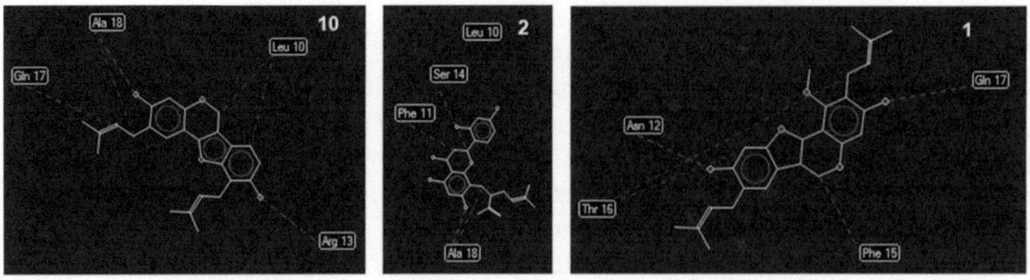

Figure 6.
Representations of the interactions between the three best ligands (compounds 10, 2, and 1) and the amino acid residues of the signal peptide TCP3 PDB id: 2I2H. Blue dashed lines represent hydrogen bonds and red dashed lines represent steric interactions.

bonds and steric interactions with Ala18 and Leu10 residues contributed to the energy reduction of these complexes, especially of the best ligands.

3.2.3 ATP binding protein ComA (PDB: 3VX4)

Quorum sensing is mediated by a signaling molecule autoinducer [53]. This system in some streptococcal species such as **S. mutans** is the ComABCDE pathway, in which inducing peptides are processed from the ComC precursor and exported to the extracellular space by ComA and ComB [43, 54]. ComA is a bifunctional ATP-binding cassette transporter comprising three domains: an N-terminal peptidase domain (PEP), a transmembrane domain, and a C-terminal nucleotide linker domain [55–57]. PEP is a peptidase belonging to the cysteine protease family [55, 58–60].

Docking with the ATP binding protein ComA PDB id: 3VX4 identified as the best ligands the compounds: licorisoflavan A (16) (Edock = −-132.56 kJ/mol), licoricidin (15) (Edock = −128.75 kJ/mol), and methoxyficifolinol (1) (Edock = −127.50 kJ/mol). When observing the interactions of the best ligands in the formed complexes, it was observed that hydrogen bonds with residues Thr568 and Ser563 and steric interactions with Lys567 are common, indicating that these interactions contributed to the reduction of the interaction energy and stabilization of the complexes (**Figure** 7).

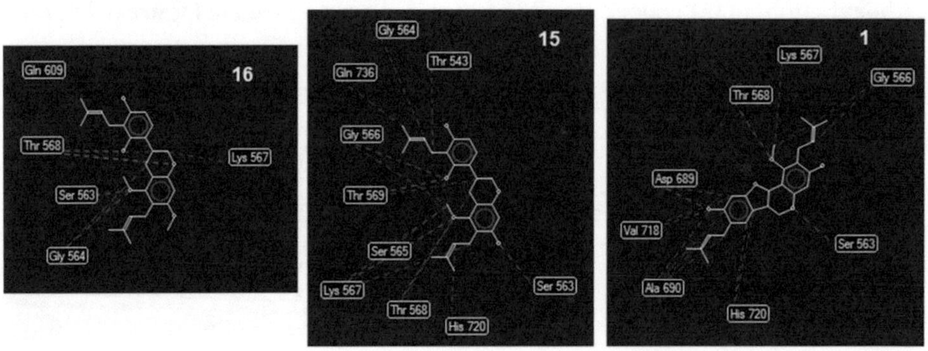

Figure 7.
Representations of the interactions between the three best ligands (compounds 16, 15, and 1) and the amino acid residues of the ATP binding protein ComA PDB id: 3VX4. Blue dashed lines represent hydrogen bonds and red dashed lines represent steric interactions.

3.3 Exoenzymes

3.3.1 Glucanosyucrase (PDB id: 3AIC)

Glucansucrases or glycosyltransferases (GTFs) are extracellular enzymes, produced by various bacteria, including **S. mutans**, that cleave sucrose into glucose and fructose and build sticky biofilm chains. The growth of the glucan chain was associated with adherence of one bacteria to another and the dental surface. Furthermore, modulate the diffusion of substances through the biofilm, which could occasionally serve as an extracellular energy reserve [61].

The glucanosucrase in *S. mutans* allows the metabolism of sucrose into lactic acid, which reduces the pH around the tooth, facilitating the dissolution of calcium phosphate from tooth enamel, which induces tooth decay [62]. These characteristics make the **S. mutans** glucanosucrase as one of the main and most studied targets for the development of new agents useful in the prevention of dental caries.

The best ligands that interacted with glucansucrase PDB id: 3AIC in the docking simulation were: erycrystagallin (10) (Edock = −145.72 kJ/mol), malvidin-3,5-diglucoside (20) (Edock = −138.84 kJ/mol), and erystagallin (11) (Edock = −136.44 kJ/mol). Hydrogen bonds with residues Asp480, Asp481, Asn537, and steric interactions with residues Leu433, Glu515, and Trp517 are common to the two best ligands and seem to be important for reducing the energy of formation of these complexes (**Figure 8**).

The docking study conducted out by Kim et al. [63] between rubusoside and **S. mutans** glucanosucrase (PDB id: 3AIC), identified residues Leu 433, Leu434, Ala478, Asp480, Glu515, Trp517, and Tyr916 as the main ones involved in the stabilization of the complex, and validated these residues as important anchoring sites for potential inhibitors of this enzyme.

Bhagavathy, Mahendiran, and Kanchana [64], performed molecular docking between seven phytochemical isolates of *Psidium guajava* and *S. mutans* glucanosucrase (PDB id: 3AIB) and demonstrated that the main residues involved in the formation of the complexes were Thr426, Ile427, Gln553, and Tyr978. These residues diverged from those identified in this study.

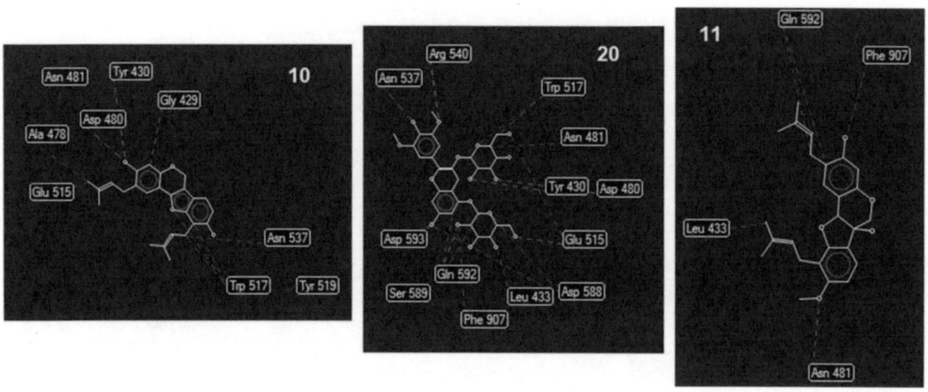

Figure 8.
Representations of the interactions between the three best ligands (compounds 10, 20, and 11) and the amino acid residues of the glucanoscarase PDB id: 3AIC. Blue dashed lines represent hydrogen bonds and red dashed lines represent steric interactions.

Opposing, Islam et al. [65] performed a molecular docking study between epigallocatechin gallate (EGCG) and the same **S. mutans** enzyme, glucanosucrase (PDB id: 3AIB). The results showed that the main interactions that stabilize the complex of the ligand (EGCG) with the enzyme occurred between the amino acid residues Glu515 and Trp517, which were the same residues identified in our work, reinforcing the importance of these residues for the stabilization of the complex.

3.3.2 Dextranase (PDB id: 3VMO)

S. mutans dextranase is an enzyme that hydrolyzes the α-1,6 bonds of dextran and produces isomalto-oligosaccharides of different sizes for metabolic use [66, 67]. This protein is composed of 850 aa residues with a molecular mass of 94.5 kDa, but it has multiple native and recombinant forms [68, 69]. According to the sequencing of several enzymes in this family, dextranases are divided into five regions: a signal peptide sequence (N-terminal with 24 aa), a variable N-terminal region (Ser25-Asn99), a conserved region (Gln100-Ala615), a glucan binding site (Leu616-Ile732), and a C-terminal variable region (Asn733-Asp850) [70, 71].

Some biochemical studies, based on the comparison of amino acid sequences with other glycosyltransferases, revealed that the Asp385 residue is essential for the catalytic reaction [72]. Besides, it was observed that Asp270 from cycloisomalto oligosaccharide glucanotransferases from *Bacillus circulans* T3040 [73] and Asp243 from endodextranase from *Thermotoga lettingae* TMO [74], corresponding to Asp385 from dextranase from **Streptococcus mutans**, were recognized as **S. mutans** residues catalytic.

Molecular docking performed with the dextranase PDB id: 3VMO identified as the best ligands: licorisoflavan A (16) (Edock = −138.02 kJ/mol), malvidin-3,5-diglucoside (20) (Edock = −136.94 kJ μg/mol), and licoricidin (15) (Edock = −129.73 kJ/mol). Compounds 15 and 16 showed steric interactions in common with residues Tyr257 and Ala559 and showed steric interactions and hydrogen bonds with the key residue Asp385 which has already been identified as essential for catalytic reaction. Diglucoside 20, on the other hand, had a lower energy conformation distinct from compounds 15 and 16 and interacted with other amino acid residues in the active site of the enzyme (**Figure 9**).

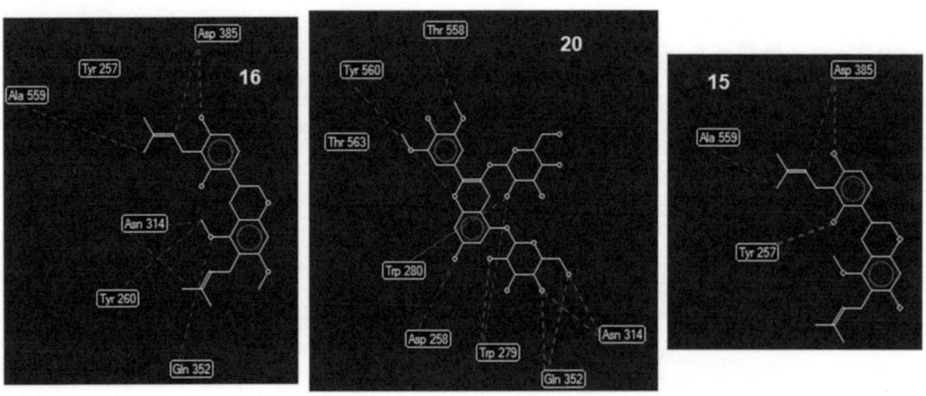

Figure 9.
Representations of the interactions between the three best ligands (compounds 16, 20, and 15) and the amino acid residues of dextranase PDB id: 3VMO. Blue dashed lines represent hydrogen bonds and red dashed lines represent steric interactions.

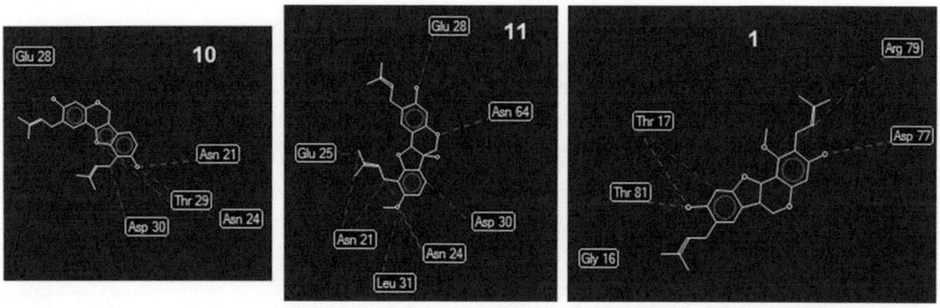

Figure 10.
Representations of the interactions between the three best ligands (compounds 10, 11, and 1) and the amino acid residues of hemolysin PDB id: 2RK5. Blue dashed lines represent hydrogen bonds and red dashed lines represent steric interactions.

3.3.3 Hemolysin (PDB id: 2RK5)

Hemolysins are exotoxins capable of promoting erythrocyte lysis. They are toxins produced by some species of streptococci [75] and contribute to the virulence process of **S. mutans** [76]. In **S. mutans**, alpha- and gamma-hemolytic strains are described [77], as well as beta-hemolytic [78].

Docking with hemolysin PDB id: 3VMO identified as the best ligands the compounds: erycristagallin (10) (Edock = −112.64 kJ/mol), erystagallin (11) (Edock = −104.10 kJ/mol), and methoxyficifolinol (1) (Edock = −100.63 kJ/mol). The steric interactions and hydrogen bonds with Asn21, Asn24, and Asp30 residues were common for compounds 10 and 11, and seem to be important for the stabilization of the complexes. Compound 1, despite belonging to the same chemical class as compounds 10 and 11, showed a more stable conformation in another position of the active site, consequently, is stabilized by interactions with different amino acid residues, but which contributed less to the stabilization of the complex (**Figure 10**).

4. Concluding remarks

In the research phase for phytochemicals with activity against *S. mutans*, carried out in the present study, no specific research was carried out for the classes of phytoconstituents. However, surprisingly, all isolated and identified chemical structures (24 compounds) belonged to the class of phenolic compounds, more specifically the class of flavonoids (2, 3, 4, 5, 6, 7, 8, 9, 12, 13, 14, 15, 16, 17, 18, 19, 20, 21, 23, 24) and isoflavonoid derivatives (1, 10, 11, and 22).

Five phytocompounds evaluated were elected as one of the three best ligands for at least three target proteins, highlighting the following compounds: 11 (erystagallin) (highlighted for 6 targets), 10 (erycristagallin) (highlighted for 5 targets), 1 (methoxyficifonilol) (highlighted for 4 targets), 20 (malvidin-3,5-diglucoside), and 2 (sophoraflavanone G), which provided indications of a possible and desirable multi-target action of these compounds.

Based on these findings, these selected compounds should have theirs *in vitro* and *in vivo* activities evaluated, to validate the efficiency of these compounds in inhibiting the virulence factors of planktonic *S. mutans* and in biofilms. The positive results in these tests will allow the incorporation of these phytoconstituents in toothpaste, mouthwashes, among others, and could be an effective alternative for the control of tooth decay.

Acknowledgements

This work was supported by National Council for Scientific and Technological Development (CNPq) [grant number 308590/2017-1], and Coordination for the Improvement of Higher Education Personnel (CAPES), Brazil [financing code 001].

Conflict of interest

The authors declare that they have no conflict of interest with this manuscript.

Author details

Diego Romário da Silva[1,2], Tahyná Duda Deps[1,2], Otavio Akira Souza Sakaguchi[3], Edja Maria Melo de Brito Costa[4], Carlus Alberto Oliveira dos Santos[4], Joanilda Paolla Raimundo e Silva[4], Bruna Dantas da Silva[5], Frederico Favaro Ribeiro[6], Francisco Jaime Bezerra Mendonça-Júnior[6] and Andréa Cristina Barbosa da Silva[7]*

1 Faipe College, Cuiabá, Mato Grosso, Brazil

2 Garça Branca Pantanal College, Cuiabá, Mato Grosso, Brazil

3 Department of Dentistry, Northern College of Mato Grosso, Guarantã do Norte, Mato Grosso, Brazil

4 Department of Dentistry, State University of Paraiba (UEPB), Campina Grande, PB, Brazil

5 Department of Dentistry, State University of Paraiba (UEPB), Araruna, PB, Brazil

6 Laboratory of Synthesis and Drug Delivery, Biological Science Department, State University of Paraiba (UEPB), João Pessoa, PB, Brazil

7 Department of Pharmacy, State University of Paraiba (UEPB), Campina Grande, PB, Brazil

*Address all correspondence to: andreacbsilva@gmail.com

References

[1] Khanna I. Descoberta de medicamentos na indústria farmacêutica: Desafios e tendências de produtividade. Drug Discovery Today. 2012;**17**:1088-1102

[2] Morgan S, Grootendorst P, Lexchin J, Cunningham C, Greyson D. The cost of drug development: A systematic review. Health Policy. 2011;**100**(1):4-17. DOI: 10.1016/j.healthpol.2010.12.002

[3] Silva DR, Sardi JCO, Freires IA, Silva ACB, Rosalen PL. In silico approaches for screening molecular targets in *Candida albicans*: A proteomic insight into drug discovery and development. European Journal of Pharmacology. 2018;**842**:64-69. DOI: 10.1016/j.ejphar.2018.10.016

[4] van de Waterbeemd H, Gifford E. ADMET in silico modelling: Towards prediction paradise? Nature Reviews. Drug Discovery. 2003;**2**(3):192-204

[5] da Silva ACB, da Silva DR, de Macedo Ferreira SA, Agripino GG, Albuquerque AR, do Rego TG. In silico approach for the identification of potential targets and specific antimicrobials for *Streptococcus mutans*. Advances in Bioscience and Biotechnology. 2014;**5**(4):373-385

[6] Ekins S, Mestres J, Testa B. In silico pharmacology for drug discovery: Applications to targets and beyond. British Journal of Pharmacology. 2007;**152**:21-37. DOI: 10.1038/sj.bjp.0707306

[7] Singla RK. Editorial: In silico drug design and medicinal chemistry. Current Topics in Medicinal Chemistry. 2015;**15**(11):971-972. DOI: 10.2174/156802661511150408110453

[8] Meng XY, Zhang HX, Mezei M, Cui M. Molecular docking: A powerful approach for structure-based drug discovery. Current Computer-Aided Drug Design. 2011;**7**:146-157. hh

[9] Xue LC, Dobbs D, Bonvin AM, Honavar V. Computational prediction of protein interfaces: A review of data driven methods. FEBS Letters. 2015;**589**:3516-3526

[10] Chen G, Seukep AJ, Guo M. Recent advances in molecular docking for the research and discovery of potential marine drugs. Marine Drugs. 2020 Oct 30;**18**(11):545. DOI: 10.3390/md18110545

[11] Kitchen DB, Decornez H, Furr JR, Bajorath J. Docking and scoring in virtual screening for drug discovery: Methods and applications. Nature Reviews. Drug Discovery. 2004;**3**:935-949

[12] Von Itzstein M, Wu WY, Kok GB, Pegg MS, Dyason JC, Jin B, et al. Rational design of potent sialidase-based inhibitors of influenza virus replication. Nature. 1993;**363**(6428):18-423

[13] Druker BJ, Lydon NB. Lessons learned from the development of an Abl tyrosine kinase inhibitor. The Journal of Clinical Investigation. 2000;**105**(1):3-7

[14] Kaldor SW, Kalish VJ, Davies JF, Shetty BV, Fritz JE, Appelt K, et al. Viracept (nelfinavir mesylate, AG 1343): A potent, orally bioavailable inhibitor of HIV-1 protease. Journal of Medicinal Chemistry. 1997;**40**(24):3979-3985

[15] Squires M, Ward G, Saxty G, Berdini V, Cleasby A, King P, et al. Potent, selective inhibitors of fibroblast growth factor receptor define fibroblast

growth factor dependence in preclinical cancer models. Molecular Cancer Therapeutics. 2011;**10**(9):1542-1552

[16] Stanzione F, Giangreco I, Cole JC. Use of molecular docking computational tools in drug discovery. Progress in Medicinal Chemistry. 2021;**60**:273-343. DOI: 10.1016/bs.pmch.2021.01.004

[17] Rarey M, Kramer B, Lengauer T, Klebe G. A fast flexible docking method using an incremental construction algorithm. Journal of Molecular Biology. 1996;**261**(3):470-489. DOI: 10.1006/jmbi.1996.0477

[18] Brooijmans N, Kuntz ID. Molecular recognition and docking algorithms. Annual Review of Biophysics and Biomolecular Structure. 2003;**32**:335-373. DOI: 10.1146/annurev.biophys.32.110601.142532

[19] Jones G, Willett P, Glen RC, Leach AR, Taylor R. Development and validation of a genetic algorithm for flexible docking. Journal of Molecular Biology. 1997;**267**(3):727-748. DOI: 10.1006/jmbi.1996.0897

[20] Venkatachalam CM, Jiang X, Oldfield T, Waldman M. LigandFit: A novel method for the shape-directed rapid docking of ligands to protein active sites. Journal of Molecular Graphics & Modelling. 2003;**21**(4):289-307. DOI: 10.1016/s1093-3263(02)00164-x

[21] Wen ZT, Yates D, Ahn S-J, Burne RA. Biofilm formation and virulence expression by *Streptococcus mutans* are altered when grown in dual-species model. BMC Microbiology. 2010;**10**:111. DOI: 10.1186/1471-2180-10-111

[22] Klein MI, Debaz L, Agidi S, Lee H, Xie G, Lin AH-M, et al. Dynamics of *Streptococcus mutans* transcriptome in response to starch and sucrose during biofilm development. PLoS One. 2010;**5**(10):e13478

[23] Loesche WJ. Role of *Streptococcus mutans* in human dental decay. Microbiological Reviews. 1986;**50**(4):353-380. DOI: 10.1128/mr.50.4.353-380.1986

[24] Michalek S, Childers NK. Development and outlook for a caries vaccine. 1990;**1**(1):37-54. DOI: 10.1177/10454411900010010401

[25] Newman DJ, Cragg GM. Natural products as sources of new drugs over the nearly four decades from 01/1981 to 09/2019. Journal of Natural Products. 2020;**83**(3):770-803. DOI: 10.1021/acs.jnatprod.9b01285

[26] Isah T. Stress and defense responses in plant secondary metabolites production. Biological Research. 2019;**52**:39. DOI: 10.1186/s40659-019-0246-3

[27] Mera IFG, Falconí DEG, Córdova VM. Secondary metabolites in plants: Main classes, phytochemical analysis and pharmacological activities. Bionatura. 2019;**4**(4):1000-1009. DOI: 10.21931/RB/2019.04.04.11

[28] Ajdic D et al. Genome sequence of *Streptococcus mutans* UA159, a cariogenic dental pathogen. PNAS. 2002;**99**(22):14434-14439. DOI: 10.1073/pnas.172501299

[29] Rodrigues KAF, Dias CNS, Néris PLN, Rocha JC, Scotti MT, Scotti L, et al. European Journal of Medicinal Chemistry. 2015;**106**:1-14

[30] Ribeiro FF. Uso de ferramentas do planejamento racional de fármacos auxiliado por computador aplicado a uma série de tiossemicarbazonas e seus bioisósteros frente à doença de chagas [Tese (doutorado)]. Recife: Universidade

Federal de Pernambuco. Centro de Biociências. Programa de Pós-graduação em Inovação Terapêutica; 2018. 153 f

[31] Koga T, Okahashi N, Takahashi I, Kanamoto T, Asakawa H, Iwaki M. Surface hydrophobicity, adherence, and aggregation of cell surface protein antigen mutants of *Streptococcus mutans* serotype c. Infection and Immunity. 1990;**58**:289-296

[32] Kelly CG, Todryk S, Kendal HL, Munro GH, Lehner T. T-cell, adhesion, and B-cell epitopes of the cell surface *Streptococcus mutans* protein antigen I/II. Infection and Immunity. 1995;**63**: 3649-3658

[33] Ma JK, Hunjan M, Smith R, Kelly C, Lehner T. An investigation into the mechanism of protection by local passive immunization with monoclonal antibodies against *Streptococcus mutans*. Infection and Immunity. 1990;**58**: 3407-3414

[34] Ma JK, Hikmat BY, Wycoif K, Vine ND, Chargelegue D, Yu L, et al. Characterization of a recombinant plant monoclonal secretory antibody and preventive immunotherapy in humans. Nature Medicine. 1998;**4**:601-606

[35] Taubman MA, Nash DA. The scientific and public-health imperative for a vaccine against dental caries. Nature Reviews. Immunology. 2006;**6**:555-563

[36] Heim KP, Sullan RMA, Crowley PJ, El-Kirat-Chatel S, Beaussart A, Tang W, et al. Identification of a supramolecular functional architecture of *Streptococcus mutans* adhesin P1 on the bacterial cell surface. The Journal of Biological Chemistry. 2015;**290**:9002-9019

[37] Larson MR, Rajashankar KR, Patel MH, Robinette RA, Crowley PJ, Michalek S, et al. Elongated fibrillar structure of a streptococcal adhesin assembled by the high-affinity association of a- and PPII-helices. Proceedings of the National Academy of Sciences of the United States of America. 2010;**107**:5983-5988

[38] Heim KP, Crowley PJ, Long JR, Kailasan S, McKenna R, Brady LJ. An intramolecular lock facilitates folding and stabilizes the tertiary structure of *Streptococcus mutans* adhesin P1. Proceedings of the National Academy of Sciences. 2014;**111**:15746-15751

[39] Heim KP, Crowley PJ, Brady LJ. An intramolecular interaction involving the N terminus of a streptococcal adhesin affects its conformation and adhesive function. The Journal of Biological Chemistry. 2013;**288**(288):13762-13774

[40] Jakubovics NS, Strömberg N, Dolleweerd CJV, Kelly CG, Jenkinson HF. Differential binding specificities of oral streptococcal antigen I/II family adhesins for human or bacterial ligands. Molecular Microbiology. 2005;**55**(5):1591-1605. DOI: 10.1111/j.1365-2958.2005.04495.x

[41] Brady LJ, Maddocks SE, Larson MR, et al. 2010. The changing faces of Streptococcus antigen I/II polypeptide family adhesins. Molecular Microbiology. 2010;**77**(2):276-286. DOI: 10.1111/j.1365-2958.2010.07212.x

[42] Liao S, Klein MI, Heim KP, Fan Y, Bitoun JO, Ahn S-J, et al. *Streptococcus mutans* extracellular DNA is upregulated during growth in biofilms, actively released via membrane vesicles, and influenced by components of the protein secretion machinary. Journal of Bacteriology. 2014;**196**(13):2355-2366

[43] Cvitkovitch DG, Li Y-H, Ellen RP. Quorum sensing and biofilm formation in Streptococcal infections. The Journal of Clinical Investigation. 2003;**112**(11): 1626-1632. DOI: 10.1172/JCI20430

[44] Li YH, Lau PCY, Lee JH, Ellen RP, Cvitkovitch DG. Natural genetic transformation of *Streptococcus mutans* growing in biofilms. Journal of Bacteriology. 2001;**183**:897-908

[45] Aspiras MB, Ellen RP, Cvitkovitch DG. ComX activity of *Streptococcus mutans* growing in biofilms. FEMS Microbiology Letters. 2004;**238**:167-174

[46] Li YH, Tang N, Lau PCY, Aspiras MB, Ellen RP, Cvitkovitch DG. A quorum sensing signaling system essential for genetic competence in *Streptococcus mutans* is involved in biofilm formation. Journal of Bacteriology. 2002;**184**:2699-2708

[47] Li YH, Hanna MN, Svensäter G, Ellen RP, Cvitkovitch DG. Cell density modulates acid adaptation in *Streptococcus mutans*: Implication for survival in biofilms. Journal of Bacteriology. 2001;**183**:6875-6884

[48] Kuramitsu HK. Virulence factors of mutans streptococci: Role of molecular genetics. Critical Reviews in Oral Biology and Medicine. 1993;**4**:159-176

[49] Kolenbrander PE, Andersen RN, Blehert DS, Egland PG, Foster JS, Parmer RJ Jr. Communication among oral bacteria. Microbiology and Molecular Biology Reviews. 2002;**66**:486-505

[50] Syvitski RT, Tian XL, Sampara K, Salman A, Lee SF, Jakeman DJ, et al. Structure-activity analysis of quorum-sensing signaling peptides from *Streptococcus mutans*. Journal of Bacteriology. 2007;**189**(4):1441-1450. DOI: 10.1128/JB.00832-06

[51] Ishii S, Fukui K, Yokoshima S, Kumagai K, Beniyama Y, Kodama T, et al. High-throughput screening of small molecule inhibitors of the streptococcus quorum-sensing signal pathway. Scientific Reports. 2017;7:4029. DOI: 10.1038/s41598-017-03567-2

[52] Garcia-Contreras R, Maeda T, Wood TK. Can resistance against quorum-sensing interference be selected? The ISME Journal. 2016;**10**:4-10

[53] Fuqua WC, Winans SC, Greenberg EP. Quorum sensing in bacteria: The LuxR-LuxI family of cell density-responsive transcriptional regulators. Journal of Bacteriology. 1994;**176**:269-275

[54] Hossain MS, Biswas I. An extracellular protease, SepM, generates functional competence-stimulating peptide in *Streptococcus mutans* UA159. Journal of Bacteriology. 2012;**194**:5886-5896

[55] Håvarstein LS, Diep DB, Nes IF. A family of bacteriocin ABC transporters carry out proteolytic processing of their substrates concomitant with export. Molecular Microbiology. 1995;**16**:229-240

[56] Lin DY, Huang S, Chen J. Crystal structures of a polypeptide processing and secretion transporter. Nature. 2015;**523**:425-430

[57] Ishii S, Yano T, Hayashi H. Expression and characterization of the peptidase domain of *Streptococcus pneumoniae* ComA, a bifunctional ATP-binding cassette transporter involved in quorum sensing pathway. The Journal of Biological Chemistry. 2006;**281**:4726-4731

[58] Ishii S, Yano T, Okamoto A, Murakawa T, Hayashi H. Boundary of the nucleotide-binding domain of Streptococcus ComA based on functional and structural analysis. Biochemistry. 2013;**52**:2545-2555

[59] Kotake Y, Ishii S, Yano T, Katsuoka Y, Hayashi H. Substrate recognition mechanism of the peptidase domain of the quorum sensing-signal-producing ABC transporter ComA from Streptococcus. Biochemistry. 2008;**47**: 2531-2538

[60] Ishii S et al. Crystal structure of the peptidase domain of Streptococcus ComA, a bifunctional ATP-binding cassette transporter involved in the quorum-sensing pathway. The Journal of Biological Chemistry. 2010;**285**: 10777-10785

[61] van Hijum SA, Kralj S, Ozimek LK, Dijkhuizen L, van Geel-Schutten IG. Structure-function relationships of glucansucrase and fructansucrase enzymes from lactic acid bacteria. Microbiology and Molecular Biology Reviews. 2006;**70**(1):157-176

[62] Featherstone JD. Dental caries: A dynamic disease process. Australian Dental Journal. 2008;**53**(3):286-291. DOI: 10.1111/j.1834-7819.2008.00064.x

[63] Kim et al. Anti-cariogenic characteristics of rubusoside. Biotechnology and Bioprocess Engineering. 2019;**24**:282-287. DOI: 10.1007/s12257-018-0408-0

[64] Bhagavathy S, Mahendiran C, Kanchana R. Identification of glucosyl transferase inhibitors from *Psidium guajava* against *Streptococcus mutans* in dental caries. Journal of Traditional and Complementary Medicine. 2018;**9**(2): 124-137. DOI: 10.1016/j.jtcme.2017.09.003

[65] Islam et al. Inhibitory potential of EGCG on *Streptococcus mutans* biofilm: A new approach to prevent cariogenesis. Microbial Pathogenesis. 2020;**143**: 104129

[66] Walker GJ, Pulkownik A, Morrey-Jones JG. Metabolism of the polysaccharides of human dental plaque: Release of dextranase in batch cultures of *Streptococcus mutans*. Journal of General Microbiology. 1981;**127**(1): 201-208. DOI: 10.1099/00221287-127-1-201

[67] Colby SM, Whiting GC, Russell RR. Inactivation of the dextranase gene in *Streptococcus mutans*. Developments in Biological Standardization. 1995;**85**: 377-381

[68] Igarashi T, Yamamoto A, Goto N. Sequence analysis of the *Streptococcus mutans* Ingbritt dexA gene encoding extracellular dextranase. Microbiology and Immunology. 1995;**39**(11):853-860. DOI: 10.1111/j.1348-0421.1995.tb03282.x

[69] Khalikova E, Susi P, Korpela T. Microbial dextran-hydrolyzing enzymes: Fundamentals and applications. Microbiology and Molecular Biology Reviews: MMBR. 2005;**69**:306-325. DOI: 10.1128/MMBR.69.2.306-325.2005

[70] Igarashi T, Asaga E, Goto N. Roles of *Streptococcus mutans* dextranase anchored to the cell wall by sortase. Oral Microbiology and Immunology. 2004;**19**:102-105. DOI: 10.1046/j.0902-0055.2003.00123.x

[71] Morisaki H, Igarashi T, Yamamoto A, Goto N. Analysis of a dextran-binding domain of the dextranase of *Streptococcus mutans*. Letters in Applied Microbiology. 2002;**35**:223-227. DOI: 10.1046/j.1472-765X.2002.01160.x

[72] Igarashi T, Morisaki H, Yamamoto A, Goto N. An essential amino acid residue for catalytic activity of the dextranase of *Streptococcus mutans*. Oral Microbiology and Immunology. 2002;**17**:193-196. DOI: 10.1034/j.1399-302X.2002.170310.x

[73] Yamamoto T, Terasawa K, Kim Y-M, Kimura A, Kitamura Y, Kobayashi M, et al. Identification of catalytic amino acids of cyclodextran glucanotransferase from *Bacillus circulans* T-3040. Bioscience, Biotechnology, and Biochemistry. 2006;**70**(8):1947-1953

[74] Kim Y, Kim D. Characterization of novel thermostable dextranase from *Thermotoga lettingae* TMO. Applied Microbiology and Biotechnology. 2010;**85**:581-587. DOI: 10.1007/s00253-009-2121-6

[75] Beruheimer AW. Hemolysins of streptococci; characterization and effects on biological membranes. In: Wannamaker LW, Matsen JM, editors. Streptococci and Streptococcal Diseases. New York: Academic Press Inc.; 1972. pp. 19-31

[76] Ajdić D, McShan WM, McLaughlin RE, Savić G, Chang J, Carson MB, et al. Genome sequence of *Streptococcus mutans* UA159, a cariogenic dental pathogen. Proceedings of the National Academy of Sciences of the United States of America. 2002;**99**(22): 14434-14439. DOI: 10.1073/pnas.172501299

[77] Facklam RR. Physiological differentiation of viridans streptococci. Journal of Clinical Microbiology. 1977;**5**:184-201

[78] Perch B, Kjems E, Raun T. Biochemical and serological properties of *Streptococcus mutans* from various human and animal sources. Acta Pathologica et Microbiologica Scandinavica. Section B. Microbiology and Immunology. 1974;**82**:357-370

Section 2

Oral Health Management and Prevention

Chapter 10

Oral Health Knowledge, Attitudes, and Behavior in Young Adults

Ljiljana Kesic, Radmila Obradovic, Milica Petrovic, Marija Bojovic, Dragoslav Lazic, Branislava Stojkovic and Simona Stojanovic

Abstract

Knowledge about the importance of oral health and oral hygiene practices, attitudes, and behavior among young adults shows the association of insufficient or irregular oral hygiene with the occurrence of gingival/periodontal diseases, caries, and consequently systemic disease occurrence including cardiovascular disease, cancer, diabetes mellitus, infections of the respiratory tract, adverse pregnancy outcomes, and neurological disorders. Public health dentists should be trained for oral health needs assessments as well as for the evaluation of community-based oral health improvement strategies among different population groups.

Keywords: oral health, oral hygiene, young adults, caries, periodontal disease

1. Introduction

Knowledge about the importance of oral health and oral hygiene practices, attitudes, and behavior among young adults shows the association of insufficient or irregular oral hygiene with the occurrence of gingival/periodontal diseases, caries, and consequently systemic disease occurrence including cardiovascular disease, cancer, diabetes, respiratory infections, adverse pregnancy outcomes, and neurological disorders [1–8].

Periodontal diseases are highly prevalent and can affect up to 90% of the worldwide population [9]. Periodontal disease is an inflammatory disease, followed by pathologic loss of tooth-supporting tissues (periodontal ligament, gingiva, cementum, and alveolar bone).

Dental caries affects approximately 36% of the worldwide population and is still one of the major causes of tooth loss and pain in industrialized countries [10–12]. Dental caries is a multifactorial disease in which the signs of carious demineralization can be seen on the hard dental tissues [13]. It could cause pain, discomfort, and anxiety, if dental caries is untreated, cause the development of infection and tooth loss [14]. This condition may not only affect an individual's ability to eat and speak properly but may also result in lost work and school hours and affect the individual's overall well-being. The crucial role that a healthy oral microbiome plays in preventing caries and promoting oral health is also being increasingly recognized. Caries prevention has traditionally relied on fluoride exposure, diet control, thorough oral hygiene, and antibacterial measures [15].

The most common forms of periodontal diseases in young adults are gingivitis and periodontitis [16]. Gingivitis is characterized by gingival inflammation, swollen and bleeding gums. In the absence of causal therapy, it may progress to periodontal disease, with the appearance of the periodontal pocket, tissue destruction, and bone resorption [17].

Dental caries, in young adults, is associated with bad oral hygiene habits, more gingivitis, higher consumption of sugar, as well as acidic beverages [18].

2. Oral biofilm

The primary etiologic factor responsible for the initiation and progression of periodontal disease, as well as dental caries, is microbial dental biofilm [19, 20].

Oral biofilm is an organic deposit, which consists of—bacteria, leukocytes, immunoglobulins, inorganic substances, mucins, fungi, desquamated epithelial cells, and low-molecular substances. The qualitative and quantitative composition of oral biofilm microorganisms is different in each person, but one gram contains up to 22×10^9 bacteria [21]. The role of microorganisms in the development of periodontitis is very important, the percent of damage of periodontal tissues is a consequence of the interaction of microbiological factors and the immune-host response [22].

The main periopathogens are *Aggregatibacter actinomycetemcomitans*, *Prevotella intermedia*, *Porphyromonas gingivalis*, *Treponema denticola*, and *Tannerella forsythensis*. Oral health is critically dependent upon the maintenance of good oral hygiene [23].

The oral biofilm is also highly resilient, and it is reorganized into remarkable similar communities following perturbations, such as daily brushing and flossing or professionally administered oral prophylaxis. It takes very large and sustained perturbations to disturb this resilience, particularly smoking, antibiotic use, and certain systemic diseases [24].

Also, ***local and systemic etiological factors*** have an impact on the initiation and progression of periodontitis. There is a number of local and general factors that have an impact on the pathological processing speed of periodontal disease [25–28].

The various local factors that facilitate and accelerate the accumulation of oral biofilm include the following:

1. Anatomical anomalies

2. Food impaction

3. Bad habits

4. Dental caries

5. Iatrogenic factors

6. Gingival lesions

The systemic factors included that reduced the general organism resistance and accelerate the action of the harmful agents of oral biofilm. Due to its effect, the destruction was much more severe. These risk factors are subdivided into two subgroups:

1. Invariant risk factors—genetic predisposition, race, and sex;

2. Variable risk factors—intercurrent diseases, use of drugs, diet, age, stress, and smoking [8, 19, 29].

The main causative agents of oral biofilm for the development of dental caries are acidogenic species *Streptococcus mutans*, including members of the mitis, anginosus and salivarius groups of streptococci, *Enterococcus faecalis*, *Actinomyces naeslundii*, *Actinomyces viscosus*, *Rothia dentocariosa*, *Propionibacterium*, *Prevotella*, *Veillonella*, *Bifidobacterium*, and *Scardovia* [30, 31].

3. Treatment

Periodontal treatment consists of—causal therapy (scaling and root planning), antiseptic rinses, and occasionally systemic antibiotics and surgical interventions. Aims at preventing further periodontal disease progression with the intention to reduce the risk of tooth loss, minimize symptoms and perception of the disease, possibly restore loss of periodontal tissue, and provide information on maintaining a healthy periodontium. Therapeutic intervention includes the introduction of techniques to change behavior, such as individually tailored oral hygiene instructions, a smoking cessation program, dietary adjustment, subgingival instrumentation to remove plaque and calculus, local and systemic pharmacotherapy, and various types of surgery.

Periodontal treatment, because of the chronic nature of the periodontal disease, is a lifelong commitment to basic therapy and intricate oral hygiene techniques, which, when properly implemented, will minimize the risk of disease initiation and progression [32, 33].

Dental caries is preventable with simple procedures, such as tooth brushing with fluoride toothpaste or professional applications of topical fluoride treatments [34]. The aim of therapy is to preserve tooth structures and prevent their further destruction. Whether the carious lesion is cavitated or noncavitated dictates the treatment plan. A dental restoration or dental filling with dental restorative material (dental amalgam, composite resin, porcelain, and gold) is used to repair the function, integrity, and morphology of missing tooth structure [35]. Also, the use of antimicrobial peptides for the prevention and treatment of dental caries is justified [36].

4. Discussion

An association between insufficient or irregular oral hygiene with the occurrence of dental caries, gingival/periodontal diseases, and consequently general diseases has been established. The frequency of brushing teeth, interdental cleaning as well as regular examinations are important determinants of periodontal health. Educational level is by far the most important factor of good oral behavior [37].

Numerous studies have been conducted on young adults around the world to assess oral hygiene habits. Interviews on oral hygiene habits were conducted and analyzed in Europe [38–43], North America [44, 45], Africa [46–49], Asia [50–63], and South America [64–66].

Muthu investigated 282 dental students (63 male and 219 female), ages 18–22, and showed the following results—of the total, 38% had never visited a dentist and brushed their teeth only once a day; 56% visited the dentist only when they were experiencing pain; 49% ignore the color of their teeth; 62% do not pay attention to the color of their gums, while 20% reported bleeding from the gums during brushing. Only 64% were satisfied with the color and appearance of their teeth and gums. Male students preferred hard toothbrushes and mouthwash [67].

Brushing twice a day is recommended in industrialized countries [68], but in some other countries, it is far from achieved [49]. Also, Rimondini et al. showed that 81.6% of Italian students used one toothbrush for less than 3 months [68], while Kirtiloğlu and Yavuz found that 49% of Turkish students used one toothbrush for less than 3 months [69]. Rimondini et al. conclude that a strategy to promote the use of dental services for prevention may be useful for improving oral health in the young Italian population [68].

Peltzer, Pengpid have conducted a survey of 3344 university students from five countries (Indonesia, Malaysia, Thailand, Vietnam, and Myanmar) [70]. The mean age of the respondents was 20.5 years. Regarding brushing, the following results were obtained—in Indonesia, 95.2% of respondents; in Malaysia 83.2%; in Thailand 93.2%; while in Vietnam 76.3% and 48.2% in Myanmar brush their teeth two or more times a day. Then, 29% of respondents never went to the dentist, 51.1% went once a year, and 19.9% more than once a year (Indonesia); 25.7% have never visited a dentist, 35.7% once a year, and 38.6% several times a year (Malaysia); 29.4% never went to the dentist, 46.5% once a year, and 24% several times a year (Thailand); 28.3% never, 47.4% once a year, 24.3% more than once a year (Vietnam); 49.8% never go to the dentist, 1.7% once a year, and 48.5% more times a year (Myanmar).

Agrawal et al. conducted a very interesting study on 223 juvenile detainees, aged 6–18 years [71]. The results showed that the detainees' oral hygiene status was poor, with only 28.1% of respondents having good oral hygiene. The findings confirmed that detainees in the juvenile detention center have poor oral hygiene and an increased prevalence of periodontal disease compared to a population of similar age in the general population.

Ohshima et al. compared periodontal health status and oral health behavior between Japanese and Chinese dental students [72]. The study was conducted on 118 students of the Faculty of Dentistry of Nihon University and 92 students of the Dental School of Nanjing Medical University. An occult blood test of saliva was performed to classify whether subjects could have periodontal disease. Further questionnaires were given to assess different lifestyles and habits of oral hygiene. The positive test rate for occult blood of saliva was 13.6% among Japanese dental students and 43.5% among Chinese dental students. Bleeding from the gingiva as a subjective symptom was as follows: Japanese 7.6%; Chinese 37.0%. Japanese dental students brushed their teeth for 13.5 min each day and Chinese students for 4.6 min. Japanese students (33.1%) used interdental means, while Chinese 7.6%. It is believed that the recorded differences between Japanese and Chinese dental students are the main reason for the appearance of periodontitis, which indicates the need to improve hygiene measures in the city of Nanjing. It is proposed to establish and strengthen education on oral hygiene, including the importance of brushing teeth for the prevention of gingival/periodontal diseases.

	Group 1 (n = 523)		**Group 2 (n = 357)**	
Do you brush your teeth?				
Depends	11	2.10%	5	1.40%
Sometimes	1	0.19%	14	3.92%
Every day	**511**	***97.71%**	**338**	**94.68%**
$\chi^2 = 18.10$, df = 2, p = 0.0001				
How many times per day do you brush your teeth??				
Once	57	10.90%	14	3.92%
Twice	**247**	**47.23%**	**191**	**53.50%**
Three times	183	34.99%	147	41.18%
After every meal	36	6.88%	5	1.40%
$\chi^2 = 30.33$, df = 3, p < 0.001				
When do you brush your teeth?				
In the morning	**503**	***96.18%**	**330**	**92.44%**
Before dinner	33	6.31%	35	9.80%
After dinner	425	81.26%	304	85.15%
Before getting out	265	50.67%	196	54.90%
$\chi^2 = 4.20$, df = 3, p = 0.2407				
Do you use teeth brush?				
Sometimes	1	0.19%	15	4.20%
Every day	**522**	**99.81%**	**342**	**95.80%**
$\chi^2 = 19.12$, df = 1, p < 0.001				
Do you use toothpaste?				
Depends	1	0.19%	4	1.12%
Sometimes	4	0.76%	1	0.28%
Every day	**518**	**99.04%**	**352**	**98.60%**
$\chi^2 = 0.37$, df = 1, p = 0.5375				
Do you use toothpaste with fluoride?				
Yes	**271**	**51.82%**	**204**	**57.14%**
No	18	3.44%	7	1.96%
Dont know	206	39.39%	121	33.89%
Sometimes	28	5.35%	25	7.00%
$\chi^2 = 5.44$, df = 3, p = 0.1426				
Does the toothpaste with fluoride could protect the teeth of caries?				
Yes	**272**	**52.01%**	**246**	*****68.91%**
No	31	5.93%	3	0.84%
Dont know	220	42.07%	108	30.25%
$\chi^2 = 32.45$, df = 2, p = p < 0.001				
Do you use: toothpicks, floss, interdental brushes?				
Never	107	***20.46%	14	3.92%
Rarely	106	20.27%	51	14.29%

	Group 1 (n = 523)		Group 2 (n = 357)	
Depends	24	4.59%	77	21.57%
Sometimes	**238**	**45.51%**	**174**	**48.74%**
Every day	48	9.18%	41	11.48%
χ^2 = 101.34, df = 4, p < 0.001				
Do you use mouthwash?				
Never	80	*15.30%	35	9.80%
Rarely	82	15.68%	67	18.77%
Depends	36	6.88%	16	4.48%
Sometimes	137	26.20%	98	27.45%
Every day	**188**	**35.95%**	**141**	**39.50%**
χ^2 = 9.00, df = 4, p = 0.0610				
Do you use electrical toothbrush?				
Never	**431**	**82.41%**	**310**	**86.83%**
Rarely	44	8.41%	24	6.72%
Depends	0	0.00%	2	0.56%
Sometimes	17	3.25%	8	2.24%
Every day	31	5.93%	13	3.64%
χ^2 = 3.81, df = 3, p = 0.2824				

Attribute variables are given as frequencies and percentages.
**p < 0.05, **p < 0.01, ***p < 0.001 (χ^2 test).*
The daily frequency of brushing teeth is 2 and 3 times more common in group 1 with statistically significant difference between the groups (p<0.001). Morning tooth brushing was statistically more represented in group 1 (p<0.05). There is a statistically significant difference between the groups in the frequency of using a toothbrush (p<0.001). The groups did not differ in the use of fluoride toothpaste, but differed in the opinion that fluoride toothpaste protects teeth from caries (p<0.001), which is a consequence of the statistically more frequent confirmatory opinion of group 2 respondents (p <0.001). Groups of respondents differ statistically significantly in the frequency of use of toothpicks, floss and interdental brushes (p<0.001). But, mouthwash, statistically more often never used by subjects of group 1 (p<0.05).

Table 1.
Oral hygiene practices among students.

Kaira et al. surveyed 111 nursing students at Rohilkhand Hospital, Bareilly, India [73]. Most of the respondents had good oral hygiene, which included brushing their teeth twice a day with a brush and toothpaste for 2–3 min. Almost 87% of them knew that oral biofilm causes gingival inflammation and consequently periodontitis. Almost half of the participants visited the dentist solely because of the pain. However, most of them gave the same importance to dental health as to general health. They concluded that the knowledge, attitude, and practice of oral health care students are adequate, but that further improvements can be encouraged.

Sharda surveyed 825 participants (577 men, 248 women) from six different professions belonging to the non-medical, paramedical, and medical categories of the survey [74]. The knowledge was significantly higher among medical students compared to those who were not. Attitude scores were significantly lower for the non-medical category compared to the other two categories. The results indicate that knowledge was not sufficient to influence oral health-related behaviors.

Bojović et al. investigation supplied a new understanding of oral health risk factors among students in the University of Niš medical programs [75]. Namely, the results of this research indicate that students in the clinical medical program have better knowledge about oral hygiene issues compared with students in the preclinical medical program. The authors suggested that it is necessary to educate preclinical students to raise awareness of the importance of oral health.

Bojović investigated risk factors for oral health conditions by examining oral hygiene practices, attitudes, and behaviors among the students in the medical program of the University of Niš, collecting data using questionnaires [76]. The study included 880 students of medicine, dentistry, pharmacy, and vocational studies. Students were divided into two groups—those who were in preclinical (group 1) and those who were in clinical subjects (group 2). Prior to the clinical examination, subjects completed an anonymous survey, which contained four aspects—(1) sociodemographic data; (2) oral hygiene habits and behaviors; (3) health risk behaviors, disorders, drug use, parafunctional habits; (4) maintaining oral health. Oral hygiene, as expected, showed that a high percentage of respondents brush their teeth daily (97.22%). The largest percentage of all respondents (45.45%) sometimes use interdental brushes/floss/toothpicks. Tooth brushing lasted 3 min in 39.39% of subjects (**Table 1**).

Today, in the world, there is a tendency to evaluate, analyze, and propose education programs for medical students, but also for students of other study programs [75–100]. Also, there is a need for other groups of the population (chronic patients, diabetics, pregnant women, patients with blood dyscrasias, oncology patients, etc.) to be educated, acquired and adopted knowledge, attitudes, and brhaviors about oral health.

5. Conclusion

Oral health education and promotion through dentists, electronic media, print media, and public health programs are needed to improve oral hygiene practices among young adults as well as the general population. Regular visits to the dentist for prevention, prophylaxis, and professional referral to oral hygiene are key to the prevention of oral diseases [75].

Public health dentists should be trained to assess the need for oral health, implement and evaluate strategies to improve oral health among different population groups.

Conflict of interest

The authors declare no conflict of interest.

Author details

Ljiljana Kesic[1*], Radmila Obradovic[1], Milica Petrovic[1], Marija Bojovic[1], Dragoslav Lazic[2], Branislava Stojkovic[3] and Simona Stojanovic[4]

1 Medical Faculty, Department of Oral Medicine and Periodontology, Clinic for Dental Medicine, University of Nis, Serbia

2 Faculty of Medicine, Department of Prosthodontic, University of Prishtina with Temporary Headquarters in Kosovska Mitrovica, Serbia

3 Medical Faculty, Department of Pediatric Dentistry, Clinic for Dental Medicine, University of Nis, Serbia

4 Medical Faculty, Department of Oral Surgery, Clinic for Dental Medicine, University of Nis, Serbia

*Address all correspondence to: kesic.ljiljana@gmail.com

References

[1] Petersen PE. Global policy for improvement of oral health in the 21st century: Implications to oral health research of World Health Assembly 2007, World Health Organization. Community Dentistry and Oral Epidemiology. 2009;**37**(1):1-8

[2] Locker D, Quiñonez C. To what extent do oral disorders compromise the quality of life? Community Dentistry and Oral Epidemiology. 2011;**39**(1):3-11

[3] Nazir MA. Prevalence of periodontal disease, its association with systemic diseases and prevention. International Journal of Health Sciences. 2017;**11**(2): 72-80

[4] Winning L, Linden GJ. Periodontitis and systemic disease: Association or causality? Current Oral Health Reports. 2017;**4**(1):1-7

[5] Chan S, Pasternak GM, West MJ. The place of periodontal examination and referral in general medicine. Periodontology 2000. 2017;**74**(1):194-199

[6] Le Bars P, Matamoros S, Montassier E, et al. The oral cavity microbiota: Between health, oral disease, and cancers of the aerodigestive tract. Canadian Journal of Microbiology. 2017;**63**(6):475-492

[7] Bui FQ, Almeida-da-Silva CLC, Huynh B, et al. Association between periodontal pathogens and systemic disease. Biomedical Journal. 2019;**42**(1): 27-35

[8] Kim J, Amar S. Periodontal disease and systemic conditions: A bidirectional relationship. Odontology. 2006;**94**:10-21

[9] Pihlstrom BL, Michalowicz BS, Johnson NW. Periodontal diseases. The Lancet. 2005;**366**(9499):1809-1820

[10] Kassebaum NJ, Bernabé E, Dahiya M, et al. Global burden of untreated caries: A systematic review and metaregression. Journal of Dental Research. 2015;**94**(5): 650-658

[11] Sheiham A. Oral health, general health and quality of life. Bulletin of the World Health Organization. 2005;**83**(9):644

[12] Frazão P. Epidemiology of dental caries: When structure and context matter. Brazilian Oral Research. 2012;**26**(Special Issue 1):108-114

[13] Selwitz HR, Ismail A, Pitts BN. Dental caries. Lancet. 2007;**369**(9555): 51-59

[14] Sheiham A, Conway D, Chestnutt I. Impact of oral diseases and oral health inequalities. In: Watt RG, Listl S, Peres M, Heilmann A, editors. Social Inequalities in Oral Health: From Evidence to Action. UCL; ISBN:978-0-9527377-6-6 2015. pp. 4-5

[15] Mathur VP, Dhillon JK. Dental caries: A disease which needs attention. Indian Journal of Pediatrics. 2018;**85**(3):202-206

[16] Research, Science and Therapy Committee Guidelines of the American Academy of Periodontology. Treatment of plaque-induced gingivitis, chronic periodontitis, and other clinical conditions. Journal of Periodontology. 2001;**72**:1790-1800

[17] Wade WG. The oral microbiome in health and disease. Pharmacological Research. 2013;**69**:137-143

[18] Hagman J, Wide U, Werner H, et al. Oral health and oral health behavior in young adults with caries disease.

BDJ Open. 2021;7:28. DOI: 10.1038/s41405-021-00084-3

[19] Petrović MS, Kannosh IY, Milašin JM, et al. Clinical, microbiological and cytomorphometric evaluation of low-level laser therapy as an adjunct to periodontal therapy in patients with chronic periodontitis. International Journal of Dental Hygiene. 2018;**16**(2):120-127

[20] Kinane DF, Stathopoulou PG, Papapanou PN. Periodontal diseases. Nature Reviews. Disease Primers. 2017;**3**:17038

[21] Curtis MA, Zenobia C, Darveau RP. The relationship of the oral microbiotia to periodontal health and disease. Cell Host & Microbe. 2011;**10**(4):302-306

[22] Wolff L, Dahlen G, Aeppli D. Bacteria as risk markers for periodontitis. Journal of Periodontology. 1994;**65**:498-510

[23] Newton JT. Effective communication with patients to improve motivation. In: Palmer RM, Ide M, Floyd PD, editors. A Clinical Guide to Periodontology. 3rd ed. London: British Dental Association; 2013. pp. 33-40

[24] Kumar PS. Microbial dysbiosis: The root cause of periodontal disease. Journal of Periodontology. 2021;**92**(8):1079-1087

[25] Cronin AJ, Claffey N, Stassen LF. Who is at risk? Periodontal disease risk analysis made accessible for the general dental practitioner. British Dental Journal. 2008;**205**(3):131-137

[26] Irwin C, Mullally B, Ziada H, Allen E, Byrne PJ. Periodontics: 2. Risk factors and susceptibility in periodontitis. Dental Update. 2007;**34**(5):270-276

[27] Gera I. Risk factors for destructive periodontitis I. Behavioral and acquired factors. Fogorvosi Szemle. 2004;**97**(1):11-21

[28] Arowojolu MO, Dosumu EB, Onyeaso CO, Lawoyin JO. Effects of some risk factors and immunodeficiencies on the periodontium—A review. African Journal of Medicine and Medical Sciences. 2002;**31**(3):195-199

[29] Wilson TG. Not all patients are the same: Systemic risk factors for adult periodontitis. General Dentistry. 1999;**47**(6):580-588

[30] Simón-Soro A, Mira A. Solving the etiology of dental caries. Trends in Microbiology. 2015;**23**(2):76-82

[31] Karpiński TM, Szkaradkiewicz AK. Microbiology of dental caries. Journal of Biology and Earth Sciences. 2013;**3**(1):21-24

[32] Graziani F, Karapetsa D, Alonso B, Herrera D. Nonsurgical and surgical treatment of periodontitis: How many options for one disease? Periodontology 2000. 2017;**75**:152-188

[33] Slots J. Periodontitis: Facts, fallacies and the future. Periodontology 2000. 2017;**75**:7-23

[34] Lenzi TL, Montagner AF, Soares FZ, et al. Are topical fluorides effective for treating incipient carious lesions?: A systematic review and meta-analysis. Journal of the American Dental Association (1939). 2016;**147**:84-91. e1

[35] Yadav K, Prakash S. Dental caries: A review. Asian Journal of Biomedical and Pharmaceutical Sciences. 2016;**6**(53):1-7

[36] Niu JY, Yin IX, Wu WK, Li QL, Mei ML, Hung CC. Antimicrobial peptides for the prevention and

treatment of dental caries: A concise review. Archives of Oral Biology. 2020;**9**:105022

[37] Gómez MV, Toledo A, Carvajal P, et al. A multicenter study of oral health behavior among adult subjects from three South American cities. Brazilian Oral Research. 2018;**32**:22. DOI: 10.1590/1807-3107bor-2018.vol32.0022

[38] Molarius A, Engström S, Flink H, Simonsson B, Tegelberg A. Socioeconomic differences in self-rated oral health and dental care utilisation after the dental care reform in 2008 in Sweden. BMC Oral Health. 2014;**14**(1): 134. DOI: 10.1186/1472-6831-14-134

[39] Sakalauskienė Z, Vehkalahti MM, Murtomaa H, Mačiulskienė V. Factors related to gender differences in toothbrushing among Lithuanian middle-aged university employees. Medicina (Kaunas, Lithuania). 2011;**47**(3):180-186

[40] Skeie M, Skaret E, Espelid I, Misvar N. Do public health nurses in Norway promote information on oral health? BMC Oral Health. 2011;**11**:23. DOI: 10.1186/1472-6831-11-23

[41] Petersen PE. Effectiveness of oral health care-some Danish experiences. Proceedings of the Finnish Dental Society. Suomen Hammaslaakariseuran Toimituksia. 1992;**88**(1-2):13-23

[42] Pacauskiene IM, Smailiene D, Siudikienė J, Savanevskyte J, Nedzelskiene I. Self-reported oral health behavior and attitudes of dental and technology students in Lithuania. Stomatologija. 2014;**16**(2):65-71

[43] Pavi E, Karampli E, Zavras D, Dardavesis T, Kyriopoulos J. Social determinants of dental health services utilisation of Greek adults. Community Dental Health. 2010;**27**:145-150

[44] Payne BJ, Locker D. Relationship between dental and general health behaviors in a Canadian population. Journal of Public Health Dentistry. 1996;**56**(4):198-204. DOI: 10.1111/j.1752-7325.1996.tb02436.x

[45] Ronis DL, Lang WP, Farghaly MM, Passow E. Tooth brushing, flossing, and preventive dental visits by Detroit-area residents in relation to demographic and socioeconomic factors. Journal of Public Health Dentistry. 1993;**53**(3):138-145. DOI: 10.1111/j.1752-7325.1996.tb02436.x

[46] Olusile AO, Adeniyi AA, Orebanjo O. Self-rated oral health status, oral health service utilization, and oral hygiene practices among adult Nigerians. BMC OralHealth.2014;**14**(1):140.DOI:10.1186/1472-6831-14-140

[47] Osuh ME, Oke GA, Asuzu MC. Dental services and attitudes towards its regular utilization among civil servants in Ibadan, Nigeria. Annals of Ibadan Postgraduate Medicine. 2014;**12**(1):7-14

[48] Carneiro L, Kabulwa M, Makyao M, Mrosso G, Choum R. Oral health knowledge and practices of secondary school Students, Tanga, Tanzania. International Journal of Dentistry. 2011. Article ID 806258. Volume 2011. 6 pages. DOI: 10.1155/2011/806258

[49] Åstrøm AN, Masalu JR. Oral health behavior patterns among Tanzanian university students: A repeat cross-sectional survey. BMC Oral Health. 2001;**1**(1):1-7

[50] Al-Shammari KF, Al-Ansari JM, Al-Khabbaz AK, Dashti A, Honkala EJ. Self-reported oral hygiene habits and oral health problems of Kuwaiti adults. Medical Principles and Practice. 2007;**16**(1):15-21. DOI: 10.1159/000096134

[51] Harada S, Akhter R, Kurita K, et al. Relationships between lifestyle and dental health behaviors in a rural population in Japan. Community Dentistry and Oral Epidemiology. 2005;**33**(1):17-24. DOI: 10.1111/j.1600-0528.2004.00189.x

[52] Asgari F, Majidi A, Koohpayehzadeh J, Etemad K, Rafei A. Oral hygiene status in a general population of Iran, 2011: A key lifestyle marker in relation to common risk factors of non-communicable diseases. International Journal of Health Policy and Management. 2015;**4**(6):343-352. DOI: 10.15171/ijhpm.2015.18

[53] Behbehani JM, Shah NM. Oral Health in Kuwait before the Gulf War. Medical Principles and Practice. 2002;**11**(1):36-43 doi.org/10.1159/000057777

[54] Bhat M. Oral health status and treatment needs of a rural Indian fishing community. The West Indian Medical Journal. 2008;**57**(4):414-417

[55] Al OM. Prevailing Oral Hygiene Habits among Urban Saudi Arabians: Tooth Brushing and Miswak Chewing Stick Practice in Relation to Age, Gender and Socio-Economic Background. Karolinska Institute Odontologiska Institutionen: Stockholm; 2003

[56] Zhu L, Petersen PE, Wang HY, Bian JY, Zhang BX. Oral health knowledge, attitudes and behaviour of children and adolescents in China. International Dental Journal. 2003;**53**(5):289-298

[57] Lian CW, Phing TS, Chat CS, Shin BC, Baharuddina LH, Che'Jalil ZBJ. Oral health knowledge, attitude and practice among secondary school students in Kuching, Sarawak. Archives of Orofacial Sciences. 2010;**5**(1):9-16

[58] Tada A, Takashi MT. Relationship between oral health behaviors and general health behaviors in a Japanese adult population. Journal of Public Health Dentistry. 2003;**63**(4):250-254

[59] Ueno M, Ohara S, Inoue M, Tsugane S, Kawaguchi Y. Association between education level and dentition status in Japanese adults: Japan public health center-based oral health study. Community Dentistry and Oral Epidemiology. 2012;**40**:481-487

[60] Vasanthakumar AH, D'Cruz AM, Samad S, Dhinda SH, Mansib SM, Nayak S. Oral hygiene practices among paramedical staff of a private dental institution in India. RSBO. 2013;**10**(3): 205-210

[61] Saito A, Kikuchi M, Ueshima F, Matsumoto S, Hayakawa H, Masuda H, et al. Assessment of oral self-care in patients with periodontitis: A pilot study in a dental school clinic in Japan. BMC Oral Health. 2009;**9**:27

[62] Al-shammari KF, Al-Ansari JM, Al-Khabbaz AK, Honkala S. Barriers to seeking preventive dental care by Kuwaiti adults. Medical Principles and Practice. 2007;**16**:413-419

[63] Kakatkar G, Bhat N, Nagarajappa R, Prasad V, Sharda A, Asawa K, et al. Barriers to the utilization of dental services in Udaipur, India. Journal of Dentistry. 2011;**8**:81-89

[64] Scarpelli AC, Oliveira BH, Teasch FC, Leao AT, Pordeus IA, Paiva SM. Psychometric properties of the Brazilian version of the early childhood oral health impact scale (BECOHIS). BMC Oral Health.2011;**11**(1):1-11.DOI:10.1186/1472-6831-11-19

[65] Afonso-Souza G, Nadanovsky P, Chor D, Faerstein E, Werneck GL,

Lopes CS. Association between routine visits for dental checkups and self-perceived oral health in an adult population in Rio de Janeiro: The Pró-Saú de Study. Community Dentistry and Oral Epidemiology. 2007;**35**:393-400

[66] Haas AN, Reis A, Lemos CA Jr, Pannuti CM, Escobar E, Almeida ER, et al. Daily biofilm control and oral health: An epidemiological challenge consensus-Brazilian advisory panel in oral health. Brazilian Journal of Periodontology. 2012;**22**(3):40-46

[67] Muthu J, Priyadarshini G, Muthanandam S, Ravichndran S, Balu P. Evaluation of oral health attitude and behavior among a group of dental students in Puducherry, India: A preliminary cross-sectional study. Journal of Indian Society of Periodontology. 2015;**19**(6):683-686. DOI: 10.4103/0972-124X.164744

[68] Rimondini L, Zolfanelli B, Bernardi F, Bez C. Self-preventive oral behavior in an Italian university student population. Journal of Clinical Periodontology. 2001;**28**(3):207-211. DOI: 10.1034/j.1600-051x.2001.028003207.x

[69] Kirtiloğlu T, Yavuz US. An assessment of oral self-care in the student population of a Turkish university. Public Health. 2006;**120**(10):953-957. DOI: 10.1016/j.puhe.2006.05.006

[70] Peltzer K, Pengpid S. Dental health status and oral health behavior among university students from five ASEAN countries. Nagoya Journal of Medical Science. 2017;**79**(2):123-133

[71] Agrawal A, Bhat N, Shetty S, Sharda A, Singh K, Chaudhary H. Oral hygiene and periodontal status among detainees in a juvenile detention center, India. Oral Health & Preventive Dentistry. 2011;**3**:281-287

[72] Ohshima M, Zhu L, Yamaguchi Y, Kikuchi M, Nakajima I, Langham CS, et al. Comparison of periodontal health status and oral health behavior between Japanese and Chinese dental students. Journal of Oral Science. 2009;**51**(2): 275-281

[73] Kaira LS, Srivastava V, Giri P, Chopra D. Oral health-related knowledge, attitude and practice among nursing students of Rohilkhand medical college and hospital: A questionnaire study. JOFR. 2012;**2**(1):20-23

[74] Sharda AJ, Shetty S. A comparative study of oral health knowledge, attitude and behaviour of non-medical, para-medical and medical students in Udaipur city, Rajasthan, India. International Journal of Dental Hygiene. 2010;**8**(2): 101-109

[75] Bojović MD, Kesić LG, Mitić AN, Kocić B, Obradović RR, Ignjatović A, et al. Oral Health-Related Risk Factors Among Students in Southeast Serbia. Medical Science Monitor. 2021;**27**: e929375-e929371

[76] Bojović MD. Analysis of oral-hygienic habits, periodontal indices and conditions of oral mucosa in the student population [Doctoral dissertation]. University of Niš; 2021

[77] Peres MA, Daly B, Guarnizo-Herreño CC, Benzian H, Watt RG. Oral diseases: A global public health challenge—Authors' reply. Lancet. 2020;**395**(10219):186-187

[78] Menegaz AM, Silva AER, Cascaes AM. Educational interventions in health services and oral health: Systematic review. Revista de Saúde Pública. 2018;**52**:52

[79] Moussa A, Ibrahim E, Esmat A, Eissa S, Ramzy M. An overview of oral health status, socio-economic and behavioral risk factors, and the pattern of tooth loss in a sample of Egyptian rural population. Bulletin of the National Research Centre. 2020;**44**(1):1-6

[80] Aly NM, Mohamed AA, Abdelaziz WE. Parenting practices and oral health status in rural areas in Egypt: A household survey. BMC Oral Health. 2020;**20**:1-9

[81] Abbass MM, Rady D, Radwan IA, El Moshy S, AbuBakr N, Ramadan M, et al. The occurrence of periodontal diseases and its correlation with different risk factors among a convenient sample of adult Egyptian population: A cross-sectional study. F1000Research. 2019;**8**

[82] Eid SA, Khattab NMA, Elheeny AAH. Untreated dental caries prevalence and impact on the quality of life among 11 to14-year-old Egyptian schoolchildren: A cross-sectional study. BMC Oral Health. 2020;**20**:83

[83] Haslach SD, Aytepe Z, Kokkari A, Azrak B, Ehlers V, Herz MM, et al. Country and gender differences in the motivation of dental students-An international comparison. European Journal of Dental Education. 2018;**22**:724-729

[84] Almutairi KM, Alonazi WB, Vinluan JM, Almigbal TH, Batais MA, Alodhayani AA, et al. Health promoting lifestyle of university students in Saudi Arabia: A cross-sectional assessment. BMC Public Health. 2018;**18**:1093

[85] Halboub ES, Al-Maweri SA, Al-Jamaei AA, Al-Wesabi MA, Shamala A, Al-Kamel A, et al. Self reported oral health attitudes and behavior of dental and medical students, Yemen. Global Journal of Health Science. 2016;**8**:56676

[86] Hamasha A, Alshehri A, Alshubaiki A, Alssafi F, Alamam H, Alshunaiber R. Gender-specific oral health beliefs and behaviors among adult patients attending King Abdulaziz medical city in Riyadh. Saudi Dental Journal. 2018;**30**:226-231

[87] Silva GMC, Borges AR, Ezequiel OS, Lucchetti ALG, Lucchetti G. Comparison of students motivation at different phases of medical school. Revista da Associacao Medica Brasileira. 2018;**64**:902-908

[88] Komar K, Glavina A, Boras VV, Verzak Ž, Brailo V. Impact of smoking on oral health: Knowledge and attitudes of Croatian dentists and dental students. Acta stomatologica Croatica. 2018;**52**: 148-155

[89] Thomas J, Kumar RV, Akhil S, Saji AM, Iype AK, Antony D. Prevalence of smoking among dental students and gauging their knowledge about tobacco cessation methods: An original study. Journal of Family Medicine and Primary Care. 2019;**8**:1562-1566

[90] Balogh E, Faubl N, Riemenschneider H, Balázs P, Bergmann A, Cseh K, et al. Cigarette, waterpipe and e-cigarette use among an international sample of medical students. Cross-sectional multicenter study in Germany and Hungary. BMC Public Health. 2018;**18**:591

[91] Gignon M, Havet E, Ammirati C, Traullé S, Manaouil C, Balcaen T, et al. Alcohol, cigarette, and illegal substance consumption among medical students: A cross-sectional survey. Workplace Health & Safety. 2015;**63**:54-63

[92] Sharareh P, Leili T, Abbas M, Jalal P, Ali G. Determining correlates of the average number of cigarette smoking among college students using count regression models. Scientific Reports. 2020;**10**:8874

[93] Shaik P, Pachava S, Palli C. Factors affecting stress among students in dental colleges of neo-capital state in India. Journal of Indian Association of Public Health Dentistry. 2019;**17**:41-47

[94] Basudan S, Binanzan N, Alhassan A. Depression, anxiety and stress in dental students. International Journal of Medical Education. 2017;**8**:179-186

[95] Ersan N, Dolekoglu S, Fisekcioglu E, Ilguy M, Oktay I. Perceived sources and levels of stress, general self-efficacy and coping strategies in preclinical dental students. Psychology, Health & Medicine. 2018;**23**:567-577

[96] Balaji NK, Murthy PS, Kumar DN, Chaudhury S. Perceived stress, anxiety, and coping states in medical and engineering students during examinations. Industrial Psychiatry Journal. 2019;**28**:86-97

[97] Halboub E, Alhajj MN, AlKhairat AM, Sahaqi AM, Quadri MFA. Perceived stress among undergraduate dental students in relation to gender, clinical training and academic performance. Acta Stomatologica Croatica. 2018;**52**:37-45

[98] Park SE, Donoff RB, Saldana F. The impact of integrating oral health education into a medical curriculum. Medical Principles and Practice. 2017;**26**:61-65

[99] Neville P, Zahra J, Pilch K, Jayawardena D, Waylen A. The behavioural and social sciences as hidden curriculum in UK dental education: A qualitative study. European Journal of Dental Education. 2019;**23**:461-470

[100] Conrad J, Retelsdorf J, Attia S, Dörfer C, Mekhemar M. German dentists' preferences for the treatment of apical periodontitis: A cross-sectional survey. International Journal of Environmental Research and Public Health. 2020;**17**:7447

Chapter 11

Upper Airway Expansion in Disabled Children

David Andrade, Joana Andrade, Maria-João Palha, Cristina Areias, Paula Macedo, Ana Norton, Miguel Palha, Lurdes Morais, Dóris Rocha Ruiz and Sônia Groisman

Abstract

Breathing is essential for life in all of its stages. Cellular, mitochondrial respiration requires an adequate supply of oxygen, provided by the air we breathe, after airway conduction, treatment by the lungs, and transport to tissues. At different stages of life, pediatric dentists and orthodontists can intervene in the upper airway, expanding it, which helps with ventilation. The greater airway space, if used, contributes in different ways to the child's development and the recovery of respiratory problems and should always be present as a weapon that physicians and the population should know. The value of the techniques becomes even more important when applied to children and young people with disabilities who can significantly improve their development and performance. Rapid Maxillary Expansion and Extraoral Traction Appliances are two important pediatric resources to treat these children. Clinical practice of the authors, is discussed, emphasizing the importance of early intervention and the need for multi and interdisciplinary collaboration in the follow-up of disabled people.

Keywords: pediatric dentistry, effects, health, development, disabled persons, syndrome, obstructive sleep apnea, neuromuscular diseases, rapid maxillary expansion, extraoral traction appliances, airway obstruction, congenital muscular dystrophy, palatal expansion technique, maxillary retrusion

1. Introduction

This chapter analyses the effects of Rapid Maxillary Expansion (RME) and Extraoral Traction Appliances (ETA) on children with a high prevalence of specific otorhinolaryngologic pathology like persistent nasal obstruction and/or repeated upper respiratory infections (three episodes over six months or four episodes in a year nasal obstruction).

This type of obstructive symptomatology is common in Down syndrome (DS) children [1] but may occur in children with other syndromes or diseases, and even in healthy persons.

Other possible causes of breathing difficulty are related to muscle weakness. If we look to the population that uses Noninvasive Ventilation (NIV), we identify the significant groups of risk, where respiratory muscles are weakened, or the airway is obstructed: Obstructive sleep apnea (OSA), Neuromuscular disorders (ND), Cystic fibrosis, Children with Obesity and Down syndrome (DS).

Upper airway obstruction may have several causes, and accumulated secretions augment the obstruction. Adenoidectomy and tonsillectomy are common to remove the obstruction, but many times, not enough. Another cause related to obstruction, often forgotten, is a constricted and/or retruded maxilla. In most cases, we find the presence of lateral crossbite and/or evidence of maxillary compression.

A diminished transverse dimension of the maxilla reduces the nasal cavities, thereby reducing the airflow into the lungs [2].

The nasal respiratory space represents a vital role in the craniofacial skeleton growth and development (the most important stimuli for the growth of the midface is ventilation by the nose).

The respiratory pattern can determine an altered mandibular posture, allowing compensatory oral ventilation. When the tongue does not occupy a stable position in the oral cavity, the entire balance that keeps the teeth in their typical situation changes, allowing the occurrence of malocclusion.

The occlusion between the maxilla and mandible is essential to choose the type of therapy to use.

Based on scientific evidence and clinical practice, this chapter supports a better understanding of these treatments that improve oral functions and the child's general development.

2. Rapid maxillary expansion

RME is a widespread orthodontic practice [3]. It is a dentomaxillofacial orthopedic treatment process commonly adopted in young patients to treat narrowed maxilla (**Figure 1**) [4]. This procedure is used for handling structural and functional problems in the middle of the face [5]. It involves applying an intraoral screw mechanism anchored on selected teeth (**Figure 2**) or bone that produces orthopedic forces to the mid palatal suture, with the forces dispersing through the circum-maxillary and cranial sutures [6].

In particular, RME enlarges the nasal cavity base and the maxilla [7, 8]. RME is used to fix the constricted transverse diameter [9], expanding the arch perimeter that will deliver more space for the correct positioning of crowded teeth and permit crossbite correction [10].

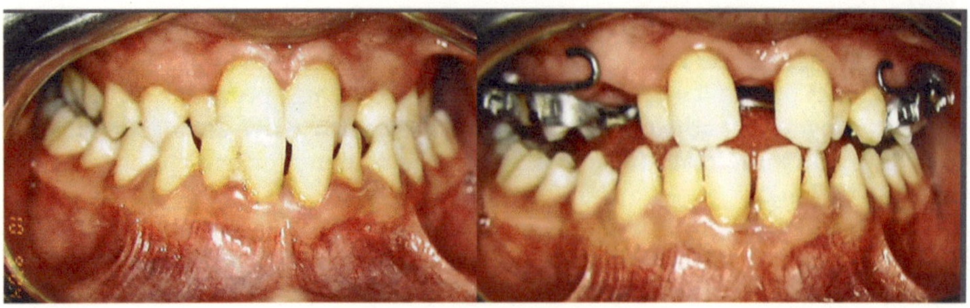

Figure 1.
Severely narrowed maxilla and first ERM appliance. Anterior and posterior crossbite before and after the first RME appliance.

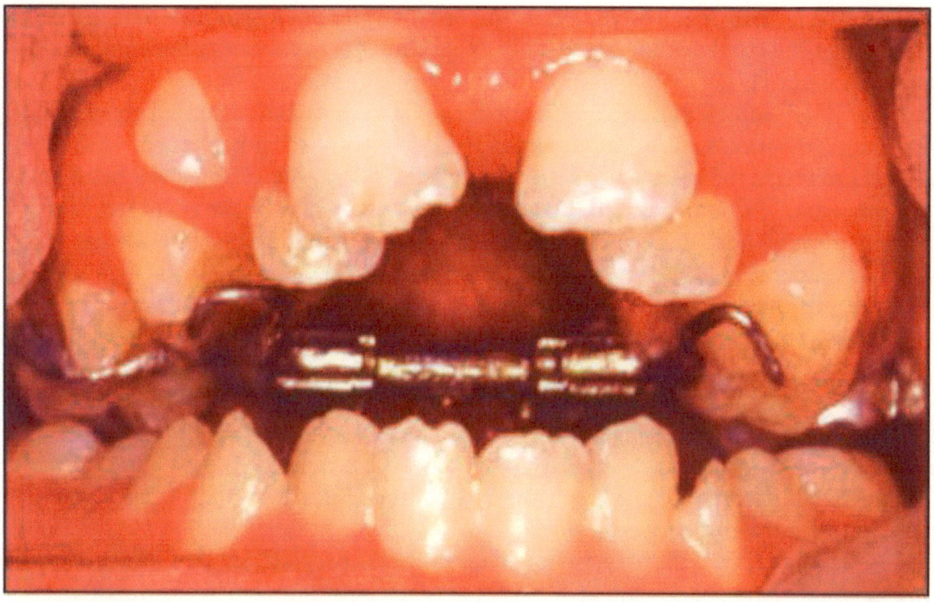

Figure 2.
After the first ERM appliance, a diastema appeared between central incisors, showing that the midpalatal suture opened.

When we open the midpalatal suture, we get a diastema between central incisors (**Figure 2**) that is closed per se without an appliance procedure.

The RME device is a fixed appliance that does not require from parents or children intense cooperation. It is easily cleaned and works in a short period, between two and four weeks [11].

Palatal enlargement in children increases nasal flow and diminishes nasal resistance [12].

The treatment of mouth breathing is multidisciplinary, and the patient should be sent to the otorhinolaryngologist as treatment should be initiated after the triggering condition of oral breathing is resolved. RME is the recommended therapy in the interception phase [13].

After RME, improved resistance and nasal flow were documented in patients in the supine position, who had a posterior and anterior obstruction. Smaller changes were observed in isolated forms of obstruction and in the orthostatic position. In nasal airway obstruction with maxillary constriction, RME has proved effective for improving nasal breathing in children via an enlargement effect on the nasopharynx [14]. Pharyngeal airway pressure during inspiration is decreased with the reduction of nasal resistance [15].

In intermaxillary, internasal, frontonasal, frontomaxillary, and maxillonasal sutures, RME produces significant width increases, whereas the zygomaticotemporal, frontozygomatic, pterygomaxillary, and zygomaticomaxillary sutures showed nonsignificant changes; forces elicited by RME affect mainly the anterior sutures (maxillary frontal nasal and intermaxillary interfaces) compared with the posterior (zygomatic interface) craniofacial structures [16]. Cephalometry showed increased maxillary width after RME [10].

The RME substantially increases interglenoid chamber distance and mandibular condyle displacement at six months in growing patients compared to a control group.

RME is effective during growth, enlarging the interglenoid fossa space and the lateral positions of the condyles and eventually expanding the nasal cavity without producing asymmetry [17].

After RME, substantial improvement in the transverse dimensions of the maxillary basal bone, the nasal cavity, and the midpalatal suture opening happened, with the highest growth in the midpalatal suture followed by nasal cavity and basal bone [18].

Considerable alterations in the space of the pharynx may be obtained in Class II patients through both RME and mandibular advancement devices with the capacity of palatal expansion [19].

RME improved the mucociliary clearance in children with maxillary narrowness, positively affecting nasal physiology and improving nasal cavity volume [20].

3. Extraoral traction appliances

There are different ETA, bone or teeth anchored (**Figure 3**) that, if used well, cause anterior traction of the upper jaw.

One can have a maxillary retrusion, a mandibular prognathea, or a mixture of the two. Respiratory problems can arise with maxillary retrusion when the maxillary is back positioned and encroaches on the nasopharyngeal airway.

Research conducted over the past decade has shown associated improvements in airway size with maxillary protraction [21].

Existing controlled clinical studies on humans show that ETA for skeletal Class III intervention might be related to broader airway proportions, mostly minor in

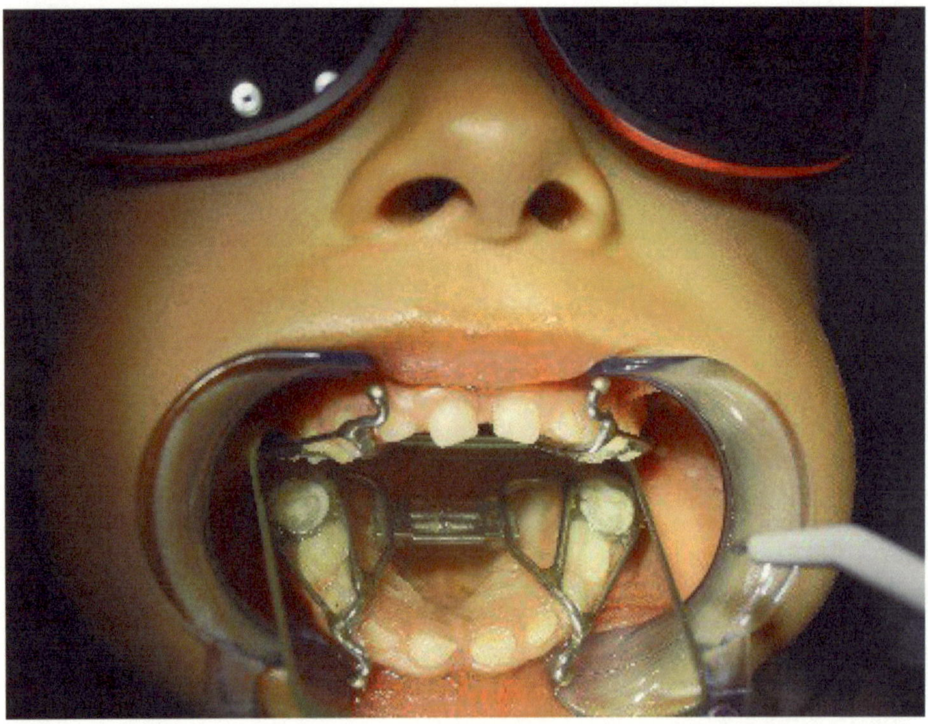

Figure 3.
Rapid maxillary expansion, prepared for traction, if necessary.

magnitude [22]. Positive stable changes in the airway dimensions of Class III subjects were obtained by treatment with RME and ETA [23].

Maxillary protraction is a complement of RME. It is used only if necessary; only those with problems in the sagittal plane may need ETA when anteroposterior dimension mismatch between the maxilla and the mandible. Most cases that require RME do not require ETA. The best time to use ETA is immediately after finishing the RME, taking advantage of the lack of union of the sutures and superior displacement of the bones, as they are less trapped.

While RME is responsible for the transverse maxillary increase, ETA becomes important in the anteroposterior dimensions.

4. Obstructive sleep apnea and obstructive sleep apnea syndrome

A small-scale upper jaw and/or mandible can predispose kids to sleep-disordered breathing, which is a continuum of gravity from snoring to OSA. Related health consequences, such as cardiovascular and neurocognitive functions, have not yet been systematically referred [24].

OSA often goes undiagnosed and affects approximately 5% of the population. Obstructive Sleep Apnea Syndrome (OSAS) is a more serious form of OSA where there is evidence of both a disruption of standard breathing patterns during sleep, and symptoms such as excessive sleepiness in the daytime. OSAS occurs in approximately a quarter of those with OSA [25, 26]. Within the upper airway, the pharynx, particularly the oropharynx and hypopharynx, is the region where most obstructive processes leading to OSAS are found [27]. It is characterized by episodes of partial or complete obstruction of the upper airway during sleep, interrupting (apnea) or reducing (hypopnea) the flow of air, followed by brief awakening that leads to the restoration of upper airway permeability. The descriptions may eventually become redundant in the context of rapid technological advances in breathing measurement and other signal acquisition [28].

OSAS prevalence is supposed to rise with the present obesity epidemic. If not treated, it is related to significant morbidities such as growth collapse, endothelial dysfunction, neurocognitive impairment, and pulmonary and systemic hypertension [29].

OSAS during infancy results in significant physical and neuropsychomotor disorders. Therefore, it must be recognized and treated as soon as possible to prevent or mitigate the chronic problems associated with OSA, harmful to child development. Adenoidectomy and, in some circumstances, continuous positive airway pressure (CPAP) have been the chosen therapies for OSAS in pediatric patients, but they are unsuccessful in ultimately improving the condition. RME in kids with OSAS seems a successful cure for this condition [5, 30, 31].

The dentist's role is pivotal in children when identified with OSA; initiating dental therapies in the course of growth can aid patients, protecting them from malocclusion, and intervening in dentofacial structural development can help escape therapies such as CPAP and different surgeries. Proper evaluation and treatment may avoid compromised quality of life, delays in treatment, morbidity, and, in some cases, mortality [32].

RME treatment positively affected kids with chronic snoring and OSA, producing growth of the nasal cavity and nasopharyngeal airway volume, with enlargement of the maxillary and nasal osseous size. Enlarged nasal width at the posterior nasal spine (PNS) plane improved nasopharyngeal volume. The enlargement of the maxillary width is directly correlated with the increase in respiratory tract volume, resulting in functional enhancement. RME treatment may reestablish and enhance a regular nasal airflow with the disappearance of OSA [33].

A better apnea-hypopnea index and lower O2 saturation were observed in OSA children treated with RME [34]. As indicated by improvement in oximetric parameters, RME would appear effective for treating slight or moderate OSA. It might be efficacious as a coadjuvant treatment to adenotonsillectomy (AT) in severe situations of pediatric patients with maxillary constriction [35].

OSA can lead, if left untreated, to severe medical complications, growth disorders, behavioral changes, and reduced quality of life. Synergy allows pediatric OSA detection, diagnosis, and treatment in an interactive and collaborative approach between ENT, orthodontists, pediatric dentists, pneumo-allergologists, sleep doctors, endocrinologists, speech-language pathologists, and myo-functional orofacial therapists to improve the short, mid, and long-term results [36].

OSAS is associated with neurobehavioral and cardiovascular abnormalities, growth, and inflammation. The treatment results in enhancements in attention, behavior, and likely improvement in cognitive skills [37]. RME can be a helpful methodology in pediatric patients with OSAS and malocclusion, as the effects of such treatment persist 24 months after the end of treatment [38].

Determining apnea-hypopnea index (AHI) per hour of sleep is essential. The greater the index, the more serious the OSA is. The onset of anomaly is 1.5AHI/h for children and 5AHI/h for adults. This syndrome has consequences far from negligible, potentially affecting mood problems, learning disabilities, growth abnormalities, and delayed neurocognitive development; it can even affect metabolism [39].

Adenotonsillar hypertrophy, in children, continues the main anatomical risk factor of OSA. AT and orthodontic treatment were more successful together than separately to cure OSA in children [40]. After undergoing both treatments, there was a more significant reduction in AHI and respiratory disturbance index and a major increase in the lowest O2 saturation and the O2 desaturation index [41].

RME devices reduce AHI in pediatric patients with OSAS making RME therapy a correct alternative treatment decision for these patients [42, 43].

RME has positive effects on nose breathing, natural head position, OSAS, nocturnal enuresis, and conductive hearing loss. RME can be considered the last treatment choice for those with normal occlusion when other possible interventions in nose breathing, nocturnal enuresis, OSAS, and conductive hearing loss have been unsuccessful [44].

Repetitive hypoxia seen in obstructive sleep apnea syndrome (OSAS) may affect bone metabolism, increasing the risk for secondary osteoporosis [45].

5. Down syndrome

In Trisomy 21, the rate of otolaryngologic infection (otitis media, amygdalitis, and adenoiditis) decreased significantly before and after RME when compared to controls, regarding breathing obstruction symptoms ($p < 0.01$), audiometric and tympanometric progress, and various factors considered by speech pathologists such as articulation of speech sounds and tongue mobility ($p < 0.01$). RME offers a considerable decrease in upper airway obstruction, hearing loss, and enhanced tongue mobility and articulation in pediatric patients [46]. RME results in decreased hearing loss, the annual rate of ENT infections, parentally considered symptoms of upper airway obstruction, and enhanced articulation, tongue mobility, and intelligibility. Breaking the cycle of mouth breathing and growing the area for nasal ventilation may deliver an answer for some respiratory issues, a decrease of tongue projection and drooling, as well as the high incidence of repeating respiratory infections and the high rates of crossbites and compression. The parents relate that RME produces an esthetic improvement. By putting the tongue in its natural place, speech is enhanced, thus enabling integration into society, because of the higher esthetics and self-confidence of the child. This appliance should be part of the recommendation to parents' organizations of children who have Trisomy 21. These outcomes are possibly associated with enlarged oronasal space due to RME [47].

After the expansion of palatal suture by RME, conductive hearing impairment enhancement was due to the renovated normal function of the openings of the auditory tubes [48].

6. Adverse effects of noninvasive ventilation

In ND, DS, and other diseases, it is frequent to use noninvasive ventilation to help children ventilation. Masks, type bilevel positive airway pressure (BiPAP), continuous positive airway pressure (CPAP), and similar are generally supported on the maxilla. However, if used in the tender bone of young children and for a long time, these appliances (BiPAP, CPAP, or similar) may produce retrusion of the face. The deleterious facial effects of noninvasive ventilation [49] are described in a girl with neuromuscular dystrophy, an example of these rare diseases (**Figure 4**). And the necessity of an interdisciplinary team is essential for successful treatment.

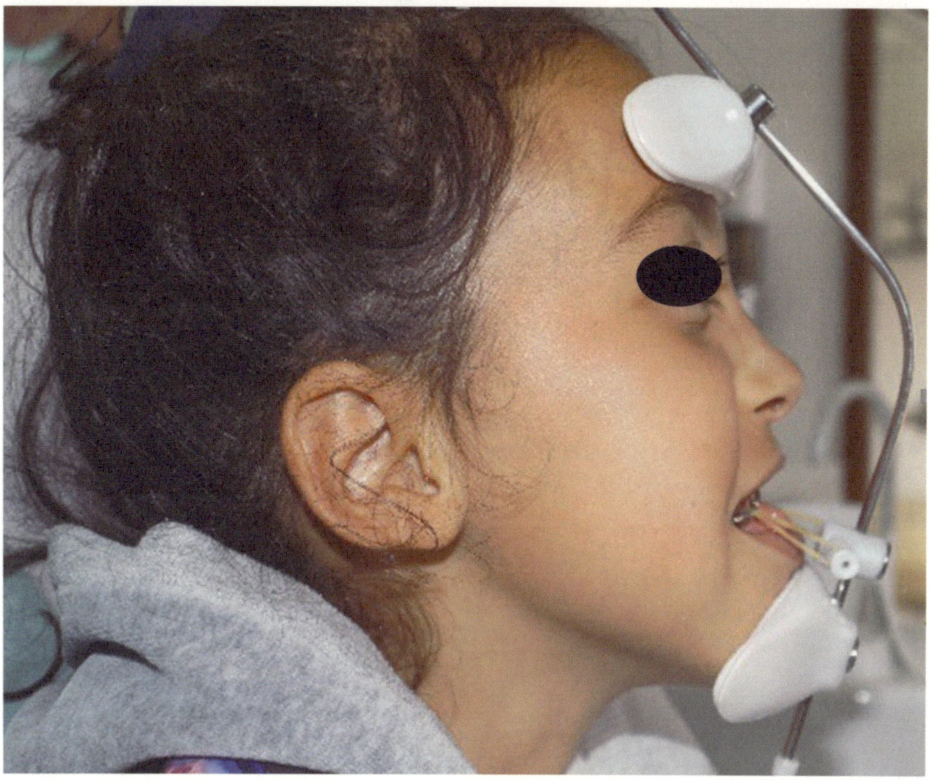

Figure 4.
Extraoral traction appliance (face mask) in a child with neuromuscular dystrophy.

In the same way, RME may be used to restore the compressed maxilla of Carey Fineman Ziter syndrome, a very rare genetic muscular disorder present at birth (congenital myopathy), and ETA may reestablish the correct relationship between maxilla and mandible. In **Figure 4**, we may find maxillary constriction in conjunction with anterior and bilateral posterior crossbites in a child with Carey Fineman Ziter syndrome that used a BiPAP from the age of four months.

Congenital nemaline myopathy is another rare disease that may benefit from pediatric dental treatment, as oral maxillofacial dystrophy is highly dysfunctional (**Figure 5**) and needs intervention and special care from birth.

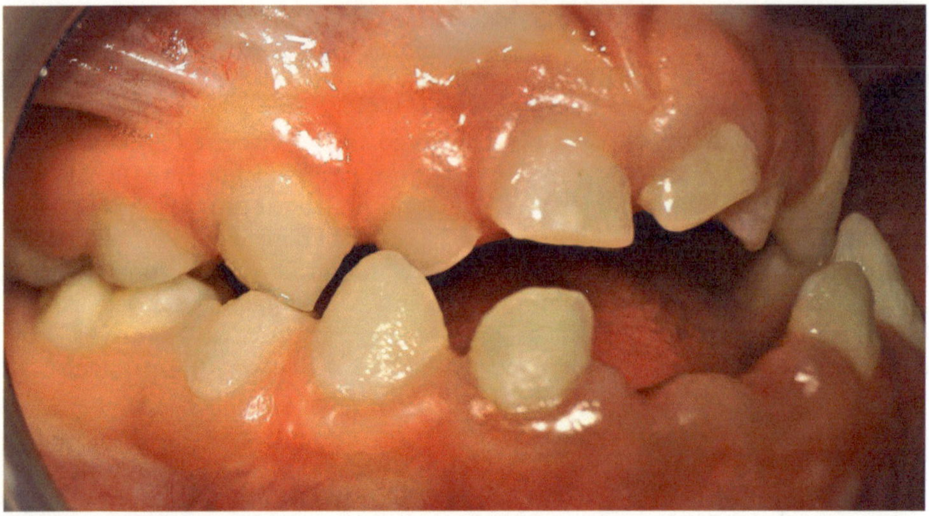

Figure 5.
Maxillary constriction in conjunction with anterior and bilateral posterior crossbites in a child with Carey Fineman Ziter syndrome that used a BiPAP from the age of 4 months.

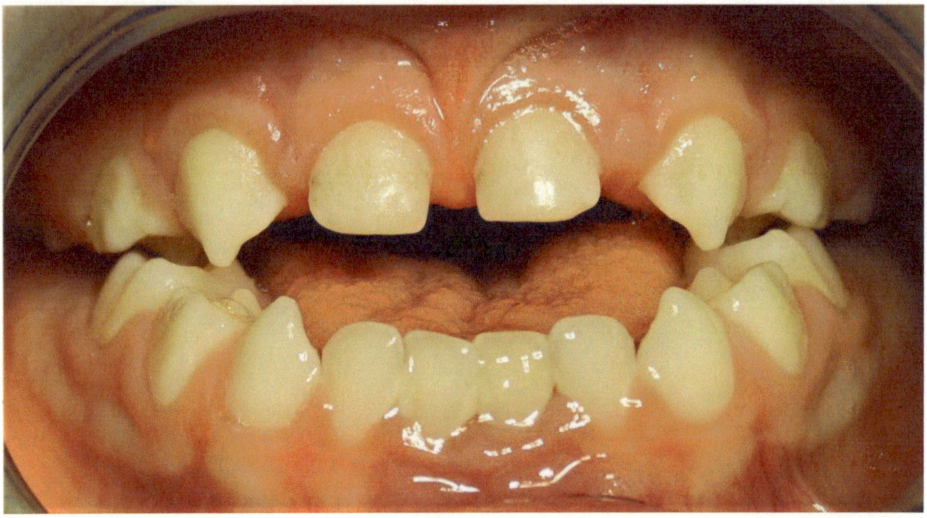

Figure 6.
Severe dentomaxillofacial pathology in a boy with congenital nemaline myopathy with one of the known mutations, nebulin. In addition to the compressed jaw, the maxilla has enormous retrusion, affecting several essential functions, from breathing to swallowing, chewing, and speaking.

Anyway, this is just one of the phases of the multidisciplinary treatment that may help oral functions in a moment of life, but that always needs to be complemented by other professionals, including pediatric surgeons, speech therapists, myofunctional physiotherapists, ENT, and others (**Figure 6**).

7. Other syndromes

RME proved to be a beneficial treatment in a patient with Turner syndrome. Followed by an esthetic rehabilitation of dental morphology proved feasible to achieve facial and smile harmony [50].

Also, in patients affected by imperfect osteogenesis and treated with bisphosphonates, RME could be performed with a standardized protocol without complications after a follow-up of one year [51].

In the case of a child with Schwartz-Jampel syndrome, severe OSA, constricted maxilla, and moderate tonsillar hypertrophy, who could not tolerate the initially prescribed CPAP, following RME therapy, as the pressure setting decreased, the patient showed better compliance with CPAP [52].

Rapid blood cell turnover and bone marrow expansion produced by beta-thalassemia (βT) lead to dentoalveolar and craniofacial abnormalities. The recent literature proposes early interceptive orthodontics to reduce dentoskeletal anomalies, severe malocclusion, and soft tissue imbalance. Therapy includes dental-maxillomandibular orthopedic and functional management with dental-maxillary treatment, preventing orthosurgical procedures later or minimizing their extent. So, an interdisciplinary approach involving a pediatrician, a hematologist, an orthodontist, and a pediatric dentist may enhance the patient's quality of life [53].

Also, ETA proved beneficial in causing significant improvement in patients having combined cleft lip and palate [54]. These children's conductive hearing loss and middle ear effusion improved significantly during RME and after six months of follow-up [55]. Also, a study showed that the correction of the palatal anatomy through RME had a positive and statistically significant effect on improving hearing and middle ear function in patients without cleft and with bilateral cleft lip and palate, with normal hearing levels and with mild conductive hearing loss. Likewise, RME significantly influenced voice quality in patients without cleft but had no significant effect in patients with bilateral cleft lip and palate [56].

8. The role of the pediatric dentist and orthodontist and the importance of early intervention

Early treatment of Class III syndrome resulted in better skeletal modifications with less dental compensation [57]. Early intervention with class III protraction facemask was less likely to need orthognathic surgery than untreated controls. Early class III ETA decreases the need for orthognathic surgery [58].

Starting orthodontic treatment as soon as symptoms occur is essential to enhance the effectiveness of therapy. Integrated medicine is necessary [5].

Besides, early intervention stimulates and improves several functions in children, young people, and adolescents.

The dentist must instruct these techniques to medical colleagues for the benefits they can bring to the general population and, specifically, to children with disabilities [1].

The dentist must check certain aspects of the child's ventilation, articulating with the pediatrician and the ventilatory difficulties team.

Pediatric dentists and orthodontists play a progressively more important role in handling breathing problems and snoring with oral appliances, including RME [59].

Overall, parent satisfaction with their children's RME therapy is significantly higher when supplied by pediatric dentists than orthodontists. Factors related to the doctor-patient relationship and situational aspects (i.e., office place and project, appointment waiting, and treatment length) substantially affected parent satisfaction [60].

9. Discussion

RME can be used to treat problems associated with the growth of the middle face and can produce positive side effects on the patient's overall health. The RME and ETA procedures allow an increase of the whole nasal pyramid, causing benefits for the oral and general health of disabled children, seen in clinical evaluation and related by caregivers. Overall, esthetics and function improve significantly (**Table 1**).

The upper airway problem may be congenital, hereditary, or acquired, interfering in the size and position of the maxilla and in the greater or lesser tonus and synchrony

Effects	
Orofacial skeletal modifications: expansion of the maxilla, the opening of the midpalatal suture, and the skeletal structures like the nasal cavity [34]. Improvement on nasal symptomatology, rhinorrhea, and allergy and increase the area for nasal ventilation (nasal width) [9–11, 21, 33, 35, 38, 61, 62]. Better airway—increase in total upper [11, 31, 33, 50, 63] airways volume [64, 65]. Improves nasal permeability, mucus drainage, better drainage of secretions [10, 11, 50]. Otologic symptomatology: resolution from the serous otitis, hearing, decreased nasal edema, reduced mucosal inflammation, and improvement of an audiogram and tympanogram [10, 11]. Progress on mouth breathing, return of nasal breathing [4, 10, 11, 30, 31, 38]. Tongue mobility and positioning, more space in the oral cavity for the tongue, reduction of tongue protrusion and drooling [10, 11, 33, 35, 50, 62, 66]. Improvement on bruxism [4] Improvement on halitosis [4] Better skin* Esthetics***	Respiratory (with better breath), better ventilation [11, 31, 33, 50, 64, 65]. Decreases the number of upper airway infections [11]. Improvement in chewing (more firmly and quickly**) [50, 66]. Improvement on swallowing [66] Drinking (faster)** [50]. Improves several parameters analyzed by speech therapists (sound modification—alteration of voice quality, word articulation, intelligibility, speech/diction) [10, 11, 50, 65, 67]. Improvement of AHI [4, 8, 31, 33, 35, 38, 40–42, 64, 68–70]. Improvement on snoring, reduced and quieter [10, 38, 70, 71]. Improvement of sleep, without nightmares and sudden waking with startle [4, 10, 38, 41]. Nocturnal sweating ceased [41, 70] Improvement on dribbling [10, 72]. Less sleepiness/fatigue during the day, irritability, tiredness, headaches, an increase of attention and activity [4, 11, 38, 41, 70]. Performance in school improved [38, 41, 70]. A smaller number of hours lost by family in medical consultations [11, 50]. Better general health and development [11, 50, 70]. The self-confidence of the individual enables his integration into society [10, 11, 66].

**Clinical experience (not published).*
***Caregivers' testimony.*
****All treatments improve esthetics.*

Table 1.
Reported effects of rapid maxillary expansion.

of the ligaments and muscles, including the vascular and nervous components of the organs in which it is integrated.

Some severe cases of respiratory disease may include the obligatory use of non-invasive ventilation during a high period of time and sometimes beginning in the first months of life. This required helpful device may have different consequences, depending on the time of use, the direction of the forces, type of appliance, place where the force takes effect, and hardness of the structure.

As we have seen, the absence of treatment for this situation can have serious consequences, and there are multiple treatment approaches. Among the different possibilities, the doctor must not forget the devices we are talking about, among many others with beneficial effects.

When we opt for any orthodontic techniques, we have to consider that the child may not be able to collaborate in the placement or use of the device, which is a limitation.

Furthermore, when expansion is achieved in children who are used to mouth ventilation, the collaboration of a myofunctional therapist may be imperative to teach and encourage nasal ventilation, meaning space is not enough. We have to train muscles to the desired function.

Usually, in children, we use tonsillectomy and adenoidectomy to free up some space so that the child breaths better. RME is an alternative treatment to AT because it reduces nasal resistance and makes air passage through the nose easier. Besides enhancing the quality of nasal breathing, RME benefits the growth of the maxillary dental arch and thus enhances the tongue position, allowing proper sealing of the lips [13, 37, 73–76].

Children submitted to RME revealed an augment in the total nasal volume from the initial symptoms to after treatment that persisted over time. Besides, RME substantially increases nasal volume, $P < 0.05$, compared to the control group; these outcomes are constant through the retention period [3].

OSA children with maxillary constriction had no clinical complaint after treatment with RME. Also, clinical evaluations (orthodontic and otolaryngological) remain normal at the 12-year follow-up period. There was a substantial reduction of the AHI and its duration and a significant increase of $SpO2$ [31, 59]. Children with OSA, with dental malocclusion and treated with RME, improved AHI significantly, respiratory symptoms and nasal resistance diminished, and nasal breathing returned in almost 80% of the children [59].

It remains crucial to understand if RME alone is sufficient for treating mild OSA if significant adenotonsillar hypertrophy is present or if surgery is necessary. When combined with the two techniques, it will not be relevant which treatment is started first as both will be necessary. Still, in some circumstances, there will be the possibility that one treatment performed first solves the problem [74].

The long-term evolution of RME treatment suggests that a reappearance of elderly symptoms is possible, so follow-up is recommended to avoid recurrence [75].

Remember that relapse is always possible and a retention period, sometimes forever (fixed contention), is necessary.

Beckwith-Wiedemann, Marfan's, Crouzon, or Down Syndrome are characterized by a specific phenotype and OSA prevalence [9–11, 40, 76–80].

Applying these techniques always requires a prior individualized study, holistically considering the patient, evaluating their ability to collaborate and the child's different family, social, cognitive, and developmental aspects. And some pathologies do not get better with ERM, like Solitary Median Maxillary Central Incisor Syndrome [81] that does not benefit from RME despite the typical nasal and maxilla anomalies.

The different conditions may present with their specifications or integrate with other pathologies, making it difficult to differentiate the treated problem. So, we need to get better definitions of each condition, which may appear as technology gets better.

If we want an increase in the oronasal and pharyngeal space, we depend on the children's occlusion before and after treatment.

The generality of studies are about mechanical effects of fixed appliances and do not aim at general health, not approaching themes such as cardiovascular risk, neurocognitive impairment or quality of life and the consequences to child's development.

The importance of the intervention of the pediatric dentist and the techniques used are poorly known among physicians and pediatricians, so its dissemination to family doctors and other specialties is essential, and hospital teams that include the different professionals should be rapidly implemented.

10. Conclusions

Despite being very well documented, this technique is often unremembered. It is vital to maintain the studies involving RME and ETA in disabled children, analyzing the differences before and after the treatment regarding clinical outcomes and personal development.

More studies need to address these positive effects on disabled children.

Regardless of the importance of this treatment for the child's development, the intervention should have an interdisciplinary team (oral, dentomaxillary, pediatric, ENT, total myofunctional rehabilitation) to improve these children's quality of life and should be mainly focused on functions.

Conflict of interest

The authors declare no conflict of interest.

David Casimiro de Andrade, Joana Andrade and Maria João Palha are responsible for the conception and design, data collection and manuscript redaction.

Cristina Areias, Paula Macedo, Ana Norton, Miguel Palha, Lurdes Morais, Dóris Rocha Ruiz and Sônia Groisman were responsible for the critical revision of its intellectual contents.

David Casimiro de Andrade was responsible for graphics and photos, the critical revision of its intellectual contents, and the final approval of the version to be published.

All authors declare that written informed consent was obtained from the patient (or other approved parties) to publish this research paper.

Author details

David Andrade[1*], Joana Andrade[2], Maria-João Palha[3], Cristina Areias[1], Paula Macedo[1], Ana Norton[1], Miguel Palha[4], Lurdes Morais[5], Dóris Rocha Ruiz[6] and Sônia Groisman[7]

1 Faculty of Dental Medicine, University of Porto, Porto, Portugal

2 Clínica Dentária de Espinho, Espinho, Portugal

3 Santa Maria Hospital, Lisbon North University Hospital Center, EPE, Avenida Professor Egas Moniz, Lisbon, Portugal

4 Child Development Centre Diferenças, Lisbon, Portugal

5 North Maternal and Child Centre from Centro Hospitalar do Porto, Porto, Portugal

6 Faculty of Medicine, University of São Paulo, São Paulo, Brazil

7 Faculty of Dentistry, Federal University of Rio de Janeiro, Rio de Janeiro, Brazil

*Address all correspondence to: casimirodandrade@gmail.com

References

[1] De Moura C, Silveira H, Andrade D, Palha M, Clemente M. Down syndrome—Otolaryngologic perspective [Trissomia 21—Perspectiva otorrinolaringológica]. Arquivos de Medicina. 2004;**18**(1-2):61-65

[2] Calvo-Henriquez C, Capasso R, Chiesa-Estomba C, Liu SY, Martins-Neves S, Castedo E, et al. The role of pediatric maxillary expansion on nasal breathing. A systematic review and metanalysis. International Journal of Pediatric Otorhinolaryngology. 2020;**135**:110139. DOI: 10.1016/j.ijporl.2020.110139

[3] Levrini L, Lorusso P, Caprioglio A, Magnani A, Diaféria G, Bittencourt L, et al. Model of oronasal rehabilitation in children with obstructive sleep apnea syndrome undergoing rapid maxillary expansion: Research review. Sleep Science. 2014 Dec;7(4):225-233. DOI: 10.1016/j.slsci.2014.11.002

[4] Villa MP, Rizzoli A, Rabasco J, Vitelli O, Pietropaoli N, Cecili M, et al. Rapid maxillary expansion outcomes in treatment of obstructive sleep apnea in children. Sleep Medicine. 2015;**16**(6): 709-716. DOI: 10.1016/j.sleep.2014.11.019

[5] McNamara JA Jr, Lione R, Franchi L, Angelieri F, Cevidanes LH, Darendeliler MA, et al. The role of rapid maxillary expansion in the promotion of oral and general health. Progress in Orthodontics. 2015;**16**(1):33. DOI: 10.1186/s40510-015-0105-x

[6] Ghoneima A, Abdel-Fattah E, Hartsfield J, El-Bedwehi A, Kamel A, Kula K. Effects of rapid maxillary expansion on the cranial and circummaxillary sutures. American Journal of Orthodontics and Dentofacial Orthopedics. 2011;**140**(4):510-519. DOI: 10.1016/j.ajodo.2010.10.024

[7] Iwasaki T, Saitoh I, Takemoto Y, Inada E, Kanomi R, Hayasaki H, et al. Improvement of nasal airway ventilation after rapid maxillary expansion evaluated with computational fluid dynamics. American Journal of Orthodontics and Dentofacial Orthopedics. 2012;**141**(3):269-278. DOI: 10.1016/j.ajodo.2011.08.025

[8] MC ADC, Macho V, Tavares P, Palha M. Effects of Rapid Maxillary Expansion in Down Syndrome Children. Hong Kong: Hong Kong International Dental Expo And Symposium (HKIDEAS); 2010

[9] de Moura CP, Vales F, Andrade D, Cunha LM, Barros H, Pueschel SM, et al. Rapid maxillary expansion and nasal patency in children with down syndrome. Rhinology. 2005;**43**(2): 138-142

[10] de Moura CP, Andrade D, Cunha LM, Tavares MJ, Cunha MJ, Vaz P, et al. Down syndrome: Otolaryngological effects of rapid maxillary expansion. The Journal of Laryngology and Otology. 2008;**122**(12):1318-1324. DOI: 10.1017/S002221510800279X

[11] Areias C, Maia B, Macho V, Norton A, Macedo P, Andrade DC. Oral health in Down Syndrome. In: Health Problems in Down Syndrome. Rijeka: Subrata Dey, Intech Open Science|Open Minds; 2015. pp. 45-68. DOI: 10.5772/60652

[12] Moura CP, Andrade D, Vales F, Cunha LM, Barros H, Clemente M. Rapid maxillary expansion and nasal patency of the down Syndrome pediatric population. Otolaryngology and Head

and Neck Surgery. 2004;**131**(2):
P252-P252. DOI: 10.1016/j.otohns.
2004.06.510

[13] Macedo P, Norton A, Guedes-Pinto E, Guedes-Pinto AC, de Andrade DC. Prevenção das Más Oclusões a Nível Odontopediátrico. In: Andrade DC, Guedes-Pinto AC, editors. Textos Escolhidos de Odontopediatria (Odontopediatria (Portuguese Edition) [Print Replica] Kindle Edition). Porto: Universidade do Porto Editora; 2017. p. 660

[14] Monini S, Malagola C, Villa MP, Tripodi C, Tarentini S, Malagnino I, et al. Rapid maxillary expansion for the treatment of nasal obstruction in children younger than 12 years. Archives of Otolaryngology—Head & Neck Surgery. 2009;**135**(1):22-27. DOI: 10.1001/archoto.2008.521

[15] Iwasaki T, Takemoto Y, Inada E, Sato H, Suga H, Saitoh I, et al. The effect of rapid maxillary expansion on pharyngeal airway pressure during inspiration evaluated using computational fluid dynamics. International Journal of Pediatric Otorhinolaryngology. 2014;**78**(8):1258-1264. DOI: 10.1016/j.ijporl.2014.05.004

[16] Negreiros PO, Freitas KMS, Pinzan-Vercelino CRM, Janson G, Freitas MR. Smile attractiveness in cases treated with self-ligating and conventional appliances with and without rapid maxillary expansion. Orthodontics & Craniofacial Research. 2020;**23**(4): 413-418. DOI: 10.1111/ocr.12383

[17] Ghoussoub MS, Garcia R, Sleilaty G, Rifai K. Effect of rapid maxillary expansion on condyle-fossa relationship in growing patients. The Journal of Contemporary Dental Practice. 2018;**19**(10):1189-1198. DOI: 10.5005/jp-journals-10024-2404

[18] Christie KF, Boucher N, Chung CH. Effects of bonded rapid palatal expansion on the transverse dimensions of the maxilla: A cone-beam computed tomography study. American Journal of Orthodontics and Dentofacial Orthopedics. 2010;**137**(4 Suppl):S79-S85. DOI: 10.1016/j.ajodo.2008.11.024

[19] Rădescu OD, Colosi HA, Albu S. Effects of rapid palatal expansion (RPE) and twin block mandibular advancement device (MAD) on pharyngeal structures in class II pediatric patients from Cluj-Napoca, Romania. Cranio. 2020;**38**(1):22-29. DOI: 10.1080/08869634.2018.1475940

[20] Babacan H, Doruk C, Uysal IO, Yuce S. Effects of rapid maxillary expansion on nasal mucociliary clearance. The Angle Orthodontist. 2016;**86**(2):250-254. DOI: 10.2319/121714-918.1

[21] Quo S, Lo LF, Guilleminault C. Maxillary protraction to treat pediatric obstructive sleep apnea and maxillary retrusion: A preliminary report. Sleep Medicine. 2019 Aug;**60**:60-68. DOI: 10.1016/j.sleep.2018.12.005

[22] Havakeshian G, Koretsi V, Eliades T, Papageorgiou SN. Effect of orthopedic treatment for class III malocclusion on upper airways: A systematic review and meta-analysis. Journal of Clinical Medicine. 2020;**9**(9):3015. DOI: 10.3390/jcm9093015

[23] Cretella Lombardo E, Franchi L, Lione R, Chiavaroli A, Cozza P, Pavoni C. Evaluation of sagittal airway dimensions after face mask therapy with rapid maxillary expansion in class III growing patients. International Journal of Pediatric Otorhinolaryngology. 2020;**130**:109794. DOI: 10.1016/j.ijporl.2019.109794

[24] Huynh NT, Desplats E, Almeida FR. Orthodontics treatments for managing obstructive sleep apnea syndrome in children: A systematic review and meta-analysis. Sleep Medicine Reviews. 2016;**25**:84-94. DOI: 10.1016/j.smrv.2015.02.002

[25] The OSA Partnership Group. Obstructive Sleep Apnoea. n.d. Available from: https://osapartnershipgroup.co.uk/osa-partnership-group-what-is-osa [Accessed: March 1, 2022]

[26] Rajesh S, Wonderling D, Simonds AK. Guideline Committee. Obstructive sleep apnoea/hypopnoea syndrome and obesity hyperventilation syndrome in over 16s: Summary of NICE guidance. BMJ. 2021;**375**(2360):n2360. DOI: 10.1136/bmj.n2360

[27] Rosen CL. Obstructive sleep apnea syndrome (OSAS) in children: Diagnostic challenges. Sleep. 1996;**19**(10 Suppl): S274-S277

[28] Riha RL. Defining obstructive sleep apnoea syndrome: A failure of semantic rules. Breathe (Sheffield, England). 2021;**17**(3):210082. DOI: 10.1183/20734735.0082-2021

[29] Tapia IE, Marcus CL. Newer treatment modalities for pediatric obstructive sleep apnea. Paediatric Respiratory Reviews. 2013;**14**(3):199-203. DOI: 10.1016/j.prrv.2012.05.006

[30] Machado-Júnior AJ, Zancanella E, Crespo AN. Rapid maxillary expansion and obstructive sleep apnea: A review and meta-analysis. Medicina Oral, Patología Oral y Cirugía Bucal. 2016;**21**(4):e465-e469. DOI: 10.4317/medoral.21073

[31] Villa MP, Malagola C, Pagani J, Montesano M, Rizzoli A, Guilleminault C, et al. Rapid maxillary expansion in children with obstructive sleep apnea syndrome: 12-month follow-up. Sleep Medicine. 2007;**8**(2):128-134. DOI: 10.1016/j.sleep.2006.06.009

[32] Moin Anwer HM, Albagieh HN, Kalladka M, Chiang HK, Malik S, McLaren SW, et al. The role of the dentist in the diagnosis and management of pediatric obstructive sleep apnea. Saudi Dental Journal. 2021;**33**(7):424-433. DOI: 10.1016/j.sdentj.2021.02.001

[33] Pirelli P, Fiaschetti V, Fanucci E, Giancotti A, Condo R, Saccomanno S, et al. Cone beam CT evaluation of skeletal and nasomaxillary complex volume changes after rapid maxillary expansion in OSA children. Sleep Medicine. 2021;**86**:81-89. DOI: 10.1016/j.sleep.2021.08.011

[34] Amat P. Troubles respiratoires obstructifs du sommeil et orthodontie: Primum non nocere [Obstructive sleep disordered breathing and orthodontics: Primum non nocere]. L'Orthodontie Française. 2019;**90**(3-4):247-262. DOI: 10.1051/orthodfr/2019039

[35] Sánchez-Súcar AM, Sánchez-Súcar FB, Almerich-Silla JM, Paredes-Gallardo V, Montiel-Company JM, García-Sanz V, et al. Effect of rapid maxillary expansion on sleep apnea-hypopnea syndrome in growing patients. A meta-analysis. Journal of Clinical and Experimental Dentistry. 2019;**11**(8):e759-e767. DOI: 10.4317/jced.55974

[36] Lê-Dacheux MK, Aubertin G, Wartelle S, Delaisi B, Iniguez JL, Tamalet A, et al. Syndrome d'apnées obstructives du sommeil de l'enfant : Une affaire d'équipe ! [Obstructive Sleep Apnea in Children: A Team effort!]. Orthod Fr. 2020;**91**(4):323-345. DOI: 10.1684/orthodfr.2020.28

[37] Marcus CL, Brooks LJ, Draper KA, Gozal D, Halbower AC, Jones J, et al. American Academy of Pediatrics. Diagnosis and management of childhood obstructive sleep apnea syndrome. Pediatrics. 2012;**130**(3):e714-e755. DOI: 10.1542/peds.2012-1672

[38] Villa MP, Rizzoli A, Miano S, Malagola C. Efficacy of rapid maxillary expansion in children with obstructive sleep apnea syndrome: 36 months of follow-up. Sleep & Breathing. 2011; **15**(2):179-184. DOI: 10.1007/s11325-011-0505-1

[39] Galievsky M, Lambert A. Sleep respiratory problems in children: Diagnosis and contribution of the orthodontist. International Orthodontics. 2017;**15**(3):405-423. DOI: 10.1016/j.ortho.2017.06.007

[40] Taddei M, Alkhamis N, Tagariello T, D'Alessandro G, Mariucci EM, Piana G. Effects of rapid maxillary expansion and mandibular advancement on upper airways in Marfan's syndrome children: A home sleep study and cephalometric evaluation. Sleep & Breathing. 2015;**19**(4):1213-1220. DOI: 10.1007/s11325-015-1141-y

[41] Templier L, Rossi C, Miguez M, Pérez JC, Curto A, Albaladejo A, et al. Combined surgical and orthodontic treatments in Children with OSA: A systematic review. Journal of Clinical Medicine. 2020;**9**(8):2387. DOI: 10.3390/jcm9082387

[42] Vale F, Albergaria M, Carrilho E, Francisco I, Guimarães A, Caramelo F, et al. Efficacy of rapid maxillary expansion in the treatment of Obstructive Sleep Apnea Syndrome: A systematic review with meta-analysis. The Journal of Evidence-Based Dental Practice. 2017;**17**(3):159-168. DOI: 10.1016/j.jebdp.2017.02.001

[43] Alexander N, Boota A, Hooks K, White JR. Rapid maxillary expansion and adenotonsillectomy in 9-year-old twins with pediatric obstructive sleep apnea syndrome: An interdisciplinary effort. The Journal of the American Osteopathic Association. 2019;**119**(2):126-134. DOI: 10.7556/jaoa.2019.019

[44] Eichenberger M, Baumgartner S. The impact of rapid palatal expansion on children's general health: A literature review. European Journal of Paediatric Dentistry. 2014;**15**(1):67-71

[45] Sies NS, Zaini AA, de Bruyne JA, Jalaludin MY, Nathan AM, Han NY, et al. Obstructive sleep apnoea syndrome (OSAS) as a risk factor for secondary osteoporosis in children. Scientific Reports. 2021;**11**(1):3193. DOI: 10.1038/s41598-021-82605-6

[46] Moura CP, Casimiro Andrade DJ, Cunha LM, Cunha MJ, Clemente MA, Pueschel SM. P147: Down syndrome: Rapid Maxillary Expansion and ENT Evolution. Toronto, 17 a 20 de setembro. Otolaryngology—Head and Neck Surgery. 2006;**135**(2_suppl):P261-P261. DOI: 10.1016/j.otohns.2006.06.1180

[47] Andrade DC, Palha M, Macho V, Pinto M, Moura C. Effects of Rapid Maxillary Expansion in Down Syndrome. O66 MH Abstracts and Proceedings book of the 10th World Down Syndrome Congress. Dublin: Down Syndrome Education International; 2009. https://www.researchgate.net/publication/320623232_Effects_of_Rapid_Maxillary_Expansion_In_Down_Syndrome_Faculdade_de_Medicina_Dentaria_da_Universidade_do_Porto_PORTUGAL

[48] Kamińska I. Efekty laryngologiczne rozsuwania szwu podniebiennego [laryngological effects of palatal suture expansion]. Annales Academiae Medicae Stetinensis. 2008;**54**(3):24-30

[49] Andrade D, Palha M-J, Norton A, Macho V, Andrade R, Palha M, et al. Deleterious facial effects caused by noninvasive ventilation mask early treatment, in congenital muscular dystrophy. In: Current Trends in Orthodontics. Rijeka: IntechOpen; 2021. DOI: 10.5772/intechopen.100161

[50] Marçal FF, Costa AC, Magalhães IA, Guerra LM, Lopes LL, Alves E, et al. Orthodontic treatment and aesthetic rehabilitation in a patient with turner syndrome: A case report. Special Care in Dentistry. 2020;**40**(5):498-505. DOI: 10.1111/scd.12495

[51] Ierardo G, Calcagnile F, Luzzi V, Ladniak B, Bossu M, Celli M, et al. Osteogenesis imperfecta and rapid maxillary expansion: Report of 3 patients. American Journal of Orthodontics and Dentofacial Orthopedics. 2015;**148**(1): 130-137. DOI: 10.1016/j.ajodo.2015.01.029

[52] Peanchitlertkajorn S, Assawakawintip T, Pibulniyom M, Srisan P, Pungchanchaikul P, Jaroenying R. Successful treatment of a child with Schwartz-Jampel syndrome using rapid maxillary expansion and CPAP. Journal of Clinical Sleep Medicine. 2021;**17**(3):601-604. DOI: 10.5664/jcsm.9028

[53] Einy S, Ben-Barak A, Kridin K, Aizenbud D. Craniofacial deformities in patients with Beta-thalassemia: Orthodontic versus surgical correction-A systematic review. Journal of Pediatric Hematology/Oncology. 2020;**42**(3): 198-203. DOI: 10.1097/MPH.0000000000001651

[54] Kumar S, Verma G, Hassan N, Anjan R, Khan RA, Shaikh S. Facemask therapy in unilateral cleft lip and palate patients. Journal of Pharmacy & Bioallied Sciences. 2021;**13**(Suppl 2): S1303-S1305

[55] Rosso C, Colletti L, Foltran M, Saibene AM, Pisani A, Stefanoni E, et al. Effects of rapid maxillary expansion on hearing loss and otitis media in cleft palate children. European Archives of Oto-Rhino-Laryngology. 2021:1-9. DOI: 10.1007/s00405-021-07187-5

[56] Singh H, Maurya RK, Sharma P, Kapoor P, Mittal T, Atri M. Effects of maxillary expansion on hearing and voice function in non-cleft lip palate and cleft lip palate patients with transverse maxillary deficiency: A multicentric randomized controlled trial. Rev Bras Otorrinolaringol (Engl Ed). 2021;**87**(3): 315-325

[57] Wendl B, Muchitsch AP, Winsauer H, Walter A, Droschl H, Jakse N, et al. Retrospective 25-year follow-up of treatment outcomes in angle Class III patients : Early versus late treatment. [Retrospektive Untersuchung von Behandlungsergebnissen bei Klasse-III-Patienten 25 Jahre nach der Therapie : Frühe und späte Behandlung im Vergleich]. Journal of Orofacial Orthopedics. 2017;**78**(3):201-210. DOI: 10.1007/s00056-016-0076-7

[58] Mandall N, Cousley R, DiBiase A, Dyer F, Littlewood S, Mattick R, et al. Early class III protraction facemask treatment reduces the need for orthognathic surgery: A multi-Centre, two-arm parallel randomized, controlled trial. Journal of Orthodontics. 2016;**43**(3):164-175. DOI: 10.1080/14653125.2016.1201302

[59] Pavoni C, Cretella Lombardo E, Lione R, Bollero P, Ottaviani F, Cozza P. Orthopaedic treatment effects of functional therapy on the sagittal pharyngeal dimensions in subjects with sleep-disordered breathing and class II malocclusion. Acta Otorhinolaryngologica Italica. 2017;**37**(6): 479-485

[60] Alwadei SH, Almotiry K, AlMawash A, Alwadei FH, Alwadei AH. Parental satisfaction with their Children's rapid palatal expansion treatment provided by orthodontists and pediatric dentists. Patient Preference and Adherence. 2021;**15**:251-258. DOI: 10.2147/PPA.S293351

[61] Ngiam J, Cistulli PA. Dental treatment for paediatric obstructive sleep apnea. Paediatric Respiratory Reviews. 2015;**16**(3):174-181. DOI: 10.1016/j.prrv.2014.11.002

[62] Pirelli P, Saponara M, Attanasio G. Obstructive Sleep Apnoea Syndrome (OSAS) and rhino-tubaric disfunction in children: Therapeutic effects of RME therapy. Progress in Orthodontics. 2005;**6**(1):48-61

[63] Guilleminault C, Monteyrol PJ, Huynh NT, Pirelli P, Quo S, Li K. Adeno-tonsillectomy and rapid maxillary distraction in pre-pubertal children, a pilot study. Sleep & Breathing. 2011;**15**(2):173-177. DOI: 10.1007/s11325-010-0419-3

[64] Pirelli P, Saponara M, Guilleminault C. Rapid maxillary expansion (RME) for pediatric obstructive sleep apnea: A 12-year follow-up. Sleep Medicine. 2015;**16**(8):933-935. DOI: 10.1016/j.sleep.2015.04.012

[65] Gozal D, Ismail M, Brockmann PE. Alternatives to surgery in children with mild OSA. World Journal of Otorhinolaryngology—Head & Neck Surgery. 2021;7(3):228-235. DOI: 10.1016/j.wjorl.2021.03.005

[66] İşcan HN, Metin-Gürsoy G, Kale-Varlik S. Functional and fixed orthodontic treatment in a child with cerebral palsy. American Journal of Orthodontics and Dentofacial Orthopedics. 2014;**145**(4):523-533. DOI: 10.1016/j.ajodo.2013.06.025

[67] Moura C, Andrade DC, Cunha L, Cunha M, Vilarinho H, Barros H, et al. Voice quality in Down syndrome children treated with rapid maxillary expansion. Interspeech. 2005. (9th European conference on speech communication and technology);**5**:1073-1076

[68] Rose E, Schessl J. Orthodontic procedures in the treatment of obstructive sleep apnea in children. Journal of Orofacial Orthopedics. 2006;**67**(1):58-67. DOI: 10.1007/s00056-006-0534-8

[69] Sinha D, Guilleminault C. Sleep disordered breathing in children. The Indian Journal of Medical Research. 2010;**131**:311-320

[70] Villa MP, Castaldo R, Miano S, Paolino MC, Vitelli O, Tabarrini A, et al. Adenotonsillectomy and orthodontic therapy in pediatric obstructive sleep apnea. Sleep & Breathing. 2014;**18**(3):533-539. DOI: 10.1007/s11325-013-0915-3

[71] Guilleminault C, Quo S, Huynh NT, Li K. Orthodontic expansion treatment and adenotonsillectomy in the treatment of obstructive sleep apnea in prepubertal children [retraction in: Sleep. 2010 Jan;33] [1] [:8. Erratum in: Sleep. 2009 Jan 1;32] [1] [:Table of contents]. Sleep. 2008;**31**(7):953-957

[72] Stark TR, Pozo-Alonso M, Daniels R, Camacho M. Pediatric considerations for dental Sleep medicine. Sleep Medicine Clinics. 2018;**13**(4):531-548. DOI: 10.1016/j.jsmc.2018.08.002

[73] Li HY, Lee LA. Sleep-disordered breathing in children. Chang Gung Medical Journal. 2009;**32**(3):247-257

[74] Gozal D, Tan HL, Kheirandish-Gozal L. Treatment of obstructive sleep apnea in children:

Handling the unknown with precision. Journal of Clinical Medicine. 2020;**9**(3): 888. DOI: 10.3390/jcm9030888

[75] Cielo CM, Gungor A. Treatment options for pediatric Obstructive Sleep Apnea. Current Problems in Pediatric and Adolescent Health Care. 2016;**46**(1):27-33. DOI: 10.1016/j.cppeds.2015.10.006

[76] Brockbank JC. Update on pathophysiology and treatment of childhood obstructive sleep apnea syndrome. Paediatric Respiratory Reviews. 2017;**24**:21-23. DOI: 10.1016/j.prrv.2017.06.003

[77] Huang YS, Guilleminault C. Pediatric obstructive sleep apnea: Where do we stand? Advances in Oto-Rhino-Laryngology. 2017;**80**:136-144. DOI: 10.1159/000470885

[78] Guilleminault C, Huang YS, Quo S, Monteyrol PJ, Lin CH. Teenage sleep-disordered breathing: Recurrence of syndrome [Erratum in: Sleep Med. 2013 Sep;14] [9] [:927-8]. Sleep Medicine. 2013;**14**(1):37-44. DOI: 10.1016/j.sleep.2012.08.010

[79] Kuroda S, Watanabe K, Ishimoto K, Nakanishi H, Moriyama K, Tanaka E. Long-term stability of LeFort III distraction osteogenesis with a rigid external distraction device in a patient with Crouzon syndrome. American Journal of Orthodontics and Dentofacial Orthopedics. 2011;**140**(4):550-561. DOI: 10.1016/j.ajodo.2009.12.038

[80] Hikita R, Kobayashi Y, Tsuji M, Kawamoto T, Moriyama K. Long-term orthodontic and surgical treatment and stability of a patient with Beckwith-Wiedemann syndrome. American Journal of Orthodontics and Dentofacial Orthopedics. 2014;**145**(5):672-684. DOI: 10.1016/j.ajodo.2013.08.019

[81] Bolan M, Derech CD, Côrrea M, Ribeiro GL, Almeida IC. Palatal expansion in a patient with solitary median maxillary central incisor syndrome. American Journal of Orthodontics and Dentofacial Orthopedics. 2010;**138**(4):493-497. DOI: 10.1016/j.ajodo.2008.09.037

Chapter 12

Oral Health and Prevention in Older Adults

Irma Fabiola Díaz-García,
Dinorah Munira Hernández-Santos, Julio Alberto Díaz-Ramos and Neyda Ma. Mendoza-Ruvalcaba

Abstract

The most prevalent oral diseases such as tooth decay and chronic periodontitis, are the main responsible for tooth loss, this causes a disability in the chewing function, which alters the selection of food, the pleasure of eating, and the state of nutrition. Even the use of total prostheses to replace this loss is not always satisfactory. In the emotional sphere, poor oral health causes discomfort and a decrease in self-esteem. Unfortunately, this continues to occur in older people despite the great scientific and technological advances in dentistry today. Health promotion, which includes health education and prevention, must be present in the course of people's lives. In the prevention of oral diseases, consider not only biological factors as the only causes, but also alleviate and modify the social determinants of the disease. All those involved in the care of the older adults must promote prevention as the most important tool in favor of oral health, and make older people enjoy life with quality. Oral health is an invaluable asset and reward at this stage of life.

Keywords: oral health, prevention, older adults, health promotion, socioeconomic determinants

1. Introduction

Population aging is a human success story. A reason to celebrate the triumph of public health, medical advancement, and economic and social development over the diseases, injuries and early deaths that have limited human life spans throughout history. Globally, there were 703 million people aged 65 and over in 2019. In the next three decades, the number of older people in the world is projected to double, reaching more than 1.5 billion in 2050. All regions will see an increase in the size of their older population between 2019 and 2050.

There are not only improvements in life expectancy at birth, but also even faster improvements in life expectancy at later ages. Globally, a 65-year-old could expect to live 17 more years in 2015-2020 and 19 more years by 2045-2050 [1]. The World Health Organization (WHO) notes that life expectancy in older age is increasing at a much faster rate in high-income countries than in lower-resource settings conditions. See **Figure 1** [2].

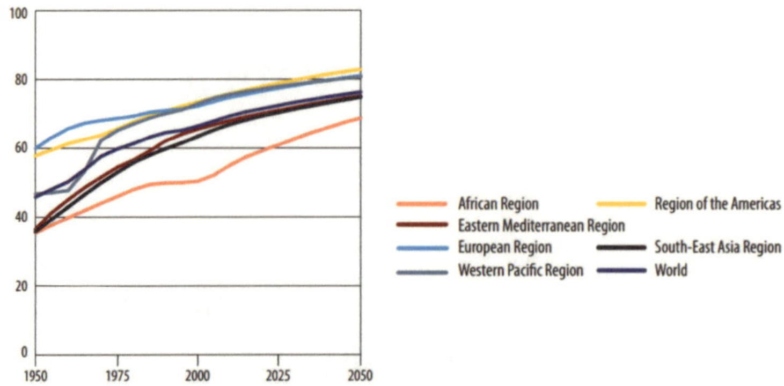

Figure 1.
Changes in life expectancy from 1950, with projections until the year 2050, by region of the WHO and worldwide [2].

This demographic transition is a major challenge for health authorities around the world, particularly as disease patterns will change at the same time. With age, the risk of losing years of healthy life is compounded by low individual resistance, poor nutritional status, chronic diseases, and adverse socio-environmental conditions [3]. Responding to this challenge requires the whole society.

One of the most important strategies we have to control and lessen the danger that this represents is the promotion of health. Health promotion uses education, prevention and health protection. This is of particular importance among developing countries where economic resources are scarce and where the largest growth in the older adult population is taking place in the world [4]. All these efforts to keep away older people from suffering and physical, emotional and social limitations as a result of disease must include the maintenance of oral health.

2. Health promotion and the prevention of health risks in older adults

In the last decades of the 20th century and the beginning of the 21st, a global agenda has been disseminated on the implementation of public policies that reduce the burden of disease in the older adults. For example, since 1995, in response to the global challenges of population aging, the WHO launched a program on aging and health. This was designed to promote knowledge about health care in old age through specific research and training activities, information dissemination, and policy development.

In 1998 in the World Health Report, WHO reported the need to strengthen health promotion among older people. The health implications of aging should be better clarified and understood. Later, in 2000, WHO reiterated the priority of older people's health through the "Aging and Life Cycle" program, which focused on the concept of "active aging". In 2002, WHO published a document entitled "Active Aging: A Policy Framework", which outlines essential approaches to achieving healthy aging. The proposed policy framework was based on three basic pillars: health, social participation and security [4].

2.1 The burden of oral diseases in old age

The WHO in its report on aging and health, 2015, emphasized: "Oral health is a crucial and often neglected area of healthy aging" [5].

In this regard, oral health is a key component in maintaining and promoting a healthy body and a high quality of life [6]. The growing body of scientific evidence confirms that good oral health is integral and essential to a person's overall health. Oral health and disease are closely related to health and disease in general. Unfortunately, older people are representative of a vulnerable population group that suffers heavily from oral diseases.

Given the comorbidities associated with the chronic disease profiles of older people, poor oral health further compromises healthy aging. The literature consistently describes oral health as a significant determinant of an individual's quality of life [7].

Health authorities around the world now face a growing public health problem, including an increasing burden of oral disease among older people. Globally, poor oral health in this age group has been shown particularly in high levels of tooth loss, decay tooth, periodontal disease, xerostomia, and oral cancer [2].

In oral health, global inequalities persist both within and between regions and societies and undermine the fabric, productivity and quality of life of many communities of the world [8]. Despite advances in prevention, restorative techniques, and dental materials, tooth loss remains a reality in both industrialized and developing countries [9]. While there have been significant improvements in oral health in the last 30 years, inequalities persist and a marked social gradient in oral health is observed similar to that of general health [8].

According to the WHO Oral Health Database, high levels of decay tooth are found in national surveys of older people; regionally, the average number of teeth affected by decay varies from an average of 9 teeth in the countries of the African region to an average of 24 teeth in Europe. In all regions, the experience of decay tooth in older people led to tooth loss, while the number of teeth treated after decay is quite limited, especially in the countries of the African region.

Regarding periodontitis, globally, surveys have reported that the percentage of older people with deep periodontal pockets is within the range of 5–30%. Data from Madagascar reported that 17.1% of people aged 65 to 74 had superficial or deep periodontal pockets, while these conditions were observed in 55.5% of Chinese older adults [10].

Poor oral health negatively affects the daily performance of older people, this condition can lead to reduced chewing performance, limited food choices, weight loss, poor communication, low self-esteem and well-being. Obviously, these conditions influence the quality of life. The increase in life expectancy without a better quality of life has a direct impact on government spending on health, and is becoming a key public health problem in the most developed countries. It will also be of great concern to developing countries and countries with high population density and emerging economies, such as China and India [2].

2.2 Oral health promotion in older adults: preventive strategies

At all ages, a healthy natural dentition and a pleasant dental appearance contribute to quality of life. Bad breath and tooth decay can promote social isolation, limit participation in social activities, and influence our judgments about personality traits [9].

Older people in good health can contribute to society, their families, their communities and economic productivity through formal or informal channels, e.g. through volunteer work, etc. [11]. Searching for effective, systematic and wide-ranging interdisciplinary solutions aimed at the current and future burden of oral diseases in our older people will be a great challenge and opportunity in the 21st century [6].

Goals in dentistry cannot be achieved solely on the basis of providing clinical treatment alone. As for any age, health promotion and self-managed disease prevention measures are important to achieve better oral health outcomes. Health promotion interventions are key to improving oral health in old age, as it encourages older people to be proactive about their health [11].

Through the Ottawa Charter, WHO, 1986, health promotion was defined as: "the process of allowing people to increase control over their health and improve it". To achieve a state of complete physical, mental, and social well-being, an individual or group must be able to identify and realize aspirations, satisfy needs, and change or cope with the environment [12].

Failure to prevent or control the progression of oral disease can increase the risk of adverse health outcomes. A recent systematic review in Cochrane found evidence that periodontal disease treatment improved metabolic control among people with type 2 diabetes. Also, it was shown that better care of oral hygiene can prevent respiratory infections and death from pneumonia. in older people in hospitals and nursing homes. Furthermore, frequent tooth brushing was reported to be associated with lower levels of cardiovascular disease [13].

The literature also indicates that health promotion activities should include the active participation of stakeholders in their planning, implementation, and evaluation. This will ensure that health promotion activities are based on the target group's own goals and needs.

Greater efforts should be made to identify opportunities for health promotion activities and the development of community models that encourage older people to improve and maintain their oral health. Ignoring health promotion and disease prevention opportunities in these groups is unfair and can increase inequalities in health standards [11].

2.2.1 Health education for older adults

Health promotion uses education, prevention and health protection. This is of particular importance among developing countries where economic resources are scarce and where the world's largest population growth is taking place [3].

Health literacy, which is within the framework of health promotion and preventive strategies, is necessary to counter oral diseases. Health literacy has been defined as "the cognitive and social skills that determine people's motivation and ability to access, understand, and use information in a way that promotes and maintains good health." In the case of older people, it is important to take into account, in addition to health literacy, functional literacy. Health professionals should consider literacy difficulties among older people than younger adults, if they associate aging with visual and/or cognitive impairments, or think that older cohorts had more likely to have missed school as children. Therefore, they need to provide clear or improved oral instruction to older people [14].

2.2.2 Preventive strategies for oral diseases, WHO recommendations

In recent years, the WHO developed a series of essential principles for the prevention of oral and general diseases and the quality of life, which must be followed by all actors involved in the health care of older people. In the report on health in the world of 2015, the strengthening of health promotion and the creation of healthy environments adapted to the older adults are highlighted in the first place. Promote a healthy diet and nutrition, especially less sugar consumption and increased consumption of fruits and vegetables, in accordance with the "WHO Global Strategy on Diet, Physical Activity and Health, and Reduction of Malnutrition."

One of the most relevant recommendations of this report is to emphasize the importance of educating caregivers about oral health knowledge, to dependent older people, in addition to involving their families, it is extended to independent older adults. As well as, to "other important people", which can be interpreted as the entire team that cares for older people. A relevant point is to ask that care models be developed thinking of older people with primary oral health care capacity. As well as, nursing homes and institutions for dependent older people in order to meet the needs of the many people neglected.

On the other hand, the economic cost of treatments is identified as a barrier to oral health care in older people. So it is requested to improve social security for this age group, and to establish health care financially fair mouthpiece for the older adults. Attention is paid to evidence-based medicine, and this report calls for the implementation of national evidence-based public health programs to achieve better oral health, general health, and quality of life. Finally, within these principles of the WHO, the surveillance of the oral health of the older adults and important risk factors is recommended [10].

2.2.3 Educational action plans

Meeting the oral health needs of the growing older population will require a diverse and capable dental workforce. A two-pronged approach is required, focusing both on (a) new entrants to the profession through dental schools and (b) existing dentists. The latter will be achieved through the continuing professional development of most dentists, but there will also be a greater need for postgraduate education and training. Undergraduate education is the hotbed of conscientious professionals, so it is important to place appropriate emphasis on oral health care for older patients in the undergraduate curriculum [15].

In this regard, the group made up of The common Task and Finish of the European College of Gerodontology (ECG) and the European Society of Geriatric Medicine (EUGMS), proposes a series of educational training actions aimed at dentists, and non-dentists in order to improve dental care for the older adults. They call this strategy "Educational Action Plans", and which in our opinion are of such importance for the prevention of oral diseases in older adults that we underline them.

According to this proposal, educational action plans should involve dental and non-dental health care providers, giving them the opportunity for interprofessional training, practical training and improvement of attitudes towards the promotion of oral health. Better training for dental professionals in oral care for frail dependent older people.

Non-dental health professionals should receive education at the undergraduate, graduate and specialty levels, in the evaluation and promotion of oral health. This includes physicians, nurses, nursing assistants, physical therapists, occupational therapists, medical assistants, pharmacists, dietitians and others. It is proposed that these health providers should recognize oral health as part of multimorbidity. Also relate medication to the impact on oral health, initially assess oral health status, and demonstrate oral hygiene measures for the older adults and their caregivers. All this by developing strategies to overcome barriers to maintaining oral health and access to dental care, deciding when to refer to the dentist, and supporting collaborative practice [16, 17].

2.2.4 Educational interventions in oral health

As the population ages, one of the main challenges for the future will be to translate existing knowledge and strong experiences in disease prevention and health promotion into appropriate programs [3]. Educational interventions on oral health in older people have shown their potential benefit to improve the level of knowledge and their application in preventive oral care measures. The most remarkable result to emerge from the data is the significant decrease in the O'Leary index and in the index of tongue coating [18].

Educational interventions have shown to significantly reduce the number of plaque-covered teeth and improve prosthetic hygiene in older people who require the care of a home health nurse. However, multiple approaches based on individual needs are required to improve the oral health of vulnerable older people, including integrating preventive dental care into the daily care plan carried out by home care nurses. It is important to consider the functional capacity and cognitive function of the older adult, as it has been associated with poorer oral hygiene [19]. Oral hygiene education programs for institutionalized older people caregivers have shown a positive impact on improving this condition of residents. The ratio of residents to caregivers should be considered, as it could play an important role in the provision of oral hygiene services, and has received little attention in the literature [20].

Unfortunately, oral health competence and attitudes towards oral care have been reported to be inadequate in nursing home care. Poor oral health has been reported for people most dependent on care, showing the need for preventive actions [21].

3. The social gradient and biological factors as causes of oral diseases

Considering only biological factors as the cause of oral diseases is not enough to explain the social differences in oral health. Consequently, addressing these factors alone, has led to reductionist approaches to prevention and treatment. Unfortunately there is a lack a sound theoretical basis and which, in general, have also failed to reduce the burden of oral diseases, and oral health inequalities [22].

In this regard, as reported by Link & Phelan, 1995, it is necessary to "contextualize risk factors" and understand the "fundamental social causes" of the disease. "Contextualize" risk factors based on the individual means that it is required (1) use an interpretive framework to understand why people become exposed to risk or protective factors and (2) determine the social conditions under which individual risk factors are related to disease [23].

3.1 Social determinants of oral diseases

In the case of oral health, there is considerable evidence of the influence of the social gradient on the oral health status of individuals. We know that many oral diseases are associated with socioeconomic status, which is linked to family income, educational level, employment status, housing, physical health, and mental health [23].

The fundamental social causes of disease essentially involve the resources that determine the degree to which people can avoid the risks of morbidity and mortality. Resources broadly can include money, knowledge, power, prestige, and the types of interpersonal resources incorporated into the concepts of social support and social network. Variables examined by medical sociologists and social epidemiologists, such as race/ethnicity and gender, are linked to resources such as money, power, prestige and/or social connection that should be considered as possible root causes of the disease [24].

3.2 Biological risk factors and the social gradient of oral disease in old age

Oral diseases share the same determinants and risk factors as the major Non-communicable Diseases (NCDs), which include heart disease, cancer, chronic obstructive pulmonary disease, diabetes, dementia, and stroke [23]. For NCDs, risk factors have been identified and many are related to lifestyle. Risk reduction is associated with smoking cessation, diet control (including reducing excessive consumption of calories, saturated fat and salt), moderate alcohol consumption, and exercise. Furthermore, many of these risk factors are important for the development of oral diseases. **Table 1**, resumes both biological and social risk factors [25].

3.2.1 Age as a risk factor

It is important to recognize that in the older adults, there are risk factors, biological and social that favor the prevalence of oral pathologies such as tooth decay and chronic periodontitis [26]. These diseases continue to appear in old age. Global data indicate that the incidence of untreated tooth decay shows an upward trend after age 60. It was suggested that this was due to the development of root decay among older people. Similarly, periodontal diseases and their sequelae are highly prevalent among older people. The age-standardized prevalence and incidence of severe periodontitis showed a slight increase worldwide during 1990-2010, with a peak incidence in the fourth decade of life [27].

From a biological perspective, the etiology of periodontal disease has consistently been related to the interaction between the microbial plaque and the host's immune response. Previous research shown, although periodontal conditions are initiated by dental plaque, the perpetuation of inflammation and the severity and progression of the disease depend on the effectiveness of the innate immune response to the bacterial biofilm. For its part, tooth decay is an essentially diet-mediated disease, in which host factors such as immune components in the microbial biofilm and saliva contribute to its progression [22].

Biological risk factors	Social risk factors
Interaction between the microbial plaque and the host's immune response Aging of oral tissues: Changes in the healing capacity of cells and tissues	Related to lifestyle: Smoking, alcohol consumption, Diet: excessive consumption of carbohydrates
Decreased salivary gland secretion; xerostomia	Socioeconomic status
Medical conditions: Disabling musculoskeletal disease Cognitive and functional impairment Frailty syndrome Depression	Educational level Ethnicity and gender

Table 1.
Biological and social risk factors of oral disease in old age.

Age can affect both oral diseases directly. When analyzing national studies of older people from the USA and Germany to observe, among other issues, the vulnerability to periodontitis and tooth decay in this population. The results showed that changes in susceptibility to periodontitis with age could be explained by exposure to pro-inflammatory conditions and changes in the healing capacity of cells and tissues [26].

The greater severity of periodontal diseases with age has been related to the length of time that periodontal tissues have been exposed to dentogingival plaque and is considered to reflect the accumulated oral history of the individual. However, the susceptibility of the periodontium to microbial plate induced periodontal degradation can be influenced by the aging process or by health problems specific to the aging patient. Differences in eating habits, increased flow of gingival exudate from the inflamed gum, and possible age-related changes in salivary gland secretions can similarly alter the conditions for growth and multiplication of microorganisms in the biofilm [28].

On the other hand, due to accumulated periodontal destruction, the number of surfaces at risk of tooth decay increases. The sequelae of restorative treatment contribute to an increased susceptibility to tooth decay development. Risk indicators for root decay include tooth decay experience, number of surfaces at risk, and poor oral hygiene [26].

With regard to tooth decay and the immune system and the impact of aging, a systematic review showed that studies are still in an early stage. A small number of studies have reported components of innate and adaptive immunity that affect the composition of dental saliva and biofilms with possible impacts on caries progression. Some conclusions could, at this stage, be considered more theoretical [29].

3.2.2 Medical conditions and their relationship with oral disease in old age

The general health of older people involves a variety of medical, cognitive and functional conditions and/or limitations that can have a direct effect on the onset and progression of oral diseases. And, by extension, the self-sufficiency of older people with respect to the performance of oral hygiene and the search for timely professional dental care [27].

3.2.3 Musculoskeletal conditions and oral health

In general, obtaining medical or dental care is known to be a problem for many older people with impaired functional status, especially those who are homebound or reside in long-term care facilities. People with disabling musculoskeletal conditions are likely to be among those affected in this way.

It is estimated that 10% of the world's population aged 60 years or older have significant clinical problems attributable to osteoarthritis, a condition that is associated with joint pain, limited movement and sensation and occurs most frequently in the knee, hip and joints of the hands [30]. While the prevalence of rheumatoid arthritis is lower, it also affects a large number of people and is associated with aging [31].

Many people with these conditions, osteoarthritis and arthritis in the hands, cannot maintain proper oral hygiene, causing plaque and stone buildup, increasing the likelihood of tooth decay and periodontal disease. The limitation of mobility resulting from these diseases, particularly in the lower extremities, makes it difficult for those affected to visit dental offices for both routine hygiene and treatment [32].

3.2.4 Cognitive and functional impairment, risk factors for oral care

Although cognitive impairment has not yet met the diagnostic criteria for dementia, people with mild cognitive impairment have been found to have poorer oral hygiene, a high gingivitis score, and more impaired root surfaces than those with intact cognition [33]. Tooth loss was reported to be independently associated with the development of cognitive impairment among older people living in the community. This finding supports the hypothesis that tooth loss may be a predictor or risk factor for cognitive decline [34].

Frail older patients in hospitals and long-term care homes, who depend on others for oral hygiene care, are at risk of poor health due to impaired functional and cognitive abilities. They are at high risk for tooth decay because foods containing sugar and refined carbohydrates remain in contact with the teeth for long periods between brushing [35].

3.2.5 Xerostomia: risk of caries and chronic periodontitis

One of the oral conditions that affect the quality of life of the older adults is xerostomia. A high prevalence of xerostomia and hypofunction of the salivary glands has been found in vulnerable older people. Etiologic factors include polypharmacy (especially with antihypertensives, antidepressants, and antipsychotics), poor general health, female sex, and advanced age. People with dry mouth require preventive measures against the consequences of the absence of saliva, including tooth decay, periodontal disease, and candidiasis [36].

3.2.6 Depression is a risk for oral care

Older people with depressive symptoms are less likely to make self-care, including oral hygiene and preventive dental care, a priority - many older people experience a chronic course of depressive symptoms. Depression in old age and depressive symptoms may be associated with poor nutrition, decreased salivary flow, distorted taste, increased oral lactobacillus counts, dental caries, advanced periodontal disease, and oral discomfort [37]. Older people with tooth loss were shown to be at increased risk of depressive symptoms [38].

3.2.7 Risk factors for oral cancer

Oral cancer poses a great threat to the health of adults and the older adults in high- and low-income countries [36]. Oral cavity cancer can be easily prevented and treated if it is diagnosed early [39].

It includes cancer of the lip, oral cavity, and pharynx, and is the eighth most common cancer worldwide. Incidence and mortality rates are higher in men than in women. The prevalence increases with advancing age, and oral cancer is of particular concern among people over 65 years of age. Variations between countries are attributable to differences in risk profiles and the availability and accessibility of health services, among others [36].

Oropharyngeal cancers, a subset of head and neck cancers, have the human papillomavirus (HPV) as a major risk factor. Modifiable lifestyle behaviors, such as smoking and alcohol use, are implicated in the etiology of oral cavity cancers. Previous studies demonstrated that smoking was associated with a 2-fold increased likelihood of oral cavity cancers among those who had never drunk alcohol and binge drinking was associated with a higher likelihood of oral cancers among those who never had they had smoked [40].

Other risk factors are the consumption of betel quid and areca nuts, poor oral hygiene, poor nutrition, a weakened immune system, genetic and immune predisposition. In most cases, it is preceded by visible painless changes in the mouth known as precancerous lesions, such as a whitish (leukoplakia) or reddish (erythroplastic) discoloration of the mucosa, an ulcer, or a swelling. The self-examination of the mouth serves for prevention and early detection. It is an easy to perform, non-invasive method, and low-cost [39].

4. Social determinants of health and life-course related to oral health

In the context of social determinants in health, as mentioned above, these have a significant influence on health inequalities. It will modulate people's health and disease during the life course. Returning to the concept of the WHO [41], which defines them as "the combination of the social conditions in which the individual is born, grows and the ages that affect his health". Cueto et al. [42] in a deeper analysis revealed two edges in this matter. In first place, older adults linked to work have less of time to go to a dentist appointment. They commonly attend when there is an emergency or pain that affects their job performance or social life. On the other hand, the older adults that are unemployed, or not perceive a pension are more likely to suffer damage to their health by the psychic instability that this condition entails, leading to a deterioration of their oral health.

An unhealthy lifestyle appears to be the most relevant SDH in older adults [43].

Kuh and Ben-Shlomo [44] defined life-course epidemiology as the "study of long-term effects on chronic disease risk of physical and social exposures during gestation, childhood, adolescence, young adulthood and later adult life". In other words, it links exposure to risk factors and consequences by considering the importance of the duration and timing of the development of the illness.

The sum in the biological systems could be influenced by independent and individual exhibitions. Specifically, the person is vulnerable to the risk factors, a series of separated situations at different phases of life and this combination increases the illness risk in later life. This is the "*accumulation risk model*". From this model follows the framework of "*chain of risk*", in which a negative or beneficial exposure guide to another negative or beneficial exposition. This version suggest a synergy between intrinsic factors (behavioral resources, self-esteem, conflict-solving abilities and coping methods) and extrinsic factors (family, sociocultural connections and material circumstances).

As stated by the WHO [45] clinically, oral diseases are caused by bad oral habits such as poor oral hygiene, high consumption of sugars, the use and abuse of alcohol and tobacco and a lack of fluoride. Moreover, it is well known that oral illnesses share behavioral risks with non-communicable diseases. For instance, a diet high in added sugars is the principal cause of dental decay and it is related to obesity and overweight.

Heilmann et al. [46] proposed a theoretical framework for oral health. In which they integrated a life course perspective, with the models of the social determinants of oral health illness and their effect on the usual risk factors that link general health and oral health. The model highlights the significance of socioeconomic factors in the infancy and adulthood, like as education and salary. These elements are affected by economic, political and social variables at the societal level. In this sense, the model shows the degree in which infancy socioeconomic status will influence adulthood socioeconomic status. For example, the advancement of dental decay over the course of life follows different patterns directions, to be specific caries levels calculated at one age predicts dental caries levels al later ages.

In 2010, Sheiham and Sabbah [47] reported in their study that the presence of caries in the infancy is a strongly precursor of caries in permanent dentition. Likewise, Hallet and O'Rourke [48] the incidence and severity of dental decay in the primary dentition is linked to the individual, together with socio-economic aspects just as income and maternal education.

However, this is not particularly surprising given the fact that the most significant outcome of enamel defects is a high susceptibility to dental decay. Seen from the *chain of risk* framework, smoking and low birth weight are an example that early stressors of life, lead to enamel defects, which are related to a higher risk to dental caries at later ages [49].

5. The relationship between oral health and general health

Caries and periodontal disease are thus more common than other chronic health conditions and increase in older age. Good oral health is an important aspect of general health and wellbeing contributing to self-esteem, dignity, social integration and nutrition.

5.1 Oral health and nutrition

Aging is a physiological process that affects in unique ways to each person. It is influenced by different factors such as social, economic, environmental conditions and lifestyle of the individual developed through the course of life. It represents a challenge for the professional due to the oral cavity is the first place of the body where the signs of the nutritional deficiencies are manifested clinically [50].

According to the WHO [51] malnutrition refers to "deficiencies, excesses or imbalances in a person's intake of energy and/or nutrients". Who enlists some of the causes that lead to malnutrition in older adults. See **Figure 2**.

It is important to highlight the fact that polypharmacy, chronic diseases and aspects associated to mental health also affect the nutritional status, circumstances that are frequently present in older adults. Poor oral health conditions in this group are associated with discomfort, pain and a reduced appetite, which lead to an inappropriate selection of aliment, with a low or none nutritional content. There is a reduced intake of harder foods, fruits, proteins, vegetables, fiber, vitamins and minerals and a high intake of cholesterol and saturated fat, which alters the nutritional status [52].

Dental loss is related to the reduction of masticatory ability, affecting the maximal biting force and leading to problems in bolus formation. As the number of teeth present in mouth diminishes, the bolus size increases, generating a swallowing dysfunction. This decline can impact seriously in older adult's health, resulting in of chronic disease like cardiovascular problems, diabetes, frailty, sarcopenia and an increased risk of malnutrition [53]. This last condition increases the risk of oral infections.

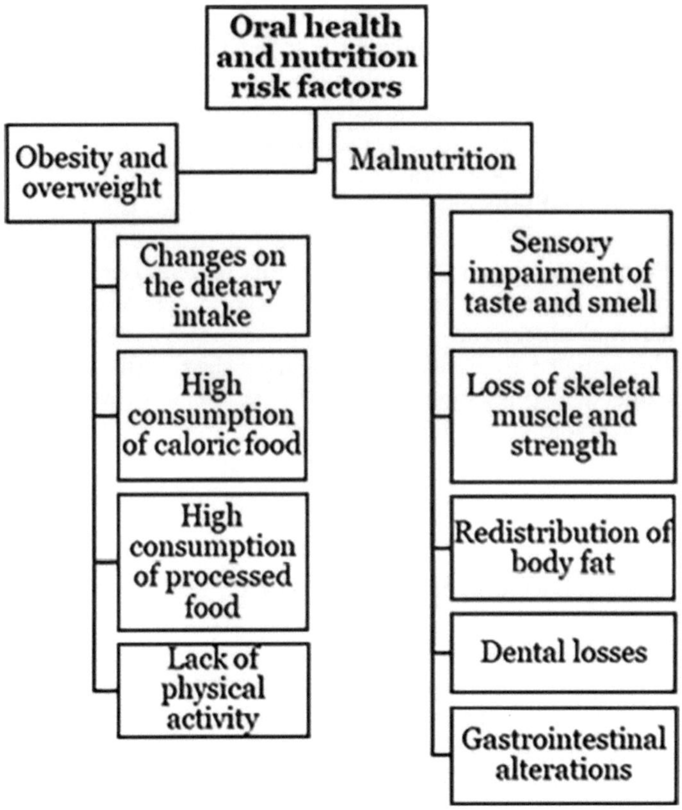

Figure 2.
Oral health and nutrition risk factors enlisted by the WHO [51].

5.2 Oral health and frailty

Frailty is defined as a state, highly prevalent in older adults, of diminished functional reserves that lead to an increased vulnerability to stressors and adverse health results. It includes falls, reduced strength, mortality, growing dependency, a reduced ability to recover from tension situations and increased health care usage [54]. When taking care for frail people is important to be aware of seemingly minor issues. Clegg et al. [55] declared "an apparently small insult (e.g. a new drug; "minor" infection; or "minor" surgery) results in a dramatic and disproportionate change in health state: from independent to dependent; mobile to immobile; postural stability to falling; lucid to delirious".

As mentioned by Castrejón-Pérez et al. [56] the relation that lies between oral health and frailty is considerable and it comes from different pathways:

- nutritional, as dentition impact the nutritional status
- biological, through the relation with chronical inflammatory answer in the body
- psychological, by the impact of oral health on depression and self-esteem.

Hakeem et al. [54] study demonstrated that frailty index was associated with periodontal disease and tooth loss in older adults. Poor nutritional status contributes to the progression of many morbidities involved in the complex and multiple etiology of frailty. This low nutritional intake leads older adults to an increased risk of oxidative stress, malnutrition, inflammation and frailty. There is a strong association between oral health and frailty. This last condition affects the oral status through loss of functions, which guide older adults to complications to take care of their oral hygiene and access to dental services [57].

6. Barriers to accessing dental care

The concept of vulnerability can be described as that subject who will not necessarily experience damage, but who is in fact more susceptible since it has higher inequalities. This condition is specially associated with individual and community situations and contexts. Aging involves an augmented risk for the development of vulnerability, since it is a process of variations that influence on life and health conditions of the individual [58].

Vulnerable groups commonly experience barriers to access oral health and are affected by oral diseases. The World Dental Federation [FDI] made a classification of this barriers [59]. See **Table 2**.

On a previous study, we found some different barriers that affect how older adults take care of their health. Lack of time, was reported as the main concern. Older adults sometimes have up to three jobs, because of their working record, since they do not count with a pension. Another example of lack of time is that some older adults (e.g. wife, mother) are caregivers of their partner or parents and therefore no time left for themselves. This is more rooted in women as part of the sociocultural inheritance and traditions; women are more tended to be a caregiver, which affects their social life and self-esteem, increasing stress factors and physical and mental fatigue.

On the other hand, education plays an important role too. Even knowing the consequences of not having good habits, older adults let the time go by without receiving oral health attention and only assist to the dentist in case of an emergency and when the pain is unbearable [60].

Moreover, is important to identify that some subjects experience accumulative challenges as they relate to simultaneous vulnerable groups. For example, an unemployed adult with physical disabilities living in a non-urban community, from a native group. In this way, more efforts are needed to facilitate access for this groups and specially be focused in address the complicated nature of the barriers meted [61].

Main causes	Examples
Individuals themselves	Low income, lack of perceived need, psychological reasons such as fear and anxiety
Dental profession	Lack of sensitivity or compassion to patient's attitude, inappropriate work team resources, difficult location access
Society	Lack of public support to healthy attitudes, low support for research and inadequate dental health work team planning

Table 2.
Barriers for access on oral health services.

7. Oral health and healthy aging

As mentioned by the WHO, healthy aging is described as "the process of fostering and maintaining the functional capacity that enables well-being in old age. Functional capacity consists of having the attributes that allow all people to be and do what is important to them" [62]. Oral health is an important element of healthy aging as the mouth influences the whole body through the course of life. A healthy mouth contributes to good nutrition, promotes a safer swallowing and prevents infections [63].

Poor oral health conditions could be inescapable in the aging process, but through prevention, patient care and education, these objectives can be achieved. Therefore, professional clinicians and researchers should work together to develop behavioral interventions for the promotion of dental health in family, community and health care settings [64].

A growing body of literature has analyzed that keeping a healthy natural dentition in old age has many benefits including the psychosocial, functional and structural point of view. Knowing this, the goals of mouth healthcare should be targeted to treat and prevent oral infection, promote oral health related to quality of life and give the resources to restore oral health function where necessary and guarantee an acceptable dental appearance [9].

8. Conclusions

Among the great challenges that humanity is facing, there is the aging population. Promoting healthy aging is a task of the whole society. Oral health is part of general health, and participates in a relevant way in the quality of life. Proper oral health promotion activities are essential to protect the oral health of the population.

Understanding the pathways through which social determinants and biological risk factors interact over the life course and shape oral health inequalities can help achieve healthy aging.

Oral health care for older people should begin with interprofessional education, and the exchange between different health care providers for older people should be expanded. The older person, and their family, should be included. Knowing the risks involved in oral diseases allows us to prevent them.

Conflict of interest

The authors declare no conflict of interest.

Author details

Irma Fabiola Díaz-García, Dinorah Munira Hernández-Santos*,
Julio Alberto Díaz-Ramos and Neyda Ma. Mendoza-Ruvalcaba
Universidad de Guadalajara, Guadalajara, Jalisco, México

*Address all correspondence to: irma.dgarcia@academicos.udg.mx

References

[1] United Nations, Department of Economic and Social Affairs, Population Division World Population Ageing 2019:Highlights (ST/ESA/SER.A/430).

[2] World Health Organization. World Report on Ageing and Health. Geneva: World Health Organization. [Internet]. 2015. Available from http://apps.who.int/iris/bitstream/10665/186463/1/9789240694811_eng.pdf.

[3] Petersen PE, Kandelman D, Arpin S, Ogawa H. Global oral health of older people--call for public health action. Community Dent Health. 2010;**27**: 257-267

[4] McGrath C, Zhang W, Lo EC. A review of the effectiveness of oral health promotion activities among elderly people. Gerodontology. 2009;**26**:85-96. DOI: 10.1111/j.1741-2358.2008.00232.x

[5] Petersen PE, Yamamoto T. Improving the oral health of older people: the approach of the WHO Global Oral Health Programme. Community Dent Oral Epidemiol. 2005;33:81-92. DOI: 10.1111/j.1600-0528.2004.00219.x. PMID: 15725170.

[6] Berkey DB, Scannapieco FA. Medical considerations relating to the oral health of older adults. Spec Care Dentist. 2013;**33**:164-176. DOI: 10.1111/scd.12027

[7] Lewis A, Wallace J, Deutsch A, King P. Improving the oral health of frail and functionally dependent elderly. Aust Dent J. 2015;60(1):95-105. DOI: 10.1111/adj.12288. PMID: 25762046.

[8] Sgan-Cohen HD, Evans RW. Whelton H, Villena RS, MacDougall M, Williams DM; IADR-GOHIRA Steering and Task Groups. IADR Global Oral Health Inequalities Research Agenda (IADR-GOHIRA(R)): A call to action. J Dent Res. 2013;**92**:209-211. DOI: 10.1177/0022034512475214

[9] Müller F, Shimazaki Y, Kahabuka F, Schimmel M. Oral health for an ageing population: the importance of a natural dentition in older adults. Int Dent J. 2017;**67**(2):7-13. DOI: 10.1111/idj.12329

[10] Petersen PE, & Ogawa H. Promoting Oral Health and Quality of Life of Older People - The Need for Public Health Action. Oral Health Prev Dent. 2018;16:113-124. DOI: 10.3290/j.ohpd.a40309. PMID: 29736489.

[11] Mariño RJ. Cultural aspects of ageing and health promotion. Aust Dent J. 2015;**60**(1):131-143. DOI: 10.1111/adj.12292

[12] Tulchinsky TH. Marc Lalonde, the health field concept and health promotion. Case Studies in Public Health. 2018:523-541. DOI: 10.1016/B978-0-12-804571-8.00028-7

[13] Griffin SO, Jones JA, Brunson D, Griffin PM, Bailey WD. Burden of oral disease among older adults and implications for public health priorities. American journal of public health. 2012;**102**:411-418. DOI: 10.2105/AJPH.2011.300362

[14] Easton P, Entwistle VA, Williams B. Health in the 'hidden population' of people with low literacy. A systematic review of the literature. BMC Public Health. 2010;**10**:459. DOI: 10.1186/1471-2458-10-459

[15] Thomsonn WM. Ma S. An ageing population poses dental challenges. Singapore Dental Journal. 2014;35:3-8. doi.org/10.1016/j.sdj.2014.10.001.

[16] Kossioni AE, Maggi S, Müller F, Petrovic M. Oral health in older people: time for action. Eur Geriatr Med. 2018;**9**:3-4. DOI: 10.1007/s41999-017-0004-4

[17] Kossioni AE, Hajto-Bryk J, Maggi S, McKenna G, Petrovic M, Roller-Wirnsberger RE, et al. An Expert Opinion from the European College of Gerodontology and the European Geriatric Medicine Society: European Policy Recommendations on Oral Health in Older Adults. J Am Geriatr Soc. 2018;**66**(3):609-613. DOI: 10.1111/jgs.15191

[18] Lee K, Choi Y, Jung E. Effectiveness of an oral health education programme for older adults using a workbook. Gerodontology. 2020;**37**:374-382. DOI: 10.1111/ger.12472

[19] Nihtilä A, Tuuliainen E, Komulainen K, Autonen-Honkonen K, Nykänen I, Hartikainen S, et al. Preventive oral health intervention among old home care clients. Age Ageing. 2017;**46**:846-851. DOI: 10.1093/ageing/afx020

[20] Portella FF, Rocha AW, Haddad DC, et al. Oral hygiene caregivers' educational programme improves oral health conditions in institutionalised independent and functional elderly. Gerodontology. 2015;32:28-34. DOI.org/10.1111/ger.12049.

[21] Bellander L, Andersson P, Nordvall D, Hägglin C. Oral health among older adults in nursing homes: A survey in a national quality register, the Senior Alert. Nurs Open. 2021;**8**:1262-1274. DOI: 10.1002/nop2.743

[22] Gomaa N, Glogauer M, Tenenbaum H, Siddiqi A, Quiñonez C. Social-Biological Interactions in Oral Disease: A 'Cells to Society' View. PloS one, 2016;11: e0146218. DOI:10.1371/journal.pone.0146218.

[23] Tellez M, Zini A, Estupiñan-Day S. Social Determinants and Oral Health: An Update. Current Oral Health Reports. 2014;**1**:148-152. DOI: 10.1007/s40496-014-0019-6

[24] Link BG, Phelan J. Social conditions as fundamental causes of disease. Journal of health and social behavior. 1995:80-94

[25] Lamster IB. Geriatric periodontology: how the need to care for the aging population can influence the future of the dental profession. Periodontol 2000. 2016;72(1):7-12. DOI:10.1111/prd.12157.

[26] López R, Smith PC, Göstemeyer G, Schwendicke F. Ageing, dental caries and periodontal diseases. J Clin Periodontol. 2017;**44**(18):S145-S152. DOI: 10.1111/jcpe.12683

[27] Al-Nasser L, Lamster IB. Prevention and management of periodontal diseases and dental caries in the older adults. Periodontol 2000. 2020;84(1):69-83. DOI:10.1111/prd.12338.

[28] Razak PA, Richard KM, Thankachan RP, Hafiz KA, Kumar KN, Sameer KM. Geriatric oral health: a review article. JIOH. 2014;**6**:110-116

[29] Preshaw PM, Henne K, Taylor JJ, Valentine RA, Conrads G. Age-related changes in immune function (immune senescence) in caries and periodontal diseases: a systematic review. J Clin Periodontol. 2017;**44**:S153-S177. DOI: 10.1111/jcpe.12675

[30] French HP, Galvin R, Horgan NF, Kenny RA. Prevalence and burden of osteoarthritis amongst older people in Ireland: findings from The Irish LongituDinal Study on Ageing (TILDA). Eur J Public Health. 2016;**26**:192-198. DOI: 10.1093/eurpub/ckv109

[31] Doherty E, O'Neill C. Estimating the health-care usage associated with osteoarthritis and rheumatoid arthritis in an older adult population in Ireland. J Public Health. 2014;**36**:504-510. DOI: 10.1093/pubmed/fdt097

[32] Kelsey JL, Lamster IB. Influence of musculoskeletal conditions on oral health among older adults. Am. J. Public Health. 2008;**98**:1177-1183. DOI: 10.2105/AJPH.2007.129429

[33] Chen X, Clark JJ, Chen H, Naorungroj S. Cognitive impairment, oral self-care function and dental caries severity in community-dwelling older adults. Gerodontology. 2015;**32**(1): 53-61. DOI: 10.1111/ger.12061

[34] Saito S, Ohi T, Murakami T, Komiyama T, Miyoshi Y, Endo K, et al. Association between tooth loss and cognitive impairment in community-dwelling older Japanese adults: a 4-year prospective cohort study from the Ohasama study. BMC Oral Health. 2018;**18**:142. DOI: 10.1186/s12903-018-0602-7

[35] Coker E, Ploeg J, Kaasalainen S, Fisher A. A concept analysis of oral hygiene care in dependent older adults. J Adv Nurs. 2013;**69**:2360-2371. DOI: 10.1111/jan.12107

[36] Gil-Montoya JA, de Mello AL, Barrios R, Gonzalez-Moles MA, Bravo M. Oral health in the elderly patient and its impact on general well-being: a nonsystematic review. Clinical Interv Aging. 2015;**10**:461-467. DOI: 10.2147/CIA.S54630

[37] Hybels CF, Bennett JM, Landerman LR, Liang J, Plassman BL, Wu B. Trajectories of depressive symptoms and oral health outcomes in a community sample of older adults. Int J Geriatr Psychiatry. 2016;**31**:83-91. DOI: 10.1002/gps.4292

[38] Kunrath I, Silva AER. Oral health and depressive symptoms among older adults: longitudinal study. Aging Ment Health. 2020:1-7. DOI: 10.1080/13607863.2020.1855104

[39] Shrestha G, Maharjan L. Mouth Self-Examination for Prevention and Control of Oral Cavity Cancer. JNMA; journal of the Nepal Medical Association. 2020;58: 360-362. DOI:10.31729/jnma.4910

[40] Akinkugbe AA, Garcia DT, Brickhouse TH, Mosavel M. Lifestyle risk factor related disparities in oral cancer examination in the U.S: a population-based cross-sectional study. BMC Public Health. 2020;20:153. DOI: 10.1186/s12889-020-8247-2.

[41] World Health Organization. Social determinants of health [Internet]. 2021. Available from: https://www.who.int/health-topics/social-determinants-of-health#tab=tab_1 [Accessed:2021-08-05].

[42] Cueto A, González RM, Batista NM. Determinantes sociales y condiciones de salud bucal de los adultos mayores. Rev Cubana Estomatol. 2019;**56**(2):1-15

[43] González RM, Cueto A, Batista NM, Rodríguez S. Oral health and social determinants in elderly adults. MOJ Gerontol Ger. 2018;**3**(1):16-20

[44] Kuh D, Ben-Shlomo Y. The life course approach to chronic disease epidemiology. 2nd ed. Oxford: Oxford University Press; 2004. 494 p. DOI: 10.1093/acprof:oso/9780198578154.001.0001.

[45] World Health Organization. Achieving better oral health as part of the universal health coverage and noncommunicable disease agendas towards 2030. [Internet]. 2020. Available from: https://apps.who.int/gb/ebwha/pdf_files/EB148/B148_8-en.pdf [Accessed:2021-08-07].

[46] Heilmann A, Tsakos G, Watt RG, Burton-Jeangros C, Cullati S, Sacker A, et al. Oral health over the life course. In: A life course perspective on health trajectories and transitions. New York: Springer; 2015. pp. 39-59. DOI: 10.1007/978-3-319-20484-0_3

[47] Sheiham A, Sabbah W. Using universal patterns of caries for planning and evaluating dental care. Caries Res. 2010;**44**(2):141-150. DOI: 10.1159/000308091

[48] Hallett KB, O'Rourke PK. (2003). Social and behavioural determinants of early childhood caries. Aust Dent J. 2003;**48**(1):27-33. DOI: 10.1111/j.1834-7819.2003.tb00005.x

[49] Phillips M, Masterson E, Sabbah W. Association between child caries and maternal health-related behaviours. Community Dent Health. 2016;**33**(2):133-137. DOI: 10.1922/CDH_3801Phillips05

[50] Hernández L, Marimón ME, Linares EM, González E. Salud oral y hábitos dietéticos en los adultos mayores no institucionalizados. RCAN. 2017;**27**(1):29-47

[51] World Health Organization. Malnutrition [Internet]. 2021. Available from: https://www.who.int/news-room/fact-sheets/detail/malnutrition [Accessed: 2021-08-03].

[52] Giraldo-Giraldo NA, Estrada-Restrepo A, Agudelo-Suárez AA. Malnutrición y su relación con aspectos de salud en adultos mayores. Nutr Clín Hosp. 2019;39(2):156-164. DOI: 10.12873/392giraldo.

[53] Azzolino D, Passarelli PC, De Angelis P, Piccirillo GB, D'Addona A, Cesari M. Poor oral health as determinant of malnutrition and sarcopenia. Nutrients. 2019;**11**(12):1-17. DOI: 10.3390/nu11122898

[54] Hakeem F, Bernabé E, Sabbah W. Association between oral health and frailty among american older adults. J. Am. Med. Dir. Assoc. 2021;22(3):559-563. DOI. https://doi.org/10.1016/j.jamda.2020.07.023

[55] Clegg A, Young J, Iliffe S, Rikkert MO, Rockwood K. Frailty in elderly people. Lancet. 2013;**381**(9868):752-762. DOI: 10.1016/S0140-6736(12)62167-9

[56] Castrejón-Pérez RC, Borges-Yáñez SA, Gutiérrez-Robledo LM, et al. Oral health conditions and frailty in mexican community-dwelling elderly: A cross sectional analysis. BMC Public Health. 2012;**12**(773):1-12. DOI: 10.1186/1471-2458-12-773

[57] Niesten D, van Mourik K, van der Sanden W. The impact of frailty on oral care behavior of older people: a qualitative study. BMC Oral Health. 2013;**13**(61):1-12. DOI: 10.1186/1472-6831-13-61

[58] Carmo ME, Guizardi FL. The concept of vulnerability and its meanings for public policies in Health and social welfare. Cad Saúde Pública. 2018;**34**(3):1-14. DOI: 10.1590/0102-311X00101417

[59] Nagarajappa R, Sanadhya S, Batra M, Daryani H, Ramesh G, Aapaliya P. Perceived barriers to the provision of preventive care among dentists of Udaipur. India. J Clin Exp Dent. 2015;7(1):e74-e79. DOI: 10.4317/jced.51770

[60] Hernández-Santos DM, Díaz-Garcia IF. Perceptions of Two Older Adults Regarding the Factors and Barriers that Influence their Oral Health Care: A Case Study. Qual Repor 2021;26(1):246-261. DOI. https://doi.org/10.46743/2160-3715/2021.4321

[61] Harnagea H, Couturier Y, Shrivastava R, et al. Barriers and facilitators in the integration of oral health into primary care: a scoping review. BMJ Open. 2017;7(9):1-17. DOI: 10.1136/bmjopen-2017-016078

[62] World Health Organization. Década del envejecimiento saludable: 2021-2030. [Internet]. 2021. Available from: https://www.who.int/es/initiatives/decade-of-healthy-ageing [Accessed: 2021-08-13].

[63] Dirks SJ, Monopoli M. Oral health and healthy aging. In: Healthy aging. Switzerland: Springer; 2019. pp. 213-226. DOI: 10.1007/978-3-030-06200-2_19

[64] Gerontological Society of America. Oral health: an essential element of healthy aging. [Internet]. 2017. Available from: https://www.geron.org/images/gsa/documents/oralhealth.pdf [Accessed: 2021-08-14].

Chapter 13

Oral Aspects and Dental Management of Special Needs Patient

Pinar Kiymet Karataban

Abstract

Individuals with special needs are the most underserved regarding healthcare needs in almost all populations. Special needs patients with intellectual disability have muscle coordination disorder, impaired oral motor function, drooling, weak muscles that cause chewing and swallowing problems. Also, soft diet consumption makes this population more prone to dental disease. They have more caries, missing teeth, orthodontic and periodontal problems. Besides more difficulties obtaining professional dental care than other segments of the population. Though many countries developed community-based systems to improve oral health for people with special needs, providing good oral health mainly depends on the effort of the families. Therefore the education of the caregiver about oral hygiene provision is also critical for the special needs patient to enjoy a lifetime of oral health the same as other members of the society.

Keywords: disability, dentistry for special needs patient, cerebral palsy, autism, down syndrome, intellectual disability

1. Introduction

According to the WHO World report on disability 2011, About 15% of the world's population lives with some form of disability, of whom 2–4% experience significant difficulties in functioning. The global disability prevalence is higher than previous WHO estimates, which date from the 1970s and suggested a figure of around 10%. This global estimate for disability is on the rise due to population aging and the rapid spread of chronic diseases, as well as improvements in the methodologies used to measure disability.

Individuals with disabilities have generally poorer health, lower education, fewer economic opportunities, and higher rates of poverty than people without disabilities. This is mainly due to the obstacles they face in their daily lives and the lack of services available to them. Regarding oral health and access to dental care, the same obstacles are of concern. Oral health is mostly ignored, oral hygiene is neglected, and dental treatments are postponed after other health issues. As a result, individuals with special needs present more dental caries, periodontal problems, orthodontic anomalies, and are more prone to dental diseases compared with the healthy population.

2. Dental management of special needs patient

2.1 Cerebral palsy

Cerebral palsy is a non-progressive movement, posture, and tone disorder characterized by the impairment of motor activities in the developing fetal or infant brain. Motor disorders are often accompanied by sensory, perception, communication, and behavioral disorders, epilepsy, and musculoskeletal problems [1]. In these patients, muscle weakness or paralysis, unbalanced and irregular gait, uncoordinated movements, sudden seizures, mental retardation, emotional disorders, learning, speech communication disorders, and weakness of swallowing, and coughing reflexes are seen. Because brain development continues during the first 2 years of life, cerebral palsy may develop as a result of brain damage occurring in the prenatal, perinatal, or postnatal periods [2]. However, more than 80% of cases are due to problems in the prenatal period.

Etiologically, in the prenatal period; maternal diseases, trauma, genetics, drug use, bleeding, consanguineous marriage, radiation, in the natal period; premature/late birth, birth trauma due to inappropriate position, low/high birth weight, cord entanglement, lack of oxygen, multiple pregnancies, difficult birth, birth trauma, in the postnatal period; febrile diseases, trauma, hyperbilirubinemia, hypoglycemia, seizure, and cerebral hemorrhage are risk factors for cerebral palsy [3].

2.1.1 Oral findings of patients with cerebral palsy

It has been reported that the rate of drooling in children with cerebral palsy is 10–58% [4]. Although drooling is normal in infants and young children, it is considered pathological after 4 years of age. Most children with cerebral palsy, who are drooling, are unable to swallow normal saliva due to oral-motor dysfunction, although not much saliva is produced. Perioral eczema, infection, and dehydration occur as a result of drooling out of the mouth [5].

Bruxism, especially in the "Spastic" type, is commonly observed in individuals with cerebral palsy [6]. It has been reported that 36.9–51% of children with cerebral palsy have bruxism. In addition to bruxism, the presence of parafunctional habits such as pacifier-finger sucking, biting objects have also been detected [7].

Periodontal diseases occur more often in children with cerebral palsy due to physical inadequacies, malocclusions, poor oral hygiene, chewing, swallowing difficulties, and consumption of soft food with high carbohydrate content. Besides, the use of phenytoin for seizure control causes gingival hyperplasia [8].

Caries formation is observed at a high rate in children with cerebral palsy. The most important reason for this situation is poor oral hygiene. Other risk factors for caries formation are mouth breathing, the effect of drugs used, and enamel hypoplasia [8]. Differences in food form, increased duration of food consumption, difficult cooperation, and structural defects in the teeth cause an increase in the prevalence of dental caries in children with cerebral palsy, and it has been reported that there are more extracted and untreated teeth compared with healthy children [9].

Malocclusions are observed two times more when compared with healthy individuals, and these patients have unilateral crossbite with excessive overbite and overjet. It has been reported that patients with cerebral palsy have a higher prevalence of malocclusion than healthy individuals, but the severity of malocclusion varies according to the degree of neurological disorder. In these individuals, musculoskeletal anomalies, altered cranial base relationships, premature tooth eruption, mouth breathing, and inadequate lip closure, as well as increased overjet and overbite, can be observed [10, 11].

It has been reported that cerebral palsy is not an etiological factor for erosion, but an increase in erosion since gastro-esophageal reflux is frequently observed in these individuals [12]. It has been reported that in children with cerebral palsy accompanied by gastro-esophageal reflux, especially in the quadriplegia type, the risk of dental erosion is considerably increased and the incidence of oral diseases is quite high [13].

2.1.2 Oral hygiene challenges for individuals with cerebral palsy

Neuromuscular problems specific to cerebral palsy affect oral health in different ways. Changes in the orofacial region cause nutritional problems as well as the development of parafunctional habits and difficulties in maintaining oral hygiene [14]. In addition, dyskinetic movements cause pathological oral reflexes such as sudden biting or nausea. Gastric reflux associated with a blended diet, often rich in sugar, further puts these patients' oral health at risk. Neuromuscular problems also prevent the patient from brushing their teeth correctly [15]. Patients with cerebral palsy have difficulty in chewing and swallowing due to changes in tongue, cheek, and lip motility. In these patients, there is an imbalance in the oral microbiota, which favors the proliferation of acidogenic bacterial species, which initiate the caries process [15].

2.1.3 Dental management of patients with cerebral palsy

Treatment sessions should be kept brief for patients with cerebral palsy. Patients may need to be moved from a wheelchair to a dental chair. The patient should be placed in the middle of the dental chair with arms and legs as close to the body as possible. After the patient is placed properly in a dental chair, the patient should be checked whether he/she is comfortable and the position of the extremities is correct. To keep the airway open, the patient should be seated at a 45-degree angle, but not in the supine position. The dental chair should be moved slowly, and the light reflector should be turned on slowly to prevent spastic muscle movements and to eliminate the risk of seizure. Myorelaxant agents should be used when necessary.

During dental treatment procedures, it is crucial to balance the patient's head at all stages. Various mouthguards should be used to control involuntary jaw movements and accidental bites. The airway should be controlled, and frequent breaks should be given to allow the patient to relax and breathe normally. To minimize the startle reflex, the patient should be warned at every stage. The use of stimuli such as sudden movements, sounds, and lights should be avoided. Efficient, fast treatment should be done, and chair time should be minimized to reduce muscle fatigue. In patients with more complex situations, sedation or general anesthesia may be an option [15–17].

2.2 Down syndrome/trisomy 21

Down syndrome, defined by Down in 1866, is an autosomal anomaly associated with the trisomy of the 21st chromosome pair. Its incidence in the population is 1/800, and it is the most common chromosomal change. There is an extra 21st chromosome (trisomy) in 95% of cases. In some cases, there are 46 normal chromosomes, but the 21st chromosome has been replaced with another chromosome [18, 19]. Mosaic Down syndrome, on the other hand, is caused by the inability of chromosomes to fully divide during cell division in the embryonic period. Some cells of the mosaic type have 47 chromosomes, while others have 46 chromosomes [19]. Individuals with Down syndrome represent learning difficulties, neuropsychiatric disorders, and behavioral problems as well as congenital cardiac anomalies, thyroid problems, seizures, visual and hearing disorders, early-onset dementia, and frequent infections. Also, some individuals with Down syndrome are hepatitis B carriers, and leukemia can be seen in patients with Down syndrome [20].

The only factor known to cause Down syndrome is the age of the mother during pregnancy, the risk increases in pregnancies over the age of 35. However, because young women, in general, have more babies, 75–80% of children with Down syndrome are babies of young mothers. There is no difference between country, nationality, or socioeconomic status [21].

2.2.1 Oral findings of patients with down syndrome

Craniofacial features of individuals with Down syndrome include brachycephaly, broad and short neck, maxillary hypoplasia, sloping palpebral fissures, short ears, midface hypoplasia, curved eyes, narrow, flat nose [22].

Palate: Compared with the mandible, the middle face of the patients shows less development. As a result, the palate has not completed its development in terms of length, height, and depth [23].

Lips and mouth opening: The corners of the lips are located below due to hypotonic muscles. Due to mouth breathing, a predisposition to angular cheilitis, chronic periodontitis, and respiratory infections develops [23].

Tongue: The tongue is fissured and hypotonic. Majority of the individuals with Down syndrome present macroglossia. With the abnormal pressure on the teeth due to macroglossia, traces of teeth in the form of a white round border can be observed on the tongue, either bilaterally or unilaterally. In addition, diastemas, tongue thrusting, tongue sucking are also observed due to macroglossia [23].

Microdontia: Microdontia is observed in the primary and permanent dentition in 35–55% of children with Down syndrome. Clinical crowns are generally conical, short, and smaller in size [23].

Hypoplasia: Hypoplastic defects are usually the result of significant systemic disease or prolonged febrile illness [23].

Dental agenesis: Congenital tooth deficiency is 10 times more common in Down syndrome patients than in the healthy population. The transfer of genetic codes is held responsible for this situation. The most prevalent teeth agenesis is the third molar, second premolar, lateral incisors, and mandibular incisors, respectively. Boys are more affected than girls, the mandible is more affected than the maxilla, and the left side of the jaws is more affected than the right side [24].

Delayed tooth eruption: Tooth eruption is usually delayed in the primary dentition, especially in maxillary and mandibular anterior teeth and first molars [25].

Dental caries: The prevalence of caries in Down syndrome children is lower than in healthy children. Many factors such as delayed tooth eruption, congenitally missing teeth, high salivary pH and bicarbonate levels, and shallow fissures on the teeth play a role in the formation of this situation [26].

Periodontal problems: Diffuse gingivitis and rapid periodontal destruction are observed in children with Down syndrome compared with healthy children with similar plaque levels. The most common periodontal diseases are as follows: marginal gingivitis, acute necrotizing ulcerative gingivitis (ANUG), aggressive periodontitis, gingival recession, horizontal and vertical bone loss, exposure of bifurcations, or trifurcations in molars, mobility and tooth loss especially in the incisor region of the mandible [27].

Occlusion: Occlusion and orthodontic problems such as Class III malocclusion, malocclusions due to mouth breathing, bruxism, shifting of the maxillary midline, anterior open bite, Temporomandibular Joint (TMJ) dysfunction, hypotonic ligaments of the mandible, and developmental disorders of the maxilla are encountered in children with Down syndrome [28].

2.2.2 Oral hygiene challenges for individuals with down syndrome

Although individuals with Down syndrome have usually a cooperative personality, providing sufficient oral hygiene depends on the family's knowledge and education level. Down syndrome children might also experience anxiety or fear of dental visits and parents are usually not aware of the dental problems of their children. Also, Down syndrome children using medical agents suffering from seizures experience dry mouth due to a decrease in the salivary flow rate, which may lead to xerostomia preparing a suitable environment for caries and periodontal problems [29, 30]. In addition, high levels of tooth wear are observed in these patients. This is mainly due to bruxism and the acidic oral environment (reflux and vomiting) [22].

2.2.3 Dental management of patients with down syndrome

The behavior management skills of the dental professional are the key factor in a child's acceptance of dental treatment [19]. Before determining the right approach to the Down syndrome child, the dentist should consider the level of the mental, emotional, and social development of the child [31]. Most Down syndrome children are affectionate and cooperative for their dental treatment and can be treated easily with the tell-show-do technique [32].

When treating Down Syndrome children, the need for prophylaxis of subacute bacterial endocarditis and the patient's compliance level should be considered [22]. During treatment, the gag reflex can be reduced by behavioral management techniques, as comforting and distracting patients. It can also be reduced by intraoral massage and pharmacological or non-pharmacological interventions [33]. The recalls should be planned frequently, and preventive dental treatments should be included in the treatment plan. The education of caregivers is crucial for sufficient oral hygiene provision and follow-ups. Mild sedation may be used in children with moderate anxiety. Extremely resistant patients may require general anesthesia [17].

2.3 Autism spectrum disorder (ASD)

Autism was first described in 1943 by an American child psychiatrist, Leo Kanner. Autism spectrum disorder (ASD) is a neurodevelopmental disorder, characterized by difficulties in communication, social relationships, and limited and repetitive behaviors [34, 35].

Individuals with ASD have characteristics such as stereotypical or repetitive motor behavior (flapping, rocking back and forth), repetitive use of objects (turning coins, putting objects in order), or making repetitive speeches. Many patients adhere to rigid routines in their lives and may have a more rigid thinking pattern. They react negatively to even minor changes or transitions [36].

No specific etiology has been identified for ASD. However, studies indicate a combination of genetical and environmental factors before and after birth, such as parental age, fetal environment (e.g., sex steroids, maternal infections/immune activation, obesity, diabetes, hypertension, or ultrasound examinations), perinatal and obstetric events (e.g., hypoxia), medication (valproate, selective serotonin reuptake inhibitors), smoking and alcohol use, nutrition (e.g., short inter-pregnancy intervals, e.g., vitamin D, iron, zinc, and copper), vaccination, and toxic exposures (air pollution, heavy metals, pesticides, organic pollutants) and low birth weight [37, 38].

2.3.1 Oral findings of patients with autism spectrum disorder

Bruxism: It has been reported that bruxism and dental wear due to bruxism are seen in one of every five children with ASD [39].

Xerostomia: One of the possible side effects of medications, such as central nervous system stimulants (methylphenidate), antihypertensives (clonidine), antidepressants (fluoxetine), anticonvulsants (carbamazepine and valproate), and antipsychotics (olanzapine and risperidone), which are often prescribed for the symptomatical relief of autism is xerostomia [40].

Delayed tooth eruption: Phenytoin is commonly prescribed for people with ASD. The tooth eruption may be delayed due to phenytoin-induced gingival hyperplasia.

Self-injury: ASD children may present self-injurious behavior and damaging oral habits such as picking at the gingiva or biting the lips; and pica—eating objects and substances such as gravel, cigarette butts, or pens. Self-injury to oral tissues results in ulcers, periodontitis, gingivitis, and self-extraction [41].

In addition, problems such as tongue thrusting, erosion, hyperactive gag reflex, and some malocclusions such as anterior open bite and maxillary retrognathia were also reported in these individuals [42, 43].

2.3.2 Oral hygiene challenges for individuals with autism spectrum disorder

Clinical conditions that ASD children present, such as sensorimotor and attention deficits, anxiety and related emotion regulation, comprehensive difficulties, and general speech disorders, create various difficulties for families, educators, and dentists in the provision of oral health care of these children [44]. Besides, parents face difficulties in brushing the teeth of the ASD children due to the sensory sensitivities of their children and the unpredictable or aggressive behavior that may require physical restraints.

In the literature, the caries experience of ASD individuals is controversial. Research reports state that ASD children are more prone to dental caries due to the consumption of sugar-containing food [45–47]. Besides, insufficient chewing and prolonged time of food staying in the mouth also increase caries formation [48]. The fact that autistic individuals are more difficult to accept oral and dental health care than healthy individuals and that their hand skills are not sufficiently developed and that they cannot perform adequate and effective tooth brushing is also effective in the formation of caries [49].

2.3.3 Dental management of patients with autism spectrum disorder

The impaired behavioral activities and complicated medical conditions make the dental management of patients with ASD challenges. Children with ASD have remarkable difficulties in establishing relationships with other people, understanding and the following information, and dentists may be insufficient in providing cooperation during the dental treatment process [40]. Furthermore, the invasive nature of dental treatment procedures along with the hypersensitivity of children with ASD to sensory stimulation (sound, touch, and light) may trigger undesired responses during dental treatment.

In the dental treatment of autistic individuals, many basic behavior management techniques such as tell-show-do, desensitization, and voice control behavior management can be successfully applied [50].

The dental treatment sessions of autistic individuals should be kept short and the sensory stimulation should be minimized. However, it has been reported that in many cases it may be necessary to use advanced behavior management techniques including sedation and general anesthesia [51, 52]. Also, a dental office filled with unpleasant smells, sounds, and colors can be an overstimulating environment for patients with autism [53].

To minimize anxiety and uncooperative behavior pattern, soothing light, rhythmic music with or without headphones, and having minimal visual stimuli on the walls should be considered. It may also be beneficial to improve cooperation by having the same dental professional in the same operating room at all sessions [54].

If traumatic ulcers or lesions are observed on oral mucosa or gingiva, a mouth guard may be prescribed for patients who have problems with self-injurious behavior or bruxism.

2.4 Intellectual disability

The term intellectual disability (ID) is generally used to describe mental retardation. The most widely used current definition of disability is the World Health Organization's (WHO) International Classification of Functioning, Disability and Health (ICF), which incorporates the complex interactions between health conditions, environmental factors, and personal factors. Regarding a person with an ID, this definition would consider how their factors, health condition, and environment affect their lives (WHO 2001). Three elements are common for people with ID:

1. Significant impairment of intelligence,

2. A resultant significant reduction in adaptive behavior/social functioning and

3. The development of the condition (which persists throughout life) before the age of 18 years.

Mental retardation is a developmental disorder that occurs before the age of 18. In addition to having significant retardation in normal functions, there is an inadequacy in the adaptive skills necessary to maintain daily life. Adaptive skills cover skill areas such as self-care skills such as feeding, dressing, bathing, home life skills such as housekeeping, speaking and understanding language, as well as communication skills, social skills, social usefulness, and professional skills [55].

Intellectual disability may be caused by a problem that starts any time before a child turns 18 years old—even before birth. It can be caused by injury, disease, or a problem in the brain. For many children, the cause of their intellectual disability is not known. Some of the most common known causes of intellectual disability—such as Down syndrome, fetal alcohol syndrome, fragile X syndrome, genetic conditions, birth defects, and infections—occur before birth. Others occur during or soon after birth. Besides, other reasons for intellectual disability do not occur until a child is older; these include serious head injury, stroke, or certain infections [56].

2.4.1 Oral findings of patients with intellectual disability

Patients with intellectual disability associated with a syndrome may present typical facial appearance; e.g., in these individuals, the tongue is placed in a protruding position due to macroglossia with micrognathia. Malocclusion, enamel defects, short conical roots, delayed eruption of teeth, congenital tooth agenesis, and tooth malformation are other common intraoral findings [57]. Due to certain genetic conditions or a history of high fever, children with disabilities may have their enamel defects or malformation and thus be more prone to dental caries.

These individuals also have inadequate lip closure, impaired tongue movement, and destabilization of the chewing muscles [55]. Salivary flow rate alterations due to the use of multiple medications along with poor oral hygiene may increase dental plaque and calculus formation, which may lead to dental and periodontal disease and halitosis.

Due to early loss of teeth, speech disorders may also be observed in these individuals [58]. Individuals with intellectual disabilities often consume a cariogenic and soft diet. Besides, individuals consuming daily medicine in the form of syrup constantly have a high risk of caries due to the high sugar content.

It has been shown that individuals with MR (mental retardation) aged 4–18 present significantly higher mean DMFT and dental erosion scores than healthy individuals [59].

2.4.2 Oral hygiene challenges for individuals with intellectual disability

Individuals with severe intellectual disability present impaired oral motor functions and weakened muscles, which cause chewing and swallowing problems. These patients often consume a soft diet including puree or semi-solid foods. In addition, individuals with an intellectual disability usually need the help of their caregivers to consume liquids and do not benefit enough from the washing and cleansing effect of liquids because they consume less liquid than healthy individuals. Oral hygiene procedures such as tooth brushing, which require manual dexterity, may not be performed adequately due to varying degrees of motor dysfunction as well as cognitive deficiencies in mentally retarded individuals [55].

2.4.3 Dental management of patients with intellectual disability

Medical history is quite essential to assess the degree and type of ID and associated medical problems [60]. Complete information should be obtained from the parents/caregivers about the medical background, the medicine consumption, the level of communication of the child, the daily functions she/he can perform individually, and if there are behavior problems at home/institution [61].

It may be helpful to familiarize patients and/or caregivers with the clinical environment without any treatment at the first appointment. Dental office and instruments should be introduced patiently, and the tell-show-do method may be also introduced.

In the next session, the dental instruments that may cause anxiety are introduced, and then treatment may start. It is essential to keep the sessions short. The treatment session should begin with the easy-to-tolerate procedures and no pain stimulus should be created during the first procedure.

Behavior management with positive direction and distraction with movies or music may be applied. Perception difficulties are observed in patients with MR. In these patients, directions and explanations should be short and simple and the instructions should be repeated. General anesthesia or sedation should be considered in patients who do not comply and cannot cooperate [55].

2.5 Physical disability

2.5.1 Hearing loss/(deaf)-visional disorder/(blindness)

Visual impairment was defined as visual acuity less than 20/40 in the better eye. Hearing impairment was defined as the pure-tone average air-conduction hearing threshold worse than 25-dB hearing level (dB HL) in the better ear, averaged over four frequencies: 500, 1000, 2000, and 4000 Hz. [62] Hearing loss can be mild, moderate, moderate, severe, or profound and can affect one or both ears.

Major causes of hearing loss include congenital or early-onset childhood hearing loss due to various chronic middle ear infections, noise-induced hearing loss, age-related hearing loss, and ototoxic drugs that damage the inner ear [62]. Hereditary hearing loss can be conductive, sensorineural, or mixed and is sometimes the result of a genetic trait passed down from a parent.

Children with hearing loss experience social isolation, loneliness, and frustration, and delayed language development due to the loss of ability to communicate with others [62].

Visual impairment is usually defined as a best-corrected visual acuity worse than 20/40 or 20/60 [63]. Visual impairment, or vision loss, is a degree of reduced vision that causes problems that cannot be corrected by general methods, such as with glasses [64]. The term blindness is used for complete or near-complete loss of vision. Physical injury risks such as falling, hitting, and traumatic injuries are reported higher in visually impaired children. Besides, their conceptual development and cognitive skills may be delayed, and they have challenges especially in skills that require abstract thinking [65].

The most common causes of visual impairment are globally uncorrected refractive error (43%), cataracts (33%), and glaucoma (2%). Refractive errors include myopia, hypermetropia, presbyopia, and astigmatism. Cataracts are the most common cause of blindness [66]. Other disorders that may cause visual problems include age-related macular degeneration, diabetic retinopathy, corneal clouding, childhood blindness, and several infections [67]. Visual impairment can also be caused by problems in the brain due to stroke, premature birth, or trauma, among others [68].

2.5.2 Oral findings of patients with hearing loss, visual impairment

Visual impairment may have a negative impact on an individual's oral hygiene. As a result of the inability to remove the microbial dental plaque appropriately, visually impaired individuals experience more dental caries, calculus, and gingivitis compared with healthy individuals [69]. Reluctance to consume solid foods due to prolonged infantile swallowing patterns and poor oral hygiene may be the main reason for the oral health problems. Besides, enamel hypomineralization has been identified as a possible oral manifestation in visually impaired children.

Visually impaired children are more prone to traumatic dental injuries, especially in the anterior teeth is also a predisposing factor. Visually impaired people generally require a high level of orthodontic treatment due to the increasing prevalence and severity of malocclusions [70].

Hard tissue anomalies such as enamel hypoplasia and higher rates of demineralization in the teeth are seen in patients with hearing impairment. Also, a high incidence of bruxism is one of the problems that occur especially when the individual has both hearing loss and visual impairment [71].

Due to the difficulties of providing oral hygiene, diet type, and problems of accessibility to the routine dental check-ups, dental caries are quite often seen in patients with hearing impairment [72]. The prevalence of gingivitis is also higher in these individuals due to poor oral hygiene and mouth breathing, and they are more prone to develop periodontitis early in life [73, 74].

2.5.3 Oral hygiene challenges for individuals with hearing loss, visual impairment

Visually impaired individuals experience difficulties maintaining oral hygiene since they cannot visualize plaque on the tooth surface and adequately assess whether dental plaque is removed effectively. This leads to the progression of dental caries and also to oral inflammatory diseases [74].

Compared with healthy children, individuals with hearing impairment may have a higher risk of experiencing oral diseases, including dental caries or periodontal disease, as they have difficulties maintaining good oral hygiene [75].

2.5.4 Dental management of patients with hearing loss, visual impairment

Individuals with hearing impairment should be informed about the procedures to be performed at the first appointment, and an individual method should be developed for the communication during treatment sessions.

The degree of hearing loss should be noted in the patient's medical history. In the first appointment, it is necessary to avoid exaggerated facial movements and mimics when communicating with the patient, not to cause difficulty to read lips. Comforting the child patient and increasing the sense of trust by smiling will help to establish confidence and healthy communication with the dental professional.

Before starting the dental treatment session, the instruments should be introduced using the show-tell-do method. If the hearing-impaired patient feels that she/he is unable to understand directions, she/he may show fear or aggression. For this reason, communication should be facilitated by reducing external sounds such as high-speed air turbines, dental aspirator, and radio or TV as much as possible. Mirrors, models, pictures, and written information should be used to establish communication [71].

In visually impaired individuals, treatment should be explained using the senses of touch, taste, and smell instead of the tell-show-do technique. The environment should be introduced, and necessary definitions should be made before each treatment. The dental professional should speak to the patient in a clear, warm tone of voice and should use a descriptive manner to explain the procedures. Also, patients should be informed about how the equipment may feel and sound and how the procedures will be performed before the instruments are inserted into the mouth.

The dental restorative materials should be placed in small pieces as the sharp taste may irritate the patient. Since such patients cannot see and remove dental plaque, tooth brushing should be explained by the dentist by holding the brush together with the patient. Oral hygiene education and motivation should be given by the doctor to whom he is accustomed to the treatment of the patient [70, 75].

3. Conclusions

Special healthcare need patients are literally special patients who need special attention by means of healthcare provision including dental care. The major challenges they have with their overall health may create barriers to access to proper oral healthcare. Oral healthcare for this special group is often neglected or down the list, and as a result, they often attend to dental clinics with emergency.

Individuals with special needs are the most underserved regarding healthcare needs in almost all populations. Due to the challenges of nutrition and insufficient oral hygiene provision, this population is usually more prone to dental caries, periodontal disease, and orthodontic problems. Besides, they face more difficulties accessing professional dental care than other segments of the population.

The field of special care dentistry is attracting more interest of pediatric dentists and general dental practitioners. The inclusion of the specialty programs in the dentistry faculty curriculum may initiate the ideal treatment procedures and regular recalls of these special patients, which may facilitate the access to sufficient dental care provision and regular check-ups for this special group.

Though many countries developed community-based systems to improve oral health for people with special needs, providing good oral health mainly depends on the effort of the families. Therefore the education of the caregiver about oral hygiene provision is also critical for the special needs patient to enjoy a lifetime of oral health the same as other members of the society.

Conflict of interest

The author declares no conflict of interest.

Author details

Pinar Kiymet Karataban
Dentistry Faculty, Pediatric Dentistry Department, BAU International University, Batumi, Georgia

*Address all correspondence to: pinar.kiymet.karataban@bauinternational.edu.ge

References

[1] Bax M, Goldstein M, Rosenbaum P, Leviton A, Paneth N, Dan B, et al. Proposed definition and classification of cerebral palsy. Developmental Medicine and Child Neurology. 2005;**47**(8):571-576

[2] Krigger KW. Cerebral palsy: An overview. American Family Physician. 2006;**73**(1):91-100

[3] https://www.tscv.org.tr/PageContent/tr/cerebral-palsy-ve-nedenleri/1001 [Accessed: August 16, 2021]

[4] Tahmassebi JF, Curzon ME. Prevalence of drooling in children with cerebral palsy attending special schools. Developmental Medicine and Child Neurology. 2003;**45**(9):613-617

[5] Dougherty NJ. A review of cerebral palsy for the oral health professional. Dental Clinics of North America. 2009;**53**(2):329

[6] Botti Rodrigues Santos MT, Duarte Ferreira MC, de Oliveira Guaré R, Guimarães AS, Lira Ortega A. Teeth grinding, oral motor performance, and maximal bite force in cerebral palsy children. Special Care in Dentistry. 2015;**35**(4):170-174

[7] Ortega AO, Guimarães AS, Ciamponi AL, Marie SK. Frequency of parafunctional oral habits in patients with cerebral palsy. Journal of Oral Rehabilitation. 2007;**34**(5):323-328

[8] Mani S, Mote N, Kathariya MD, Pawar KD. Adaptation and development of dental procedure in cerebral palsy. Pravara Medical Review. 2015;**7**:17-22

[9] Grzić R, Bakarcić D, Prpić I, Jokić NI, Sasso A, Kovac Z, et al. Dental health and dental care in children with cerebral palsy. Collegium Antropologicum. 2011;**35**(3):761-764

[10] Franklin DL, Luther F, Curzon ME. The prevalence of malocclusion in children with cerebral palsy. European Journal of Orthodontics. 1996;**18**(6): 637-643

[11] Winter K, Baccaglini L, Tomar S. A review of malocclusion among individuals with mental and physical disabilities. Special Care in Dentistry. 2008;**28**(1):19-26

[12] Polat Z, Akgün Ö, Turan İ, Polat GG, Altun C. Evaluation of the relationship between dental erosion and scintigraphically detected gastroesophageal reflux in patients with cerebral palsy. Turkish Journal of Medical Sciences. 2013;**43**:283-288

[13] Guaré RO, Ferreira MC, Leite MF, Rodrigues JA, Lussi A, Santos MT. Dental erosion and salivary flow rate in cerebral palsy individuals with gastroesophageal reflux. Journal of Oral Pathology & Medicine. 2012;**41**(5):367-371

[14] Kırzıoğlu Z, Bayraktar C. Serebral palsili çocuklarda sık rastlanan oral problemler, ağız dışına salya akışı ve tedavi önerileri. Süleyman Demirel Üniversitesi Sağlık Bilimleri Dergisi. 2018;**9**(2):156-162 (Article in Turkish)

[15] Cardona-Soria S, Cahuana-Cárdenas A, Rivera-Baró A, Miranda-Rius J, Martín de Carpi J, Brunet-Llobet L. Oral health status in pediatric patients with cerebral palsy fed by oral versus enteral route. Special Care in Dentistry. 2020;**40**(1):35-40

[16] Sehrawat N, Marwaha M, Bansal K, Chopra R. Cerebral palsy: A dental

update. International Journal of Clinical Pediatric Dentistry. 2014;7(2):109-118

[17] Mc Donald, Dean A. Dentistry for the Child and Adolescents. 'Dental Problems of Children with Special Health Care Needs' James A. Weddell, Brian J. Sanders and James E. Jones, 9th ed. Elsevier Publication; 2011:460-486

[18] Alio JJ, Lorenzo J, Iglesias C. Cranial base growth in patients with Down syndrome: A longitudinal study. American Journal of Orthodontics and Dentofacial Orthopedics. 2008;**133**(5): 729-737

[19] Hennequin M, Faulks D, Veyrune JL, Bourdiol P. Significance of oral health in persons with Down syndrome: A literature review. Developmental Medicine and Child Neurology. 1999; **41**(4):275-283

[20] Demir D, Güler Y. Down Sendromlu Çocuklarda Ağız-Diş Sağlığı. Atatürk Üniversitesi Diş Hekimliği Fakültesi Dergisi. 2013;**23**(2):274-281 (Article in Turkish)

[21] https://www.downturkiye.org/down-sendromu-nedir [Accessed: August 16, 2021]. (Article in Turkish)

[22] Mubayrik AB. The dental needs and treatment of patients with down syndrome. Dental Clinics of North America. 2016;**60**(3):613-626

[23] Desai SS. Down syndrome: A review of the literature. Oral Surgery, Oral Medicine, Oral Pathology, Oral Radiology, and Endodontics. 1997;**84**(3):279-285

[24] Townsend GC. Dental crown variants in children and young adults with Down syndrome. Acta de odontologia pediatrica. 1986;7(2):35-39

[25] Sterling E. Oral and dental considerations in Down syndrome. In: Lott I, McCoy E, editors. Down Syndrome Advances in Medical Care. New York: Wiley-Liss; 1992. pp. 135-145

[26] Chan AR. Dental caries and periodontal disease in Down's syndrome patients. University of Toronto Dental Journal. 1994;7(1):18-21

[27] Shaw L, Saxby MS. Periodontal destruction in Down's syndrome and juvenile periodontitis. How close a similarity? Journal of Periodontology. 1986;**57**(11):709-715

[28] Borea G, Magi M, Mingarelli R, Zamboni C. The oral cavity in Down syndrome. The Journal of Pedodontics. 1990;**14**(3):139-140

[29] Abdul Rahim FS, Mohamed AM, Marizan Nor M, Saub R. Dental care access among individuals with Down syndrome: A Malaysian scenario. Acta Odontologica Scandinavica. 2014;**72**(8):999-1004

[30] Allison PJ, Hennequin M, Faulks D. Dental care access among individuals with Down syndrome in France. Special Care in Dentistry. 2000;**20**(1):28-34

[31] Yilmaz S, Ozlü Y, Ekuklu G. The effect of dental training on the reactions of mentally handicapped children's behavior in the dental office. ASDC Journal of Dentistry for Children. 1999;**66**(3):188-155

[32] Jeng W, Wang T, Cher T, et al. Strategies for oral health care for people with disabilities in Taiwan. J Dent Sci. 2009;**4**(4):165-172

[33] Abanto J, Ciamponi AL, Francischini E, Murakami C, de Rezende NP, Gallottini M. Medical problems and oral care of patients with Down syndrome: A literature review. Special Care in Dentistry. 2011;**31**(6): 197-203

[34] Kanner L. Autistic disturbances of affective contact. Acta Paedo psychiatrica. 1968;**35**(4):100-136

[35] Amaral DG, Schumann CM, Nordahl CW. Neuroanatomy of autism. Trends in Neurosciences. 2008;**31**(3): 137-145

[36] Vahia VN. Diagnostic and statistical manual of mental disorders 5: A quick glance. Indian Journal of Psychiatry. 2013;**55**(3):220-223

[37] Tchaconas A, Adesman A. Autism spectrum disorders: A pediatric overview and update. Current Opinion in Pediatrics. 2013;**25**(1):130-144

[38] Bölte S, Girdler S, Marschik PB. The contribution of environmental exposure to the etiology of autism spectrum disorder. Cellular and Molecular Life Sciences. 2019;**76**(7):1275-1297. DOI: 10.1007/s00018-018-2988-4

[39] Monroy PG, da Fonseca MA. The use of botulinum toxin-a in the treatment of severe bruxism in a patient with autism: A case report. Special Care in Dentistry. 2006;**26**(1):37-39

[40] Friedlander AH, Yagiela JA, Paterno VI, Mahler ME. The neuropathology, medical management, and dental implications of autism. Journal of the American Dental Association. 2006;**137**(11):1517-1527

[41] Vogel LD. When children put their fingers in their mouths. Should parents and dentists care? The New York State Dental Journal. 1998;**64**(2):48-53

[42] Loo CY, Graham RM, Hughes CV. The caries experience and behavior of dental patients with an autism spectrum disorder. Journal of the American Dental Association. 2008;**139**(11):1518-1524

[43] Orellana LM, Silvestre FJ, Martínez-Sanchis S, Martínez-Mihi V, Bautista D. Oral manifestations in a group of adults with autism spectrum disorder. Medicina Oral, Patología Oral y Cirugía Bucal. 2012;**17**(3):e415-e419

[44] Lai B, Milano M, Roberts MW, Hooper SR. Unmet dental needs and barriers to dental care among children with autism spectrum disorders. Journal of Autism and Developmental Disorders. 2012;**42**(7):1294-1303

[45] Klein U, Nowak AJ. Characteristics of patients with autistic disorder (AD) presenting for dental treatment: A survey and chart review. Special Care in Dentistry. 1999;**19**(5):200-207

[46] Bandini LG, Curtin C, Phillips S, Anderson SE, Maslin M, Must A. Changes in food selectivity in children with autism spectrum disorder. Journal of Autism and Developmental Disorders. 2017;**47**(2):439-446

[47] Akbaş M. Otizm spektrum bozukluğuna sahip 0-6 yaş arasi çocuklarda ağiz ve diş sağliği hizmetlerinin planlanmasi: Precede-proceed modeli kapsaminda öneriler. Uluslararası Sağlık Yönetimi ve Stratejileri Araştırma Dergisi. 2020;**6**(3):551-562 (Article in Turkish)

[48] Eronat N, Koparal E. Dental caries prevalence, dietary habits, tooth-brushing, and mother's education in 500 urban Turkish children. Journal of Marmara University Dental Faculty. 1997;**2**(4):599-604

[49] Jaber MA. Dental caries experience, oral health status, and treatment needs of dental patients with autism. Journal of applied oral science: Revista FOB. 2011;**19**(3):212-217

[50] Kamen S, Skier J. Dental management of the autistic child. Special Care in Dentistry. 1985;**5**(1): 20-23

[51] Davila JM, Jensen OE. Behavioral and pharmacological dental management of a patient with autism. Special Care in Dentistry. 1988;**8**(2):5 8-60

[52] Pisalchaiyong T, Trairatvorakul C, Jirakijja J, Yuktarnonda W. Comparison of the effectiveness of oral diazepam and midazolam for the sedation of autistic patients during dental treatment. Pediatric Dentistry. 2005; **27**(3):198-206

[53] Stein LI, Polido JC, Cermak SA. Oral care and sensory over-responsivity in children with autism spectrum disorders. Pediatric Dentistry. 2013;**35**(3):230-235

[54] Shapiro M, Melmed RN, Sgan-Cohen HD, Parush S. Effect of sensory adaptation on anxiety of children with developmental disabilities: A new approach. Pediatric Dentistry. 2009;**31**(3):222-228

[55] Kömerik D, Kırzıoğlu P, Efeoğlu D. Zihinsel engele sahip bireylerin ağız sağlığı: karşılaşılan güçlükler ve çözüm önerileri. Atatürk Üniversitesi Diş Hekimliği Fakültesi Dergisi. 2012;**2012**(1):105-107 (Article in Turkish)

[56] https://www.cdc.gov/ncbddd/childdevelopment/facts-about-intellectual-disability.html [Accessed: August 16, 2021]

[57] Cumella S, Ransford N, Lyons J, Burnham H. Needs for oral care among people with intellectual disability not in contact with Community Dental Services. Journal of Intellectual Disability Research. 2000;**44**(Pt 1):45-52

[58] Ningrum V, Bakar A, Shieh TM, Shih YH. The oral health inequities between special needs children and normal children in Asia: A systematic review and meta-analysis. Healthcare (Basel, Switzerland). 2021;**9**(4):410

[59] Aşıcı N, Doğan C, Odabaş M, Alaçam A. Zihinsel Engelli Çocuklarda Diş Erozyonu ve DMFT Değerlendirilmesi-Pilot Çalışma. Gazi Üniversitesi Diş Hekimliği Fakültesi Dergisi. 2003;**20**(2):15-20 (Article in Turkish)

[60] Nirmala SVSG, Saikrishna D, Nuvvula S. Dental concerns of children with intellectual disability—A narrative review. Dental, Oral and Craniofacial Research. 2018;**4**. DOI: 10.15761/DOCR.1000266

[61] American Academy of Pediatric Dentistry. Guideline on caries-risk assessment and management for infants, children, and adolescents. Pediatric Dentistry. 2012;**34**:118-125

[62] Chia E, Mitchell P, Rochtchina E, Foran S, Golding M, Wang JJ. Association between vision and hearing impairments and their combined effects on quality of life. Archives of Ophthalmology. 2006;**124**(10):1465-1470. DOI: 10.1001/archopht.124.10.1465

[63] Maberley DA, Hollands H, Chuo J, Tam G, Konkal J, Roesch M, et al. The prevalence of low vision and blindness in Canada. Eye (London, England). 2006;**20**(3):341-346

[64] Change the Definition of Blindness (PDF). World Health Organization. Archived (PDF) from the original on July 14, 2015

[65] Kizar, O. Farkli Branşlardaki Görme Engelli Sporcularin Yalnizlik Düzeylerinin Karşılaştirilması, Elaziğ, Fırat Üniversitesi,

Yüksek Lisans Tezi. (Msc Thesis Dissertation in Turkish). 2012

[66] Sabel BA, Flammer J, Merabet LB. Residual vision activation and the brain-eye-vascular triad: Dysregulation, plasticity, and restoration in low vision and blindness–A review. Restorative Neurology and Neuroscience. 2018; **36**(6):767-791

[67] https://www.who.int/blindness/GLOBALDATAFINALforweb.pdf [Accessed: August 16, 2021]

[68] Lehman S. Cortical visual impairment in children: Identification, evaluation and diagnosis. Current Opinion in Ophthalmology. 2012;**23**(5):384-387

[69] Greeley CB, Goldstein PA, Forrester DJ. Oral manifestations in a group of blind students. ASDC Journal of Dentistry for Children. 1976;**43**(1):39-41

[70] SVSG Nirmala and Degala Saikrishna. Oral health and dental care of children with visual impairment—An overview. EC Dental Science. 2019;**18**(5):848-853

[71] Fabiana CMH, Frederick SR, Jacqueline CHM. Managing dental patient with auditory deficit: Literature review. International Journal of Oral and Dental Health. 2018;**4**:058

[72] De la Teja E, Durán A, Espinosa L, Ramírez JA. Manifestaciones estomatológicas de los trastornos sistémicos más frecuentes en el Instituto Nacional de Pediatría. Revisión de la literatura y estadísticas del instituto. Acta Pediátrica de Méx. 2008;**29**:189-199

[73] Jain M, Mathur A, Kumar S, Dagli RJ, Duraiswamy P, Kulkarni S. Dentition status and treatment needs among children with impaired hearing attending a special school for the deaf and mute in Udaipur, India. Journal of Oral Science. 2008;**50**(2):161-165

[74] Sandeep V, Vinay C, Madhuri V, Rao VV, Uloopi KS, Sekhar RC. Impact of visual instruction on oral hygiene status of children with hearing impairment. Journal of the Indian Society of Pedodontics and Preventive Dentistry. 2014;**32**(1):39-43

[75] Bimstein E, Jerrell RG, Weaver JP, Dailey L. Oral characteristics of children with visual or auditory impairments. Pediatric Dentistry. 2014;**36**(4):336-341

Chapter 14

Oral Health Problems of Thai People Reported by Khon Kaen University Staffs during 1984 to 2020

Amornrat Ratanasiri, Thitima Nutravong, Supaporn Chatrchaiwiwatana, Arisara Poosari, Thawalrat Ratanasiri and Kanokporn Wongchalee

Abstract

To improve the efficiency of the dental care service system in Thailand. To synthesize content from Khon Kaen University (KKU) staffs and students' research and presentations from 1984 to 2020 about oral health hygiene and related diseases. Sixteen publications and presentations by KKU staffs and their students about oral health problems and management were retrieved, reviewed and analyzed. Poor oral health of people in the northeast of Thailand is found in every age group: children, adults and the aging, both male and female. There are still many oral health problems of Thai people in the northeast. KKU Field Works, Projects and Research were able to help reduce these oral health problems. An appropriate preventive oral health program needs to be developed and implemented in Northeastern Thailand.

Keywords: Oral health problems, Oral health management, Khon Kaen University, Dental care service

1. Introduction

Khon Kaen University (KKU), Thailand has carried out field work to improve the health, including oral health of the population in the northeast of Thailand and other rural areas. KKU has an important mission to produce graduates with essential knowledge, skills and attitudes to be able to help in national development, especially in the northeast of Thailand, and has been actively pursuing this duty and responsibility since 1984.

The KKU field practice course began in 1984 for health sciences students in KKU and the College of Asian Scholars. These students will have direct experience in solving problems in rural areas under the supervision of our staffs in related fields. They gain the experiences of working together with other students for sustainable health development.

2. Objective

The objective of this study was to synthesize knowledge about oral health hygiene and related diseases from KKU staffs and their students' projects and research presentations during 1984 to 2020.

3. Methodologies

The populations were 16 publications and presentations by KKU staffs and their students during 1984 to 2020 (**Tables 1** and **2**). The researches reviewed was approved by the Ethics Committee for Human Research at Khon Kaen University, Thailand [HE522167, HE532173, HE571074, HE591188, HE591199, and HE621269]. Most of the research was secondary data. Those who volunteered had signed a consent form.

Data and results about oral health problems and management were retrieved from 16 paper publications and presentations by KKU staffs and their students during 1984 to 2020 (**Tables 1** and **2**).

Study No.	Title	Ref.	Study Design	Age Group (year old)	Sample size (Sex) (Data from)	Findings	Year of pubn.
1[N.]	Betel Quid Chewing and Oral Health of Women	[1]	Descriptive Study and Analytical Study	31–86 women	2,253 F Data from (1992–1994)	Betel Quid Chewing associated with Periodontitis, Tooth Loss and Aging	2007
2 [I.]	ECO and Smoking Status	[2]	Cross-Sectional Study and Analytical Study,	15–70 smokers	420 Adults	ECO for Older =7 ppm, ECO For Younger = 8 ppm	2008
3 [I.]	ECO an Oral Health Status in Smokers active and passive smokers	[3]	Cross-sectional Analytical Study	30–72 workers	296 Adults (Data from 2007)	No Relationship between ECO and smoking	2011
4 [I.]	Periodontitis, ECO Level and Oral Health	[4]	Cross-sectional Analytical Study	30–89 rural 33–86 rural	625 (M) (1990–1991) 1,218 (M) (1992–1994) Adults	Tobacco smoking as a risk indicator for Periodontitis	2009
5 [I.]	Tooth Loss due to Dental Carries	[5]	In-depth Interview and Cross-sectional Analytical Study	19–53 workers	457 Adults [283 (M),174 (F)] 11 for in-depth interview	Causes from Lack of Knowledge & Time, Negative Attitudes, Inability to support cost of dental treatment	2012

Study No.	Title	Ref.	Study Design	Age Group (year old)	Sample size (Sex) (Data from)	Findings	Year of pubn.
6 [I.]	Dental and Jaw Injuries	[6]	Descriptive and Analytical Study	Thai boxing rural, urban	260 (M) (2009–2010)	Muay Thai boxing lead to dental & jaw injuries	2016
7 [I.]	Factors related to Tooth Loss	[7]	Descriptive Study and Analytical Study	19–25 urban	1,500 Adults [621 M,879F] (data from 2014)	62.2% had Tooth Loss, 60.0% Tooth Loss caused by Dental Carries	2017
8 [I.]	ECO and Age	[8]	Descriptive Study Analytical Study and ECO Level measured	16–70 workers	875 volunteers [584Non Smokers, 291Smokers] (data from 2009)	Smokers: Mean ECO Level = 11.24 ppm Non Smokers: Mean ECO Level = 2.25 ppm Optimal ECO Cut-Off Level varied by age	2017
9 [I.]	Smoking status and best ECO cut-off level and oral health conditions	[9]	Descriptive Study, Analytical Study, ECO Level Measured	19–53 workers	455 workers (data from 2009 to 2010)	Direct association between ECO Level > = 4 ppm and Periodontitis	2018

I, index journal; N, non-index journal; P, poster presentation; lr, literature review; Rw, research waiting for publication.

Table 1.
Summary of Oral health problems related to diseases from KKU staff and their students' publications and presentations during 1984–2020.

Study No.	Title	Ref.	Study Design	Age Group (years old)	Sample size (Sex) (Data from)	Findings	Year of pubn.
10 [R]	Dental Clinic at PCU Samliaum of Srinagarind Hospital	[10]	In-depth Interviews and Descriptive Study	Age above 18	400 Adults	Most of villagers need to have a dental care clinic at PCU Samliaum of Srinagarind Hospital and were able to pay dental care treatment at 1,000 Baht on each visit.	2011
11 [I.]	Dental care services at industrial estates	[11]	Analytical Study	Age 19–25	1,500 Workers from 16 Factories [621 M, 879F]	Only 36.1% used Dental care services while 63.9% could not in previous year	2015

Study No.	Title	Ref.	Study Design	Age Group (years old)	Sample size (Sex) (Data from)	Findings	Year of pubn.
12 [I.]	Health Consciousness to be Young Dentist	[12]	Descriptive Study	Students Grade11 from two Schools in Kalasin Provn.	660 Students (During 2010)	320 were Peer leaders. The peer leader scores were higher than Non-peer leaders in all domain.	2013
13 [I.]	Youth Participation Towards health promotion	[13]	Mixed Methods 1. Situations Analysis 2. Model Synthesis 3. Model Effectiveness	Students Grade 9–11	1,192 Samples for Analytical Study 35 Subjects for In-depth Interview	103 of them were Peer volunteers. The CHANYA Model was supporting youth participation towards oral health promotion	2017
14 [P]	Poster Presentation: "Maelong Volunteer for Long Term Care"	[14]	Trained the Health Volunteers and Evaluated of their KAP	Health Volunteers at Maelong Village	28 Health Voluntrs. [1 (M), 27 (F)]	Increase awareness of "Long Term Care" Gain more knowledge Need repeat training every year	2018
15 [Ir]	Masticatory Function and related effects	[15, 16]	Literature Reviews	Paper publishing and Textbooks	36 Papers and Textbooks	One paper [16] presented that 83% of dentures were still in use after 5 years, Only 50% were still in use after10 years	2020
16 [Rw]	Chronic Gingival Inflammation leads to Esophageal Cancer	[17]	Analytical Study	105 EC 105 Control	Case [M = 60%, F = 40%], Control [M = 47%, F = 53%] (2007–2017)	*Campylobacter* infection, tobacco smoking and poor oral health were associated with esophageal cancer in Northeastern, Thailand	2020

I, index journal; N, non-index journal; P, poster presentation'; lr, literature review; Rw, research waiting for publication.

Table 2.
Summary of Oral health care management by KKU staff and their students during 1984–2020.

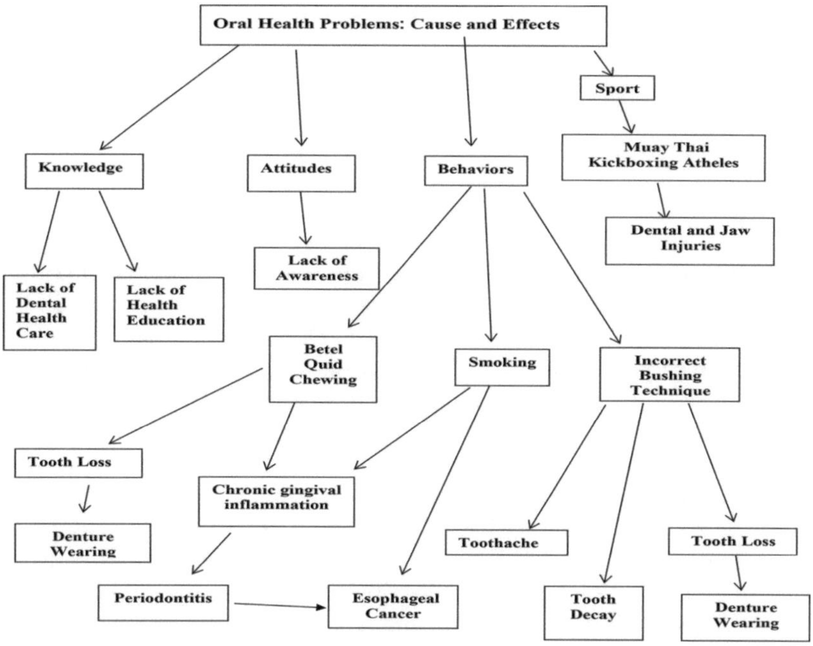

Figure 1.
Oral health problems: Causes and effects leading to related diseases.

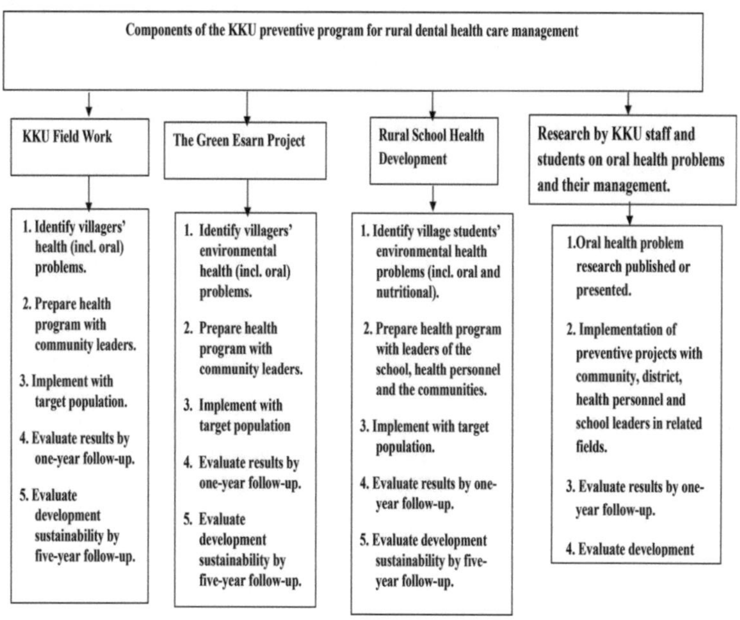

Figure 2.
Procedure for the KKU preventive program for rural dental health care management of people in the Northeast of Thailand.

To synthesize oral health problems and related diseases, included in the programs of health prevention and promotion from the 16 publications and presentations by KKU staffs and their students, we use two diagrams as follows:

1. Oral health problems: Causes and Effects leading to related diseases (**Figure 1**).

2. Procedure for the KKU preventive program for rural dental health care management of people in the Northeast of Thailand (**Figure 2**).

4. Results

In thirty-seven years of KKU field practice and research, it has been found that most students and staff had a good attitude towards practice in the community with other students and staff from various faculties. Each year, more than six hundred students and sixty staff participate in KKU field work. They provide oral health care and other health promotion work to the people in villages, and follow- up the work with those villagers after five years. Reports of follow-up studies have indicated that people in those communities have better health awareness, and the community leaders have discussed with KKU staff about other projects to implement in their community in later years. The KKU field practice has achieved its aim in equipping students with essential competency in sustainable health development for rural communities, while lessons learned had been discussed and distributed widely to the public [18–23].

Besides KKU field practice, the Department of Community Medicine, KKU has performed much more researches to develop the health status of the people in villages. Maternal and Child Health research studied children below 5 years and their mothers in two villages (Ban Had and Ban Nongtao) of Khon Kaen province [24].

Another two "excellence" projects have involved KKU staff which were 1) The Green Esarn Project which studied KAP of villagers in BanSum village, Mahachanachai district, Yasothorn province about oral health related to their environment [25], and 2) The Rural School Health Development Project: The School of the Royal Initiative of Her Royal Princess Mahachakri Sirindhorn studied KAP of villagers and dental treatment of the students in Nong Song Hong School, Khon Kaen province [26].

The results of these various studies show that poor oral health hygiene, smoking habits, betel quid chewing, and Muay Thai kickboxing of the Thai population still lead to many problems in all age groups (children, adults, workers, smokers, women who chew betel quids, Muay Thai kickboxing athletes, and the aging), both male and female. The studies indicates that bad oral hygiene leads to diseases such as oral health problems, exhaled carbon monoxide (ECO) levels, dental carries, tooth loss, and chronic gingival inflammation leading to esophageal cancer, and insufficient dental treatment (**Figure 1**).

The KKU Projects and other related projects show that after the projects had been performed by KKU staffs and their students from 1984 to 2020, the villagers had more awareness of their oral hygiene than in the previous year.

From **Figure 1**, we see that oral health problems: have 4 included variables; sport, knowledge, attitudes, and behaviors as follows:

1. Sport:

It was seen that 23.5% of 260 Thai boxing athletes had dental and jaw injuries. The popularity of this sport is still increasing in Thailand [6].

2. Knowledge:

In particular, people lacked knowledge of dental care and lacked health education. The results showed that 63.9% of 1,500 workers did not use dental care services during the previous year, mostly because they had no time to see the dentist and were unable to pay the cost of dental treatment [11].

3. Attitudes:

It was found that 62.2% of 457 adults had tooth loss due to dental carries. From in-depth interview of 11 subjects, this was caused by 1) Lack of time to visit the dentist, 2) Negative attitude towards dental treatment, and 3) Inability to support the cost of dental treatment [7].

4. Behaviors:

Betel Quid Chewing:

It was found that most aging women in Thailand chew betel quid during the day. The results from 2,253 women, aged 31–86 years old showed that there was an association between betel quid chewing and periodontitis, and also tooth loss [1].

Incorrect Brushing Technique:

It was found in Nong Song Hong School that 75% of 67 students had oral health problem such as toothache and 58.5% of them were absent from class because of toothache, 17.9% had dental carries, but none of them had tooth loss [26].

Smoking:

Findings from multivariable logistic regression showed that tobacco smoking was a risk indicator for periodontitis from 1,218 males, aged 33–86 years residing in rural areas of Khon Kaen Province during 1990–1991 [4].

Chronic Gingival Inflammation leading to Esophageal Cancer Findings of multivariable logistic regression indicated that *Campylobacter* infection, tobacco smoking, and poor oral health were associated with esophageal cancer in people in the northeast of Thailand [17].

5. Discussions

Dental Carries is believed to be a rapidly increasing oral health problem in developing countries. KKU Studies of tooth loss due to dental carries [5], factors related to tooth loss [7], dental care services at PCU [10], and dental care services at industrial estates [11] were similar to the study of Ahlberg et al. [27], which suggests that there should be dental services in industrial estates in order to prevent dental carries and its sequelae. Our finding suggest that utilization of dental care services varies by person, place, and time. It can be categorized into two factors e.g. economic factors and non-economics factors. The economic factors indicated the ability to pay for dental care treatment. Non-economic factors present awareness of oral health problems. People who use dental care services regularly will not have tooth decay.

Findings of KKU studies of ECO and smoking status [2], ECO and oral health status in active and passive smokers [3], ECO and age [8], and smoking status and best ECO cut-off level and oral conditions [9] were similar to prior studies [28, 29], which supports that the level of carbon monoxide in the exhaled breath might be used as an indicator of smoking status.

Findings of periodontitis associated with tobacco smoking [4] were similar to prior studies [30, 31], which found that tobacco smoking was related to periodontitis. Our findings from both data sets suggest that tobacco smoking is directly associated with periodontitis, and thus enhances the possibility of increased tooth extraction.

Results of KKU studies about betel quid chewing and oral health problems [1] were similar to Mehta et al. [32], which found the relationship of betel leaf chewing and periodontal disease. Our findings indicated that although betel quid chewing may reduce dental caries, betel quid chewing is a risk indicator of periodontitis enhancing the risk of increasing tooth loss.

KKU reports of dental and jaw injuries [6] were similar to the prior studies [33, 34], which have reported occurrences of injuries to the body as well as to oral cavity and jaw. We found that the location of boxing camps in the upper northeast of Thailand as well as boxing camps in rural area were directly related to dental trauma and injuries among these Thai boxing athletes.

6. Conclusions

The results from those projects and research indicate that these projects were successful because of the co-operation from the leaders of the schools, the leaders of the communities, health care providers in their districts, health volunteers in the villages, awareness of the students and the villagers, follow-up studies by KKU staffs and their students at least twice, one-year follow-up for evaluation of the outcome of villagers' health and oral health, as well as a five-year follow-up to evaluate the sustainability of the development under the supervision and funding support from the director of Khon Kaen University and all Faculties related in KKU and the College of Asian Scholars.

From the KKU projects and research above it was seen that Thai people faced oral hygiene and oral health problems. The KKU field practice course is useful to reduce this problem. There should be a policy of protection programs for Muay Thai athletes by the Muay Thai Committees. There should be a dental clinic provided near communities which can give them oral health education programs. Services and welfare for dental treatment should be provided, or there should be a dental clinic in the workplace eg. on an Industrial Estate. Preventive programs should be established to stop people chewing betel quids.

KKU field works, projects and research by KKU staffs and their students were able to assist the public and the related organizations that have the duty to deal with these problems. Some of them are effective in reducing oral health problems of students and villagers eg. PCU Samliaum of Srinagarind Hospital, Khon Kaen province, Nong Song Hong School, Khon Kaen province, and Ban Sum village, Yasothorn province.

Acknowledgements

The authors thank all of the respondents for their valuable contribution to our studies, the Cancer Unit of Faculty of Medicine, the Faculty of Dentistry, Khon Kaen University and the College of Asian Scholars staffs and their students for data support and funding support, Ajarn Ian Thomas for grammatical corrections.

Conflict of interest

All authors declare that they have no conflicts of interest.

Author details

Amornrat Ratanasiri[1*], Thitima Nutravong[2], Supaporn Chatrchaiwiwatana[3], Arisara Poosari[2], Thawalrat Ratanasiri[2] and Kanokporn Wongchalee[3]

1 Department of Community Medicine, Faculty of Medicine, Khon Kaen University, Khon Kaen, Thailand

2 Faculty of Medicine, Khon Kaen University, Khon Kaen, Thailand

3 Faculty of Dentistry, Khon Kaen University, Khon Kaen, Thailand

*Address all correspondence to: amorat@kku.ac.th

References

[1] Chatrchaiwiwatana S, Ratanasiri A, Kuhilunyaratn P, Muktabhant B. Association between Betel Quid Chewing and Oral health among females in rural Khon Kaen: Phase II Study. Thai Dental Public Health J. 2007; 12(1):27-37.

[2] Supaporn Chatrchaiwiwatan, Amornrat Ratanasiri. Exhhaled Carbon Monoxide Level and Smoking Status in Urban Khon Kaen Adults. J Med Assoc Thai 2008; 91(11):1669-1676.

[3] Supaporn Chatrchaiwiwatana, Amornrat Ratanasiri. Association between exhaled carbon monoxide and oral health status in active and passive smokers. J Med Assoc Thai 2011; 94(5): 601-609.

[4] Supaporn Chatrchchaiwiwatana, Amornrat Ratanasiri. Periodontitis associated with tobacco smoking among rural Khon Kaen Thai males: analysis of two data sets. J Med Assoc Thai 2009; 92(1):1524-1531.

[5] Supaporn Chatrchaiwiwatana, Amornrat Ratanasiri, Jeeratip Jaidee, Surasak Soontorn. Factors Related to tooth loss due to dental caries among workers in an industrial estate in Thailand. J Med Assoc Thai 2012; 95 (Suppl 11): S1-S6.

[6] Supaporn Chatrchaiwiwatana, Khanidtha Hongsawat, Mookda Siritapetawee, Amornrat Ratanasiri. Dental and Jaw injuries among Muay Thai Kickboxing Athletes. J Med Assoc Thai 2016; 99 (Suppl 5) S120-S126.

[7] Jeerateep Jaidee, Supaporn Chatrchaiwiwatana, Amornrat Ratanasiri. Factors related to tooth loss among industrial workers in Prathum Thani, Thailand. Southeast Asian J Trop Med Public Health 2017; 48(1):253-264.

[8] Supaporn Chatrchaiwiwatana, Amornrat Ratanasiri. Exhaled carbon monoxide levels among tobacco smokers by age. Southeast Asian J Trop Med Public Health 2017; 48(2):429-437.

[9] Supaporn Chatrchaiwiwatana, Amornrat Ratanasiri. Determination of Smoking status among Thai employees by the best exhaled carbon monoxide cut-off level and association with oral health conditions. Southeast Asian J Trop Med Public Health 2018; 49(1):165-174.

[10] Amornrat Ratanasiri. Independent Study of Dental Clinic at PCU Samliaum of Srinagarind Hospital for MBA (Hospital and Health Care Management), Under Supervision of Professor Dr Narin, Hirunsuthikul Chulalongkorn University, Bangkok, Thailand. 2011.

[11] Jeeratip Jaidee, Amornrat Ratanasiri, Supaporn Chatrchaiwiwatana, Surasak Soonthon. Prevalence and factors associated with the utilization of dental care services among factory workers in Nava Nakorn industrial estate, Pathumthani province, Thailand. *J Med Assoc Thai* 2015; 98(Suppl): S73-S80.

[12] Terachote C, Kessomboon P, Ratanasiri A, Koju R. Improving health consciousness and life skills in young people through peer–leadership in Thailand. Kathmandu Univ Med J 2013; 11(1): 41-44.

[13] Chanya Teerachote, Supaporn Chatrchaiwiwatana, Amornrat Ratanasiri, Suteera Pradubwong, Bowornsilp Chowchuen. Development of youth participation supportive model for oral health promotion in secondary school: a case study of understanding for cleft lip-cleft palate. J Med Assoc Thai 2017; 100 (Suppl 6) S102-S108.

[14] Thawalrat Ratanasiri, Poster presentation of the community project title "Maelong volunteer health services are fascinatingly and dependable project". for family medicine study, under supervision of Assoc. Prof. Dr. Peerasak Lerttrakarnnon and Dr. Krid Thongbunjob, Chiang Mai University, Chiang Mai, Thailand. 2018.

[15] Kanokporn Wongchalee, Literature reviews of Masticatory function and related effects. Proposal presentation for DDS thesis, Faculty of Dentistry, Khon Kaen University, Khon Kaen, Thailand, 2020.

[16] Th. Kerschbaum, KH, R. Teeuwen, F, J. Faber. Survival rate of full dentures. Deutsche Zahnarztliche Zeitschrift 2007.62:252-257.

[17] Arisara Poosari, Report of chronic inflammation lead to Esophageal Cancer under Supervision of Asst. Prof. Dr. Thitima Nutravong. Faculty of Medicine, Khon Kaen University, Khon Kaen, Thailand, 2020.

[18] Amornrat Ratanasiri, Paisan Suwannoi, Pichet Leungtongkum, Supreeda Adulyanon. The Comparison of Staff Lecturers' Knowledge, Attitude and Behavior to Participate in Health Sciences Branch of KKU Field Practices during the academic Year 1991-1992. *Srinagarind Med J*. 1992; 7(1):68-79.

[19] Amorn Premgamon, Sompong Srisanpang, Prasert Thavorndulsatit, Varanuch Pitipa, Patcharee Jearanaikul, Ploenplit Viyatas, et al. The Evaluation of the Six Faculty Joint-Filed Work: Comparison of the Marks and Attitudes of Students with Differences in Skill Level. Srinagarind Med J. 1993; 8(4):191-196.

[20] Orawan Buranruk, Amornrat Ratanasiri, Chanchai Jarupatch. Survey the Opinion of health science students and staff towards the webpage for learning and teaching activities in co-operative community health science 2000. JLTC. 2001; 10 (2): 17-27.

[21] Nithi Srisukhumchai and the Committee of Khon Kaen University Field Practice. Report the prevalence of Students Understanding Folkways After Khon Kaen University Community Fieldwork, Khon Kaen; Khon Kaen University, 2007.

[22] Amornrat Ratanasiri, and the Committee of Khon Kaen University Field Practice, 1984-2008. Khon Kaen University Field Practice: Practice with problems and rural situations for sustainable health development. Poster presentation on Thailand Research Expo 2008 during September 16-18, 2008. Bangkok Convention Center, Thailand, 2008.

[23] Tarinee Arkaravichien, Amornrat Ratanasiri. Students' Reflection on Community Medicine Field Work: A Preliminary Study. Srinagarind Med J. 2015; 30(6):572-576.

[24] Pichet Leungtongkum, Somdej Piniwatsoontorn, Prapimporn Somnasang, Manop Kanato, Amornrat Ratanasiri, Srinoi Maskasam, et al. Study groups of mother or relatives whose level of education are higher than Prathom 4 which normally look after children better than the Similar groups who have Prathom 4 education or lower, and study different factors which influence the growth of preschool children. Srinagarind Med J, 1987; 2(1):23-29.

[25] Amornrat Ratanasiri, Nasinee Sri-akajun, Pissamai Homjumpa, Somsong Na Nakorn, Pattapong Kessombo, Watana Ditstapornchoren, et al. The promotion of health care and health environment in target populations

(women, children and aging people) at Mooban Sum, Amphur Mahachanachai, Yasothorn province, Khon Kaen Agric J; 1992;20(4):213-221.

[26] Ratanasiri A, Sumlak S, Chatrchaiwiwatana S, Muktabhant B, Kunaratanaprk K, Kettowit K, et al. The Rural School Health Development Project: The School of the Royal Initiative of Her Royal Princess Mahachakri Sririndhorn, Poster Presentation on October 25, 2008, at Faculty of Medicine, Khon Kaen University, Khon Kaen, Thailand, 2008

[27] Ahlberg J, Tuominen R, Murtomaa H. Subsidized dental care improves carries status in male industrial workers. Community Dent Oral Epidemiol 1996; 24(4):249-252.

[28] Deveci SE, Deveci F, Acik Y, Ozan AT. The measurement of exhaled carbon monoxide in healthy smokers and non-smokers. Respir Med 2004; 98(6):551-556.

[29] Middleton ET, Morice AH. Breath carbon monoxide as an indication of smoking habit. Chest 2000; 117(3): 758-763.

[30] Bergstrom J, Eliasson S, Preber H. Cigarette smoking and periodontal bone loss. J Periodontol 1991; 62: 242-246.

[31] Haber J, Wattles J, Crowley M, Mandell R, Joshipura K, Kent RL, Evidence for cigarette smoking as a major risk factor for periodontitis. J Periodontol 1993; 64: 16-23.

[32] Mehta FS, Sanjana MK, Barretto MA, Doctor R. Relation of betel leaf chewing to periodontal disease. J AM Dent Assoc 1955; 5: 531-536.

[33] Bledsoe GH, Li G, Levy F. Injury risk in professional boxing. South Med J 2005; 98: 994-998.

[34] Zazryn TR, McCrory PR, Cameron PA. Injury rates and risk factors in competitive professional boxing. Clin J Sport Med 2009; 19:20-25.

Chapter 15

Management and Prevention Strategies for Treating Dentine Hypersensitivity

David G. Gillam

Abstract

The clinician faces numerous challenges when confronted with patients complaining of oro-facial pain, which can involve both dental and non-dental causes. Perhaps one of the most enigmatic clinical conditions that a clinician may encounter is that of dentine hypersensitivity (DH), dentine sensitivity (DS) or root sensitivity (RS), which is both problematic to identify and difficult to treat and may have a major effect on the patient's quality of life (QoL). Ideally, the clinician needs to prevent or minimize these effects to reduce any unnecessary discomfort for the patient and this may be accomplished through preventive strategies, the provision of the required information about the procedures both pre- and post-treatments as well as reassuring the patient in the event of any subsequent discomfort. Furthermore, it is important for the clinician to be able to correctly diagnose the exact cause of the patient's discomfort and have the confidence to successfully manage the problem. This chapter aims to cover the relevant aspects for both diagnosing and managing DH with an emphasis on adopting a preventive strategy that will attempt to minimize or eliminate the problem, thereby enabling the patient to have an improved quality of life.

Keywords: dentine hypersensitivity, management, in-office (professionally applied), over-the-counter (OTC) (at home), prevention strategies, quality of life (QoL)

1. Introduction

According to Gillam [1], one of the challenges facing the clinician when examining a patient complaining of different types of dental pain is that the patient may be suffering from both physical or emotional discomfort. This may be very traumatic to them in terms of being unable to cope, resulting in the loss of sleep and work as well as in an economic cost to the health care provider [2–4]. This in turn may present difficulties for the clinician in determining a correct diagnosis of the cause of the patient's pain. The importance of differentiating these different types of oro-facial pain based on the patient's presenting clinical features and a thorough medical and dental history is a key to the successful management of the patient's pain [1]. Furthermore, it should be recognized that pain is subjective in nature and is pertinent to the individual's own perception of pain, which may also be influenced by several factors such as a previous history of pain, anticipation, or fear of the proposed dental treatment. Although dentine hypersensitivity (DH) may not be as severe as some of the other oro-facial conditions, it is a relatively common condition, which has an impact on the individual patient's well-being and quality of life (QoL) [5]. There have been concerns regarding the awareness and confidence of clinicians to diagnose and successfully manage DH [1, 6, 7]. To address these concerns, several management and preventive strategies have been suggested to provide practical guidelines for clinicians [6, 8–10]. These guidelines include identifying the cause of the patient's presenting problem based on a good medical and dental history with a thorough clinical examination using the appropriate diagnostic tests when distinguishing DH from other forms of oro-facial pain. Recommendations for the management of DH also included the importance of removing the aetiological and pre-disposing features to prevent further episodes of pain associated with DH to alleviate the impact on the patient's QoL. The use and/or recommendations of the appropriate in-office (professionally applied) or over the counter (OTC; at-home) products and/or techniques depending on the severity of the problem should also be included in the clinician's management strategy. The importance of a management plan that includes both a preventive strategy to reduce further damage to both the hard and soft tissues of the mouth, and with a monitoring component within the plan cannot be overstated [10]. This chapter, therefore, covers the relevant aspects for diagnosing and managing DH with an emphasis on adopting a preventive strategy that will attempt to minimize or eliminate the problem, thereby enabling the patient to have an improved QoL.

2. Prevalence and awareness of dentine hypersensitivity

2.1 Prevalence of dentine hypersensitivity

The published prevalence figures for dentine hypersensitivity range from approximately 1% to over 70% depending on how the figures are collected. For example, data from questionnaire studies report a higher prevalence of the condition, whereas data from clinical studies that examine the patient provide lower prevalence figures. The information from these types of studies may also depend on the location (university or hospital clinics, general dental practice, or specialist practice such as restorative or periodontics) and the country or culture of the population. For example, the traditional prevalence figures for DH *per se* are estimated to be 10% with an average of 33% across studies as reviewed by Cuhna-Cruz and Watana [11], whereas the prevalence figures for root sensitivity (RS) due to periodontal disease or its treatment is considerably higher (60–98% [12, 13]). DH/RS may therefore affect individuals over all age groups; however, from the literature, the peak prevalence is between the ages of 30 and 60 years with females numerically more affected than males [12]. There is also evidence from the published studies that the buccal (facial) tooth surfaces are most likely to be affected and there appears to be an association between DH/DS and gingival recession. According to the West et al.'s [14] study in young European adults aged 18 to 35 years, there is a link between a so-called healthy erosive diet, lifestyle and tooth wear with DH/RS.

2.2 Awareness of dentine hypersensitivity by clinicians

According to the findings of the Canadian Advisory Board on Dentin Hypersensitivity [6], 14 knowledge gaps were identified from the survey of participating clinicians, and these were classified as relating to either the causes and diagnosis or the management of the condition. It was evident from these findings that the prevalence of DH was underestimated, and this was due in part to the lack of routine screening for the condition by clinicians. Less than 50% of the participants considered a differential diagnosis to eliminate other dental conditions with similar pain characteristics to those of DH. There was also confusion regarding the nature of the predisposing factors associated with DH as well a misunderstanding of how desensitizing products work (mechanism of action). Furthermore, about 50% of the participants indicated that they lacked confidence in treating DH effectively with a similar percentage indicating that they would try to modify any predisposing factors prior to further treatment. A recent review of questionnaire studies on the awareness of DH by clinicians indicated that there are still areas of concern in the understanding of the underlying principles involved in the management of DH [7].

3. Mechanisms, aetiology, predisposing factors, and clinical features of dentine hypersensitivity

3.1 Mechanisms

The currently accepted mechanism associated with DH as proposed by Brännström and Åström is hydrodynamic in nature [15]. This theory relies on minute fluid movements within the dentinal tubules in response to an external stimulus such as cold air or water to initiate pain in the dental pulp. There is also *in vitro* evidence that in areas of clinically identified sensitive dentine there are a greater number of open dentinal tubules compared to non-sensitive areas. Underpinning this theory is the presence of open dentinal tubules on the exposed root surface (cervical area), which in turn affects the degree of fluid flow through the tubule. This theory promotes two basic approaches for treatment: (1) by occluding the exposed open dentine tubules in the cervical region of the exposed root surface, which in turn reduces any stimulus-evoked fluid movements within the dentinal tubules and effectively prevents the transmission of the external stimulus (such as a cold stimulus) to the pulp, and (2) by potassium ion diffusion within the dentinal tubule to reduce intra-dental nerve excitability and prevent any nerve activation [16]. The question whether the hydrodynamic theory is also associated with root sensitivity has been questioned due to the presence of dental plaque on the root surface, which may encourage the ingress of bacteria within the dentinal tubules [12, 16].

3.2 Etiology and predisposing factors

The etiology of DH/RS is multifactorial in nature, and it is evident that the structure of dentine is altered because of a combination of the associated pre-disposing factors, which may include anatomical factors such as tooth position, quality of the buccal plate, and so on. For example, once the overlying hard and soft tissues have been removed exposing the underlying dentine surface through gingival recession, tooth surface loss through attrition, abrasion and possibly abfraction, over-zealous toothbrushing techniques, the effects of periodontal disease and its subsequent treatment, then these factors may play a part in widening the open dentinal tubules through erosion with the combination of over-zealous toothbrushing techniques. An epidemiological study in a population of young adults aged 18–35 years by West et al. [14] reported that there was a link between a healthy erosive diet and lifestyle and toothwear with DH.

3.3 Clinical presentation

Pain associated with DH is considered transient in nature and once the initiating stimulus, such as cold air from a dental air syringe or a cold drink, has been removed, the problem will have been resolved. The clinical features of DH as reported in the published literature primarily deal with the features associated with DH in patients with a well-maintained oral hygiene rather than clinical features associated with RS *per se*. It is reasonable, however, to acknowledge that some of the aetiological and predisposing factors will be similar (**Figure 1**). For example, the combination or synergistic effects with attrition, abrasion, erosion, and so on, together with over-zealous tooth brushing on exposed dentine in the cervical/root area of a tooth may accelerate the tooth wear process. The loss of gingival tissue due to the impact of the above factors or because of periodontal disease and/or periodontal therapy may also expose the underlying dentine resulting in DH/RS. The importance of the underlying bone texture, thickness of the buccal plate as well as the thickness of the gingival (periodontal) biotype may also result in gingival recession (loss of attachment), particularly following scaling procedures in shallow pockets (≤4 mm). Although DH/RS may affect any tooth or tooth surface, the intra-oral distribution involves the buccal (facial) surfaces of incisor, canine, premolar, and molar teeth RS, which may also affect the interdental, palatal, and lingual surfaces. Non-carious cervical lesions (NCCL) with or without DH/RS may also be present.

3.4 History taking and clinical evaluation

It is important to recognize that two broad categories of patients attend a dental clinic: (1) patients who are regular attenders and have an established relationship with the clinician, and (2) patients who have not been previously attending a dental practice but may have decided to attend due to a dental problem such as toothache, esthetic concerns, or other dental problems which have arisen. In the first category of patients, the clinician will be aware of their personal medical and treatment history and to some extent, the consultation period including the examination may be straightforward. For example, a patient who has recently received dental treatment such as restoration

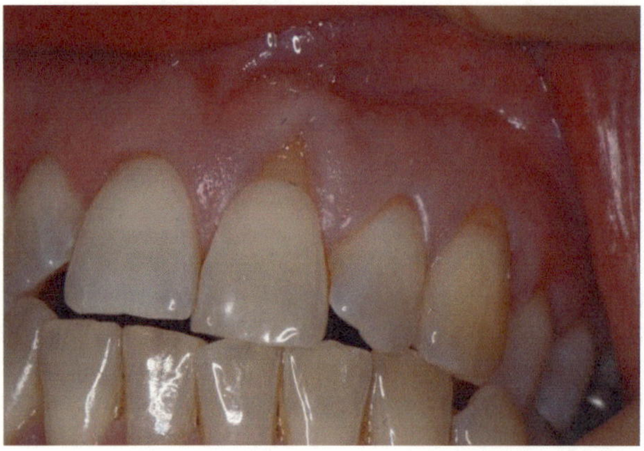

Figure 1.
Clinical features of a patient with gingival recession and dentine hypersensitivity (Acknowledgement N. Pandya [17]).

of a tooth or had their teeth professionally cleaned may be experiencing discomfort from these procedures and such a problem can be swiftly identified and treated [16]. Patients who have not previously attended a dental practice, however, may require a more prolonged consultation to obtain the relevant medical, dental, and social history prior to the clinical examination and subsequent diagnosis of DH.

For patients with a more obscure orofacial problem, a persistent idiopathic facial pain (PIFP) may require a more extensive examination and it is advisable for the clinician to refer these patients to a Specialist Oral Medicine/Pain clinic [16].

Prior to a clinical examination, the clinician should obtain medical, dental, social, and dietary histories to supplement the information collected during the clinical examination and any subsequent tests such as radiographs. During the initial consultation, it is important to ask the patient why they have arranged the appointment. Toothache is one of the most common of oro-facial pains that prompts a patient to visit a dentist and where possible the clinician should determine the nature of the problem, the location of the pain (if the patient is able to pinpoint the exact location), duration, intensity, and any factors that may intensify or relieve the pain. For example, the clinician can ask if the patient is able to continue their daily activities such as eating, drinking, brushing their teeth without any discomfort. One suggestion would be to use visual analogue scale (VAS) scores (0-10), verbal descriptors, or Quality of Life Questionnaires (QoL) to determine the severity of the discomfort the patient is experiencing, and any impact DH/RS may have the patient's QoL [5]. The clinical examination will involve a thorough evaluation of the patient's oral status including a Basic Periodontal Examination (BSP) and a Basic Erosive Wear Assessment (BEWE) to determine the degree of tooth surface loss [10].

During the clinical examination, clinicians will use a dental explorer probe and air from a triple air syringe to screen any sensitive areas on the exposed cervical/root region. If the patient is prone to DH, then this mechanical or evaporative/thermal stimulus will elicit a response from the patient [1]. The response to these stimuli will be varied depending on the individual's pain threshold and subjective perception of pain. This pain should be transient in nature, in that once the stimulus has been removed, the pain will be resolved. If the pain, however, is continuous in nature, then this may indicate that the problem is related to other dental problems such as dental caries, which will require more extensive testing using an ice stick, ethyl chloride, pulp testers, and so on to evaluate the status of the dental pulp (pulp vitality testing). A simple test at this stage of the initial evaluation for DH is to (1) ask the patient to indicate their perception of the pain they are experiencing with DH following blowing cold air on the tooth (or teeth) in question using a VAS score, (2) apply a varnish to the affected site of the identified tooth (or teeth), and (3) retest the tooth (or teeth) in question using cold air from a dental air syringe and ask the patient to indicate their pain perception using a VAS score. If there is an improvement in the VAS scores, then this may indicate that the initial diagnosis of the patient's problem was DH (see management section).

3.5 Diagnosis and differential diagnosis of Dentine hypersensitivity

3.5.1 Diagnostic evaluation including special investigations

According to Gillam [7], there are a variety of methodological approaches used in the dental clinic to identify (diagnose) DH such as tactile, evaporative, and thermal stimulation using cold air from a dental triple syringe as well as the patient's self-reporting (VAS, patient history, etc.). An example of the range of methodological approaches recommended or used by clinicians can be observed in **Figure 2** [18]. The use of these methodological approaches may, however, be difficult to justify [19].

A useful device to aid clinicians in determining both a provision and definitive is the use of mnemonics such as 'LOCATE' or 'SOCRATES'. This will help to ascertain the relevant information to identify the patient's problem by asking the following questions:

- Pain characteristics: What were the symptoms relating to pain experienced by the patient?

- Location of the pain: Was the pain localized or generalized in nature and can the patient point to the site of the problem?

- Pain onset: Was the patient able to relate to the clinician when the pain started?

- Pain duration: Was the pain transient or long lasting in nature?

- Pattern of pain: Was the patient able to recall the pattern of the pain?

- Pain severity: What was the severity of pain and did it vary?

- Relieving factors: Are there factors that relieve or worsen the pain such as the application of cold or heat, medication, changing position (lying down), and so on?

- Associated factors: Are there any other factors that you might be aware of when you are experiencing pain?

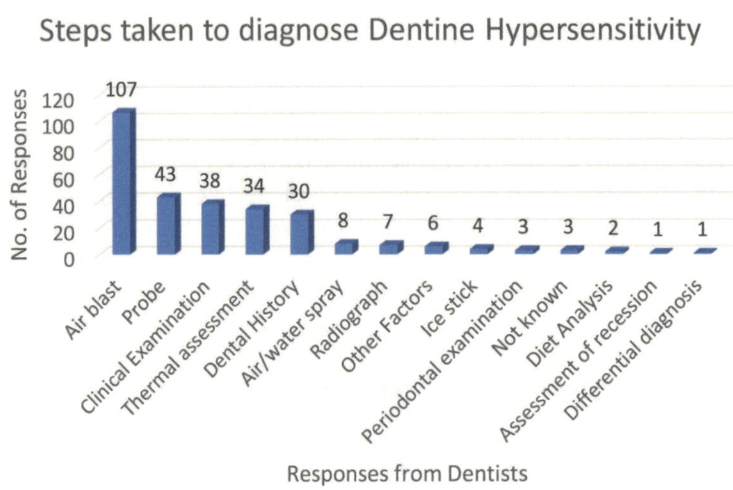

Figure 2.
Diagnostic steps used by clinicians to identify DH (Acknowledgement Exarchou et al. [18]).

The clinician, however, should be aware that depending on the longevity and severity of the patient's pain, and particularly from severe toothache, they may have difficulties recalling some of these features due to being unable to cope with pain before attending the clinic [2].

3.5.2 Diagnosis of dentine hypersensitivity

The classic definition of DH was based on specific wording as 'pain derived from exposed dentine in response to chemical, thermal tactile or osmotic stimuli which cannot be explained as arising from any other dental defect or disease' [6]. In other words, DH is in essence a diagnosis of exclusion based on both the history of the problem and a clinical examination to exclude other forms of oro-facial pain and as such a thorough clinical examination together with a medical and dental history of the patient should enable the clinician to come to a correct diagnosis [1, 20].

There are, however, several problems facing the clinician when investigating oro-facial pain, for example, the time taken to identify the areas in the mouth causing the discomfort as well as the highly subjective nature of the pain response [20]. The clinician is, therefore, reliant not only on the patient's self-reporting of the history of DH but also on the information that they have accumulated through their own analysis of the problem (medical, dental, and social history together with a thorough clinical examination, which may require further evaluation). For example, patients who have recently received restorative, bleaching, and periodontal procedures within the last few weeks before attending the clinic may in fact be suffering from post-operative sensitivity and this should be relatively easy to identify and reassure the patient that the pain should resolve within 4-6 weeks and if not to return for further investigation. For new patients or those with a recent complaint of DH, the clinician will spend more time discussing the problem with the patient, trying to determine the history of the problem using some of the diagnostic tests indicated in **Figure 2**. The clinician should be aware that as DH is an exaggerated response of the normal pulp-dentine, the patient may only be aware of the problem once an external stimulus such as a cold stimulus (cold air from a dental triple syringe, suction from a high-volume suction, etc.). The evidence identified during this process may enable to provide a provisional diagnosis of DH.

3.5.3 Differential diagnosis of dentine hypersensitivity

According to the Canadian Advisory Board on Dentin Hypersensitivity [6], there is a major problem in the diagnosis of DH where ≤50% of the clinicians participating in the survey considered using a differential diagnosis to eliminate other dental conditions with similar pain characteristics to those of DH. Other studies have also reported on the apparent reluctance by clinicians to consider in this aspect of the management of DH [7].

One of the reasons for this reluctance in making a definitive diagnosis of DH may be the complexity and time required to eliminate the other dental conditions that have similar pain characteristics to DH such as reversible and irreversible pulpitis, dental abscess, cracked tooth syndrome, periodontal disease, pericoronitis, idiopathic oral facial pain, and post-operative sensitivity [18] (**Figure 2**). It is, therefore, important for the clinician to make a definitive diagnosis of DH before undertaking any treatment of the patient's problem. A useful summary of selected oro-facial conditions with their pain characteristics and presenting features is shown in **Table 1** [20].

Aetiology	Pain character and timing	Pain intensity	Proving factors	Relieving factors	Associated features
Dentine hypersensitivity	Sharp, stabbing, stimulation evoked	Mild to moderate	Thermal, tactile, chemical, osmotic	Removal of the stimulus	Attrition, erosion, abrasion, abfraction
Atypical odontalgia (persistent dentoalveolar pain)	Continuous, no paroxysmal, dull, aching and throbbing but occasionally sharp	Mild to moderate	Touch, heat and ccld	Sleep and rest Topical agents: lidocaine, capsaicin. Systemic agents: antidepressants	May have no obvious clinical features
Reversible pulpitis	Sharp, stimulation evoked	Mild to moderate	Hot, cold, sweet	Removal of the stimulus	Caries, restorations
Irreversible pulpitis	Sharp, throbbing, intermittent/ continuous	Severe	Hot, chewing, lying flat	Cold in the late stages	Deep caries
Cracked tooth syndrome	Sharp intermittent	Moderate to severe	Biting, 'rebound pain'	—	Trauma, parafunction
Periapical periodontitis	Deep, continuous boring	Moderate to severe	Biting	Removal of trauma	Periapical redness, swelling, mobility
Lateral periodontal abscess	Deep continuous aching	Moderate to severe	Biting	—	Deep pockets redness and swelling
Pericoronitis	Continuous	Moderate to severe	Biting	Removal of trauma	Fever, malaise, imprint of upper tooth
Dry socket (acute alveolar osteitis	Continuous 4–5 days post-extraction	Moderate to severe	—	Irrigation	Loss of clot, exposed bone

Table 1.
Differential diagnosis of dental pain (modified acknowledgement Aghabeigi [20]).

4. Clinical management of dentine hypersensitivity

Once a definitive diagnosis has been determined, the clinician can then formulate a management strategy to treat the condition. The complexity of this treatment plan will depend on (1) on the extent and severity of the problem, (2) the willingness of the patient to comply with the recommendations provided by the clinician, and (3) the ability of the clinician to successfully diagnose the problem and provide the appropriate treatment including preventative strategies. Broadly speaking, the initial treatment will be either (1) professionally applied (in-office treatment) such as a fluoride varnish or more invasive strategy (composite, laser, periodontal surgery) for localized severe DH, or (2) patient applied/at home [over the counter treatment (OTC)] such as an OTC toothpaste for a mild-moderate discomfort (see **Table 2** for examples). The clinician should also be aware of the impact of DH on the QoL of the patient and it is important for the clinician to monitor whether the recommended treatment has improved the patient's QoL. For example, can the patient continue their daily routine of eating, drinking and oral hygiene practices without any interruption to their daily activities.

Several investigators have recommended treatment algorithms to help the clinician mange DH successfully [6, 8, 10]. An example of one of these algorithms is displayed in **Figure 3** based on the recommendations from a UK Guidelines workshop, London, UK [10]. An important aspect of these guidelines was the recognition that

Gingival recession	Tooth wear	Periodontal treatment
Clinical evaluation • Clinical measurement of the Gingival Recession defect • Take study casts and clinical photographs to monitor condition over time • Check and Monitor periodontal health • Identification and correction of predisposing or precipitating factors • Use of pain scores to assess and monitor DH (e.g., visual analogue scores)	Clinical evaluation • Identify cause of tooth wear (enamel loss) • Record severity of lesions, if possible, using a recognized index (Smith & Knight 1984, Bartlett et al. 2008) • Take study casts and clinical photographs to monitor condition over time • Check and Monitor periodontal health. • Use of pain scores to assess and monitor DH (e.g., visual analogue scores)	Clinical evaluation • Periodontal disease or periodontal treatment as the primary cause of exposure of dentine and associated DH. • Check and Monitor periodontal health (6-point pocket charting) • Use of pain scores to assess and monitor DH (e.g., visual analogue scores)
Patient education (including preventive advice) • Show patient the affected site(s) • Explain probable cause for recession. • Explain factors triggering sensitive teeth episodes • Encourage patients to modify their oral hygiene regimen in order to reduce damage to gingivae (e.g., reducing brushing force, correction of toothbrush technique) • Reduce excessive consumption of acid foods and drinks	Patient education (including preventive advice) • Show patient the site(s) and explain probable cause of the tooth wear lesion(s) • Recommend an oral hygiene regimen to minimize risk of further tooth wear. • Where appropriate recommend reducing frequency of consumption of acidic food & drink.	Patient education (including preventive advice) • Reinforce the need for good oral hygiene • Show patient the site(s) affected by periodontal disease and explain probable cause of the exposed dentine • Guide the patient to improve 'at home' oral hygiene regimen. • Instruction on measures of reducing periodontal risk factors for example diabetes, smoking, obesity.

Gingival recession	Tooth wear	Periodontal treatment
Corrective clinical outcomes • Reduce excessive consumption of acid foods and drinks • Manufacture of silicone gingival veneers • Orthodontic treatment • Restorative correction of recession defect and sub-gingival margins of fillings and crowns • Polymers: Sealants/varnishes/resins/dentine bonding agents • Laser obturation of dentinal tubules • Use of Desensitizing polishing pastes • Pulpal extirpation (root canal treatment)	Corrective clinical outcomes • Provide high fluoride remineralizing treatment (pre-emptive phase) • Provide professional desensitizing treatment to relieve DH • Encourage patient to seek advice from medical practitioner, if tooth wear caused by working environment or reflux/excessive vomiting (Psychiatric evaluation may also be appropriate) • Restorative correction in the form of composite build-up, crowns may also be appropriate	Corrective clinical outcomes Initial phase Non-surgical periodontal procedure(s). DH treatment (including desensitizing polishing pastes/ Fluoride varnishes) Re-evaluation Follow-up assessment on periodontal status and dentine hypersensitivity Corrective phase • Surgical periodontal procedure(s), for example, guided tissue regeneration, Coronally Advanced Flap + Enamel Matrix Derivatives, Connective Tissue Graft (flap), Free Gingival Graft (acellular dermal matrix allograft) • DH treatment (including desensitizing polishing pastes/ Fluoride varnishes) Follow-up management Maintenance phase • Supportive periodontal therapy • Ongoing monitoring of periodontal health • Dentine hypersensitivity treatment (including desensitizing polishing pastes/Fluoride varnishes) • Oral hygiene advice
Recommendations for home use (including toothpaste/mouth rinses) • Oral hygiene implementation as per recommendation • Strontium chloride/strontium acetate • Potassium nitrate/chloride/citrate/ oxalate • Calcium compounds: • Calcium carbonate and arginine and Caesin Phosphopeptide+Amorphous Calcium Phosphate • Bioactive glass • Nano/hydroxyapatite • Fluoride in higher concentration (2800/5000 ppm F[prescription]) • Amine/sodium/sodium monofluorophosphate/ stannous fluoride	Recommendations for home use (including toothpaste/ mouth rinses) • Oral hygiene implementation as per recommendation • Toothpastes and mouth rinses (see Recommendations for gingival recession)	Recommendations for home use (including toothpaste/mouth rinses) • Oral hygiene implementation as per recommendation • Regular brushing with an antibacterial toothpaste to aid plaque control. • Short period, the use of a 0.2% chlorhexidine solution for plaque control • Use of a desensitizing mouth rinse twice daily for DH control (when appropriate)

Table 2.
Overall management strategy options for treating DH (Acknowledgement Gillam et al. [10] modified).

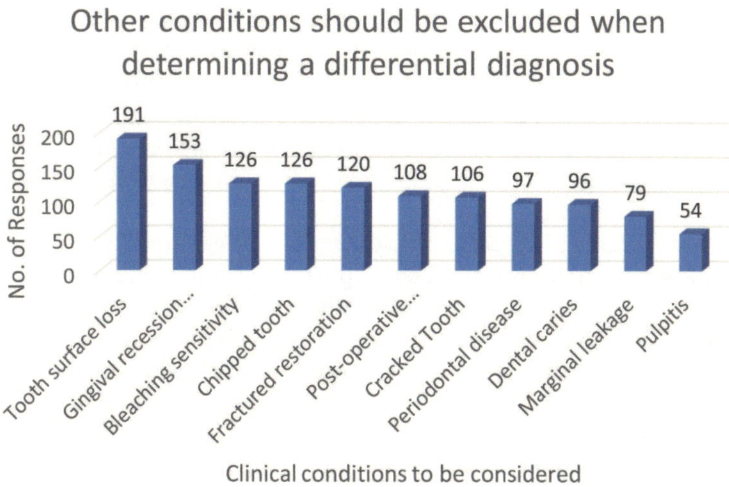

Figure 3.
Selected responses from participants on what other dental conditions should be excluded when determining a differential diagnosis (Acknowledgement Exarchou et al. [18]).

the management of DH should be based on the presenting features of the problem rather than simply providing a blanket treatment plan to cover all aspects of DH. For example, three categories were presented for the clinician to consider: (1) patients with gingival recession in a well-maintained mouth, (2) patients with a tooth wear problem, and (3) patients with a periodontal problem (**Table 2**) [10]. This concept was utilized and developed by Gillam and Koyi [21] covering six clinical case scenarios in dealing with oro-facial pain with specific clinical presentations.

The management of DH can therefore involve both simple and complex cases to treat and it is important that the clinician is aware of both their expectations of success and the patient's expectation of resolving their pain. There may be times when this aspiration can only be partially met to the satisfaction of both parties. The clinician should avoid simply handing out or recommending a treatment or technique without identifying the aetiological factors that initiated the problem in the first place. One of the concerns from the Canadian Advisory Board on Dentin Hypersensitivity [6] was whether clinicians had the confidence in the products that they recommended for treatment. This concern has also been highlighted by several investigators and it appears that this issue is still a matter of concern [7, 19].

Depending on the severity of the problem, the following products and techniques can be suggested (see **Table 2**). The question as to whether these products or techniques are effective in the treatment of DH has been the subject of several systematic reviews and meta-analysis [22–25].

5. Preventive strategies

The importance of a preventive strategy for minimizing further episodes of DH cannot be overstated. It is not enough to simply provide a patient with a treatment such as a toothpaste or composite restoration without first eliminating or at least minimizing the aetiological or predisposing features that initiated the problem in the first place. This aspect will involve reviewing the clinical features implicated with the condition such as patients with a healthy mouth or patients with a periodontal or restorative problems. For example, patients with a healthy, plaque-free mouth may be over-zealous, or an enthusiastic brusher with a healthy diet that may include acidic drinks will need advice on modifying their tooth brushing technique and minimizing the effects of dietary acids. The patient with a periodontal or restorative problem will require more extensive and prolonged treatment and perhaps one way of initially alleviating post-operative pain following this treatment would be to apply a desensitizing polishing paste or dental varnish [16].

Traditionally, clinicians expect their patients to change their health behavior, which is a philosophy based on a top-down approach (clinician directed) where the patient was provided information that was considered beneficial to them by the clinician. This philosophy, however, not only failed to empower the patient but was also ineffective in motivating the patient to initiate any behavior changes to improve their health and well-being. It is, therefore, important for the clinician to adopt management strategies and goals that will effectively encourage the patient to take individual responsibility to initiate these behavioral changes in the lifestyle of their patients. According to Gillam and Ramseier [26], the introduction of patient-centred approaches such as Motivational Interviewing is ideal for motivating patients in dental practice. It is acknowledged, however, that for many clinicians, this approach may be difficult to implement, due to time constraints, although the process could be continued over several visits as in the periodontal maintenance phase [27]. There are several factors to consider when developing a strategy using this approach, for example, (1) the extent and severity of the patient's problem, (2) acquiring the patient's permission to discuss any proposed changes, (3) the availability of the patient and their willingness to engage with the consultation process, (4) the rapport between the patient and clinician, (5) the willingness of the patient to reflect on the proposed changes and to weigh up the advantages/disadvantages and decide whether to accept or reject these proposals, (6) the patient's motivation to initiate these changes and subsequently adhere (comply) to the recommended changes to their behavior, and (7) the frequency of monitoring during the maintenance phase and subsequent reinforcement strategy in monitoring the patient's progress [26, 27].

6. Summary and take-home message

According to Gillam ([20] modified), the following key points may be useful in ascertaining whether a patient has DH and how much it impacts on their QoL and should enable the clinician not only to manage the problem in a structured manner but also to encourage to take personal ownership of their oral health by making the necessary changes/modifications in their behavior.

- Ask patients if they have a history of DH
- Ask patients if it is a current problem
- Does it impact on their QoL? If 'Yes', ask them to elaborate on the extent and severity of the problem
- Examine the patient for DH, particularly the buccal (facial) surfaces of the standing teeth using a probe and an air-blast from a dental triple syringe.

- A good history of the complaint is important, listen to the patient and examine areas where the dentine is exposed, identify any aetiological and predisposing factors. Listen to the patient; they will give you the diagnosis.

- The use of diet sheets will help in identifying potential risk factors in the diet (diet analysis).

- Have a basic understanding of the mechanisms associated with dentine hypersensitivity, in particular, the Hydrodynamic Theory and its importance in choosing a suitable OTC/professionally applied product when treating the patient.

- Educate the patient, indicating where they can reduce the impact of DH on their QoL, modifying their toothbrush technique, using a less abrasive toothpaste and avoiding consuming acidic food and drinks particularly around the time of brushing.

- Encourage the patient to take ownership of their oral health to allow for any behavior changes to reduce the impact of DH on the QoL when undertaking their day-to day activities (Consider the use of Motivational Interviewing).

- Remember there is no one treatment or procedure that will resolve all your patient's problems and that simply providing a toothpaste or in-office procedure alone without correcting or modifying any underlining predisposing features that initiated the problem will not resolve the problem in the long term.

- Apply the guidelines outlined in this chapter; in your practice, monitor patients DH within your practice's recall procedure(s), avoid simply handing out or recommending dental products expecting the problem to resolve, without any further intervention by the clinician.

- Use the algorithm (or similar examples; see references) illustrated in this chapter to aid you in the management of DH. It may be that despite all your efforts the patient still has oro-facial pain. The steps outlined in the algorithm will enable you to revisit the diagnosis of DH, which may result in further investigations to determine the cause (reversible/irreversible pulpitis) or a referral to a specialist oral medicine clinic if the problem is of a non-dental origin such as idiopathic facial pain (PIFP).

7. Concluding remarks

DH is an enigmatic dental condition that is often discounted or underdiagnosed by clinicians who may fail to appreciate its impact on the QoL of their patients, and therefore, screening for the problem should be included in a clinical examination.

Clinicians should recognize it is a diagnosis of exclusion and all other possible causes of the pain should be ruled out. This will require the clinician to collate the relevant medical, dental, social, and diet history from the patient, which will supplement the clinical examination. It is important for clinicians to acknowledge that the management is not just based on providing or recommending OTC products or in-office therapies and procedures but on the removal or modification of any predisposing feature together with involving the patient to make changes in their own behavior to minimize the impact of DH on their QoL.

Conflict of interest

The author declares no conflict of interest.

Author details

David G. Gillam
Oral Bioengineering, Institute of Dentistry, Barts and the London School of Medicine and Dentistry QMUL, London, UK

*Address all correspondence to: d.g.gillam@qmul.ac.uk

References

[1] Gillam DG. Current diagnosis of dentin hypersensitivity in the dental office: An overview. Clinical Oral Investigations. 2013;**17**(1):S21-S29. DOI: 10.1007/s00784-012-0911-1

[2] Pau AK, Croucher R, Marcenes W. Perceived inability to cope and care-seeking in patients with toothache: A qualitative study. British Dental Journal. 2000;**189**(9):503-506. DOI: 10.1038/sj.bdj.4800812

[3] Ayo-Yusuf IJ, Naidoo S. Social gradient in the cost of oral pain and related dental service utilisation among South African adults. BMC Oral Health. 2016;**16**:117. DOI: 10.1186/s12903-016-0313-x

[4] Breckons M, Shen J, Bunga J, Vale L, Durham J. DEEP study: Indirect and out-of-pocket costs of persistent orofacial pain. Journal of Dental Research. 2018;**97**(11):1200-1206. DOI: 10.1177/0022034518773310

[5] Gillam DG. The impact of dentine hypersensitivity on the quality of life: An overview. Clinical Oral Science and Dentistry. 2021;**4**:1

[6] Canadian Advisory Board on Dentin Hypersensitivity. Consensus-based recommendations for the diagnosis and management of dentin hypersensitivity. Journal of the Canadian Dental Association. 2003;**69**(4):221-226

[7] Gillam DG. Clinician's Awareness of the management of dentine hypersensitivity: An Overview. Adv Jr Dent and Stom: AJDS-101. DOI: 10.37722/AJDS.2021101

[8] Addy M, Urquhart E. Dentine hypersensitivity: Its prevalence, aetiology and clinical management. Dental Update. 1992;**19**(10):407-408

[9] Pashley D, Tay FR, Haywood VB, Collins MA, Drisko CL. Consensus-based recommendations for the diagnosis and management of dentin hypersensitivity. Compendium of Continuing Education in Dentistry. 2008;**29**(8):1S-35S

[10] Gillam D, Chesters R, Attrill D, Brunton P, Slater M, Strand P, et al. Dentine hypersensitivity—Guidelines for the management of a common oral health problem. Dental Update. 2013;**40**(7):514-516

[11] Cunha-Cruz J, Wataha JC. The burden of dentine hypersensitivity. In: Robinson PG, editor. Dentine hypersensitivity: Developing a person-centred approach to oral health. Oxford, UK: Academic Press, Elsevier Inc.; 2014. pp. 34-44

[12] Gillam DG, Orchardson R. Advances in the treatment of root dentine sensitivity: Mechanisms and treatment principles. Endodontic Topics. 2006;**13**:13-33

[13] Lin YH, Gillam DG. The prevalence of root sensitivity following periodontal therapy: A systematic review. International Journal of Dentistry. 2012;**2012**:1-12. DOI: 10.1155/2012/407023

[14] West NX, Sanz M, Lussi A, Bartlett D, Bouchard P, Bourgeois D. Prevalence of dentine hypersensitivity and study of associated factors: A European population based cross-sectional study. Journal of Dentistry. 2013;**41**:841-851

[15] Brännström M, Åström A. The hydrodynamics of the dentin; its possible relationship to dentinal pain. International Dental Journal. 1972;**22**:219-227

[16] Gillam DG, Chatzopoulou D. Post-Operative Pain Following Non-Surgical and Surgical Periodontal Procedures, Periodontology and Dental Implantology. Rijeka: IntechOpen; 2018. DOI: 10.5772/intechopen.78728

[17] Pandya N, Turner W, Gillam DG. Description of a minimally invasive technique to correct a gingival margin defect: A case report. Advances in Dentistry & Oral Health. 2020;**13**(1). DOI: 10.19080/ADOH.2020.13.55585

[18] Cunha-Cruz J, Wataha JC, Zhou L, Manning W, Trantow M, Bettendorf MM, et al. Treating dentin hypersensitivity: Therapeutic choices made by dentists of the Northwest PRECEDENT network. Journal of the American Dental Association. 2010;**141**(9):1097-1105

[19] Exarchou C, Betsani I, Sakellari D, Chatzopoulou D, Gillam D. A survey of dentists in the management of dentine hypersensitivity: A questionnaire-based study. European Journal of Dentistry. 2019;**13**(03):383-390. DOI: 10.1055/s-0039-1694306

[20] Gillam D. Diagnosis of Dentine Hypersensitivity. 2020. Available from: https://www.dentistry.co.uk/2020/11/30/diagnosis-dentine-hypersensitivity/

[21] Gillam D, Koyi B. Dentin Hypersensitivity in Clinical Practice. India: JP Medical; 2019

[22] Lin PY, Cheng YW, Chu CY, Chien KL, Lin CP, Tu YK. In-office treatment for dentin hypersensitivity: A systematic review and network meta-analysis. Journal of Clinical Periodontology. 2013;**40**:53-64

[23] He S, Wang Y, Li X, Hu D. Effectiveness of laser therapy and topical desensitising agents in treating dentine hypersensitivity: A systematic review. Journal of Oral Rehabilitation. 2011;**38**(5):348-358

[24] Sgolastra F, Petrucci A, Severino M, Gatto R, Monaco A. Lasers for the treatment of dentin hypersensitivity: A meta-analysis. Journal of Dental Research. 2013;**92**(6):492-499

[25] Hu ML, Zheng G, Lin H, Yang M, Zhang YD, Han JM. Network meta-analysis on the effect of desensitizing toothpastes on dentine hypersensitivity. Journal of Dentistry. 2019;**88**:103170. DOI: 10.1016/j.jdent.2019.07.008

[26] Gillam DG, Ramseier CA. Chapter 10: Advances in the management of the patient with dentine hypersensitivity: Motivation and prevention. In: Gillam DG, editor. Dentine Hypersensitivity: Advances in Diagnosis, Management, and Treatment. Switzerland: Springer International Publishing; 2015. pp. 143-156. DOI: 10.1007/978-3-319-14577-8

[27] Gillam DG, Yusuf H. Brief motivational interviewing in dental practice. Dental Journal. 2019;7:51. DOI: 10.3390/dj7020051

Chapter 16

Preventive Methods and Treatments of White Spot Lesions in Orthodontics

Elif Nadide Akay

Abstract

The aim of orthodontic treatment is to improve the esthetics of the teeth and face, to provide a beautiful smile, and an adequate and permanent chewing function. In individuals with insufficient oral hygiene, demineralization begins in the mouth with a very low pH value, and as a result, white spot lesions formed by decalcification of the enamel layer can be seen during orthodontic treatment. Since lesions are the first stage of caries formation, it is possible to stop caries development at this stage. Many methods, such as improving oral hygiene, regulating diets, fluoridated agents, laser, casein phosphopeptide, and microabrasion, are used in the treatment of white spot lesions. Preventive methods are of great importance in terms of preventing future tooth loss and reducing the treatment process. The purpose of this article is to manage white spot lesions in orthodontic treatment and to examine risk factors and preventive methods based on the latest evidence.

Keywords: white spot lesion, orthodontic treatment, conservative methods, demineralization

1. Introduction

The improvement of modern living conditions, the increase in life expectancy, and the propensity of looking younger and more beautiful have led to an increase in the need for esthetic treatments. Thanks to the orthodontic treatment, as long as the periodontal tissues are healthy, an esthetic smile can be served in all age groups of individuals. Regarding the esthetic involvement in the orthodontic practice as well as the treatment outcomes metallic colored brackets, tooth-colored brackets, lingual brackets, and aligner treatments have been performed in the clinical practice. Attachments and appliances used in the treatment create an area for plaque involvement at various levels.

Enamel discoloration and initial caries lesions are the most prominent clinical problems in patients undergoing orthodontic treatment. As a result of the decrease in the oral pH value, the diffusion of calcium and phosphate ions from the enamel becomes easier and a color change occurs on the enamel surface as a result of decalcification. Irregular surfaces of brackets, wires, bands, and other attachments limit naturally occurring self-cleaning mechanisms, such as the movement of saliva and its intraoral muscles. Increased incidence of these lesions has been found in patients after orthodontic treatment due to long-term plaque accumulation and inadequate oral hygiene [1]. In order to prevent the formation of white spot lesions that cause both demineralization and discoloration of the teeth, and to prevent their progression by treating them at an early stage, it is recommended to take the necessary precautions before and during the treatment and to choose the appropriate diagnostic methods and apply the necessary treatment methods [2].

2. Etiology of demineralization

2.1 Oral hygiene

The presence of orthodontic attachments in the mouth paves the way for plaque formation on the tooth surface and makes tooth cleaning more difficult [3]. The plaque develops as a result of bacterial infection, modified from dietary carbohydrates and saliva. In the presence of carbohydrates, demineralization begins when the pH of the mouth drops below 5.5 and creates white spot lesions. *Streptococcus mutans* and lactobacilli bacteria are mainly effective in colonization and also caries development [4]. The plaque on the tooth surfaces prevents the remineralization of the enamel layer with calcium and phosphate ions. In addition, it facilitates the production of acid from the sugar taken with food. It is observed that the amount of decalcification is also higher in the brackets and near the gingiva, where plaque accumulation is greater in orthodontic patients [5].

2.2 Diet

It has been stated that frequent consumption of carbohydrate-rich, sugary foods and beverages facilitates the formation of caries. During 20 minutes following sugar intake, the pH of the plaque drops below the critical level of 5.5°. In addition, another factor is the difficulty in removing food residues from the teeth due to orthodontic attachments [6].

2.3 Appliance type and design

The larger the area covered by orthodontic attachments on the enamel surface, the more difficult it is to clean the remaining tooth surface. Archwire design also affects the accumulation of plaque and food debris [7].

In a study evaluating the difference in white spot lesion (WSL) formation between conventional bracket treatments and aligner treatments, it was reported that approximately 1.2% of aligner patients developed WSL compared to 26% of conventionally treated patients. The number of developing WSL is also significantly ($P < 0.001$) less in aligner patients. In patients treated with conventional braces, moderate or poor pretreatment oral hygiene, worsening of hygiene during treatment, preexisting WSL, and longer duration of treatment ($P < 0.05$) significantly increased the risk of developing WSL during the treatment [8].

In a randomized prospective controlled study, aligner and conventional bracket treatments were compared with quantitative light-induced fluorescence. According

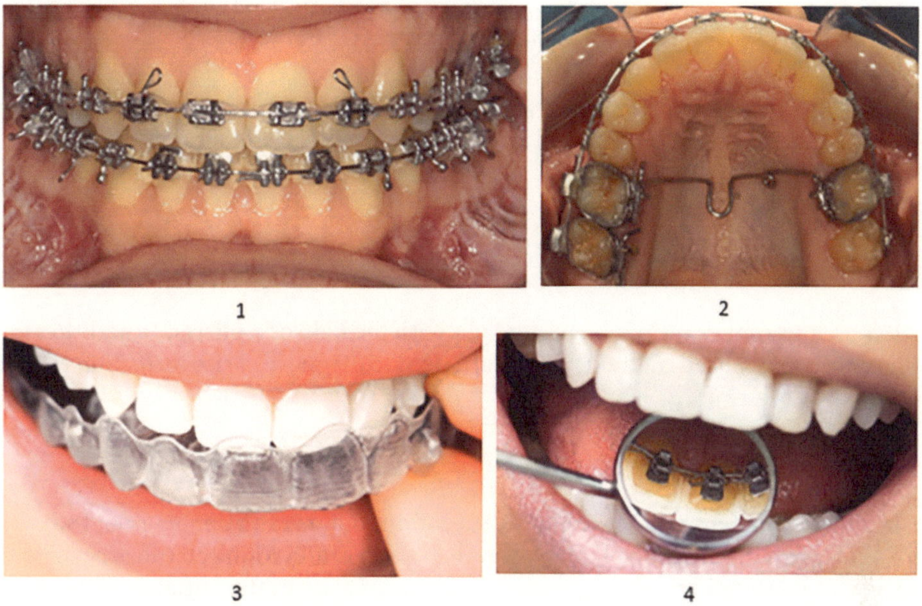

Figure 1.
Different appliance designs used in orthodontic treatment. (1) Traditional buccal metallic brackets, (2) transpalatal arch appliance, (3) clear aligner, and (4) lingual brackets.

to the results, WSL formation was observed in both treatments. In aligner treatments, the lesions are shallower and cover a larger area. Traditional braces had deeper lesions, but their area was smaller. Plaque accumulation is also greater with conventional brackets [9].

According to a study examining the difference in WSL between lingual brackets and labial conventional brackets, patients treated with lingual brackets had significantly less development of WSL [10].

Figure 1 shows different orthodontic appliances.

2.4 Bonding technique

Composite resin remaining around orthodontic attachments prepares the ground for plaque accumulation. Therefore, the composite resin around the bracket must be cleaned [7, 11].

3. Diagnostic methods

It is very important to detect enamel demineralizations associated with orthodontic treatment at an early stage. Pitts [12] stated that the tools and methods used in the diagnosis of caries lesion should be easy to apply, reliable, reproducible, and noninvasive.

Diagnostic methods can be classified as follows [13]:

1. Traditional methods: visual inspection, Sonde examination, and radiographic examination.

2. Current technologies: laser fluorescence, digital radiography, electrical conductivity, and fiber-optic transillumination (FOTI).

3. Newly developed technologies: alternating current impedance spectroscopy, quantitative laser light-induced fluorescence, and ultrasonography.

3.1 Traditional methods

3.1.1 Visual inspection

It is an intraoral examination under light with the help of a mirror. In addition to being a frequently used method, it is insufficient to diagnose caries formations at the initial stage [14].

3.1.2 Examination with probe

In addition to light and mirror, it is the examination made by contacting the caries surface with the probe [15]. However, probe examination can cause iatrogenic damage by accelerating the progression of occlusal caries in the initial stage or by carrying caries-causing bacteria from the infected area to other areas. Probing with light pressure could cause cavitation in white, opaque lesions. The use of blunt-tipped periodontal probes is recommended to control the surface structure of the lesion [16].

3.1.3 Radiographic examination

Caries lesions can be easily recognized at an early stage due to the increase in radiological density on X-ray [17]. Panoramic X-ray examination before orthodontic treatment is shown in **Figure 2**.

3.2 Current technologies

Today's diagnostic methods measure physical signals. These physical signals are X-rays, laser light, visible light, electrical current, ultrasound, surface changes, etc., which can be obtained using the following methods [18].

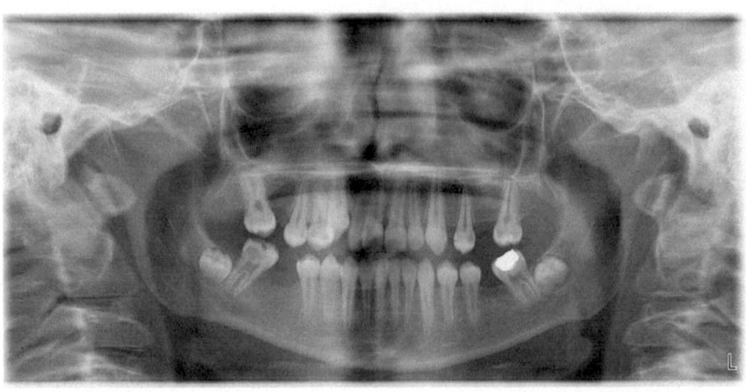

Figure 2.
Decayed tooth that can be identified on panoramic X-ray.

3.2.1 Digital radiography

Digital radiographs have been indicated as an effective method in the diagnosis of caries without a cavity. In addition, the radiation dose received by the patient is reduced, archiving and reproducing images becomes easier [14].

3.2.2 Laser fluorescence

Developed to detect and numerically measure occlusal caries. Working with the laser fluorescent method, the commonly known brand is DIAGNOdent (DD) (KaVo Dental Corporation, East Main Street Lake Zurich, IL) [19].

3.2.3 Electrical conductivity

This technique is based on the difference in conductivity in healthy and decayed tooth tissues. The electrical conductivity of the tooth tissue is sensitive enough to vary even in the case of demineralization but no loss of material on the surface [20]. Electronic caries monitor (ECM) and caries meter L devices operating based on electrical conductivity have been developed [14].

3.2.4 Fiber-optic transillumination (FOTI)

With the fiber-optic transillumination device, light scattering is prevented, and the tooth can be examined in detail due to the use of strong white light. DIFOTI (digital fiber-optic transillumination; Electro-Optical Sciences, Irvington, New York) method is a method in which FOTI and digital camera are combined to reduce the shortcomings of FOTI. DIFOTI includes two handpieces. One of them is used for caries detection on occlusal surfaces and the other on flat surfaces. Although it cannot be used to determine the depth of lesions, it gives as good results as radiographs in detecting approximal caries [21].

3.3 Newly developed technologies

3.3.1 Alternating current impedance spectroscopy

This method measures with a large number of frequency sweeps. It is reported that it has 100% sensitivity even in the diagnosis of enamel lesions without cavitation due to the use of the electrical property of the tooth [22].

3.3.2 Quantitative light-induced fluorescence

Benedict was the first to state in his research that the organic components of human teeth show fluorescent properties. In addition, he also mentioned the difference between the fluorescent properties of healthy and carious enamel in his studies [23]. The purpose of the QLF device is to determine caries at an early stage. This device can also be used for imaging lesions in remineralization treatments. The resulting image can be saved by transferring it to the computer. On the other hand, it is insufficient in imaging lesions in the approximal area [24].

3.3.3 Ultrasonografi

The basic principle of ultrasound is the application of high-frequency waves (1–20 MHz) generated by the device to the biological tissue, the returning waves are absorbed and converted into electrical impulses and detected as echoes. Each tissue has a unique internal echo level. Changes recorded at the echo level of the tissue indicate that pathological changes have occurred in the tissue [25]. It has been shown by studies that ultrasonic methods give good results in the diagnosis of early caries [26].

4. Studies evaluating the prevalence of white spot lesions

According to the first studies in this area, buccal and lingual surface lesions were found to be higher in individuals who received orthodontic treatment than in individuals who did not receive treatment. On the other hand, no significant difference was observed in the number of caries [27].

In another study, it was stated that the prevalence of decalcification among patients ranged from 2 to 96%. The reason for this great difference; the variety of methods used to assess the presence of decalcification, the presence of idiopathic lesions, and the use of a fluoride agent during treatment are indicated. Because in cross-sectional study design (orthodontic patients after treatment compared with another group of patients who have not had orthodontics), it is difficult to differentiate between idiopathic white spots and decalcification, which artificially increase the prevalence [7].

Though Zachrisson et al. [28] was the one who examined newly formed white spot lesions with the prevalence ranging from 15 to 89. In the study using photo reviews in assessment [29, 30], the prevalence of WSL was found to be 0–24%. The distribution of affected teeth has been studied [31] and has found that the maxillary incisors and the mandibular first molars to be the teeth with the highest prevalence. In another study [32], it has been stated that the lesions are concentrated in the cervical and middle third of the vestibule surface. In another study, the prevalence of WSL was found to be highest in permanent first molar teeth [33]. Contrary to these findings, in another study [34], it was stated that maxillary lateral and canines were affected too much.

In the literature, the effect of the material used to bond orthodontic bands on enamel has been investigated, but it has been stated that the main reason for WSL formation is the loss of cement integrity and the accumulation of bacteria in the area [35].

Gorelick et al. conducted a study on the incidence of white spot lesions at 6 and 12 months in patients undergoing orthodontic treatment. In their study using the visual examination technique, they reported that 50% of the patients had one or more BNL at the end of the treatment [31]. Boersma et al. [36] investigated the prevalence of white spot lesions after orthodontic treatment using quantitative light fluoroscopy and reported that 97% of patients had one or more lesions. A total of 38% of the patients had BNL 6 months after the treatment. It was stated that this rate increased to 46% in the 12-month group. Only 11% of the control group had at least one occurrence of WSL. Most patients undergoing orthodontic treatment had at least one white spot lesion in a mild form, however, a few patients presented with moderate or severe demineralization.

5. Preventive and therapeutic methods of white spot lesion

After the completion of the orthodontic treatment process, demineralization is expected to slow down. Although demineralized enamel surfaces may partially remineralize after treatment, white spot lesions have been noted to be irreversible. **Figure 3** shows white spot lesions after orthodontic treatment. However, WSL formation can be prevented by ensuring the oral hygiene of the patients during the treatment [2]. Once WSL is diagnosed, it is important to treat the cause. Social, medical, and dental histories of the patients should be taken, and caries risk assessment should be done.

While taking anamnesis; systemic and topical fluoride intake, dietary habits, snacking frequency and foods consumed between meals, bottle use, reflux, vomiting and eating disorders, salivary flow, drugs used by the person or the effect of health status on saliva flow, socioeconomic status, information status about dental diseases, dental treatment needs, value given to oral health, efforts to change habits, dental history, regular check-ups, and the amount of caries should be evaluated [37].

Numerous studies have been conducted to ensure oral hygiene of patients undergoing orthodontic treatment and to increase the resistance of teeth to demineralization. In these studies, fluorine mouthwashes, fluorinated gels and polishes, chlorhexidine mouthwashes, chlorhexidine polishes, and gels, fluorine or non-fluoride sealants covering the enamel surface around the bracket, xylitol lozenges, fluorine-releasing elastomers, and fluorine-releasing bracket bonding materials were used [38–40].

In the study investigating the effects of resin-based sealant, fluorine-containing sealant, fluorine polish, and glass ionomer cement on the initial caries lesions and the proximal surface of the adjacent tooth, it was determined that the most effective material was glass ionomer cement. The effectiveness of the other materials was determined as fluorine polish, fluorine-containing sealants, and sealants, in order from most effective to less effective [41].

The risk of enamel demineralization in patients undergoing fixed orthodontic treatment can be reduced or prevented by the following:

1. Plaque control methods

    - Mechanical plaque control methods and improving the patient's oral hygiene
    - Chemical plaque removal
    - Reducing plaque retention by the appliance

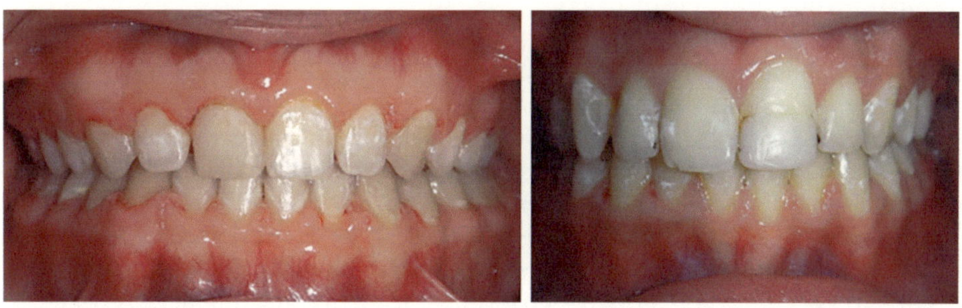

Figure 3.
White spot lesion in individuals after orthodontic treatment.

2. The use of various agents containing fluoride

   - Mouth rinsing
   - By increasing enamel resistance to microbial acid with topical fluoride
   - Fluoride containing etchant
   - Fluoride containing bonding adhesives
   - Fluoride releasing modules

3. Teeth whitening

4. Pit and fissure sealers

5. Argon-laser tooth enamel surface weakening

6. Microabrasion

7. Use of amorphous calcium phosphate of casein phosphopeptides [7].

5.1 Plaque control methods

5.1.1 Mechanical plaque control

It is very important to use the right brushing technique to control dental plaque. Flossing as a modification of the standard toothbrush can help patients achieve oral hygiene. Compared to a manual toothbrush, using an electric toothbrush in conjunction with a manual toothbrush or regular washing with water could be a more effective way to prevent dental plaque. On the other hand, no evident superiority has been found for electric brushing [42, 43].

Bracket attachment with direct attachment exposes proximal surfaces to enamel demineralization due to the difficulty of maintaining oral hygiene with the archwires in place. Flossing has been proven to be helpful in interproximal cleaning. The floss threader would also be used to thread the floss under the archwire. The soft rubber interdental stimulator could also be helpful in interproximal cleaning and massaging the interproximal areas [44].

5.1.2 Chemical plaque removal

The material to be used for plaque removal by the chemical method should not support resistant microorganisms and should not be toxic in order not to disturb the balance of the oral microflora. Chlorhexidine antiseptic, one of the chemical plaque prevention methods, is the most effective, because of its absorption onto the acquired pellicle, which prolongs its presence and effect in the mouth.

Given these stringent requirements, it is surprising that any product has been developed as a chemical antiplaque agent. However, long-term use of chlorhexidine causes brown staining on the teeth.

Lundstrom and Krasse (1987) investigated the effect of chlorhexidine mouthwash on *Streptococcus mutans* in patients receiving fixed orthodontic treatment and stated that they found the use of chlorhexidine less beneficial [45].

5.1.3 Reducing plaque retention by the appliance

The larger the area covered by orthodontic attachments on the enamel surface, the more difficult it is to clean the remaining tooth surface. Archwire design also affects the build-up of plaque and food debris [5].

5.2 The use of various agents containing fluoride

5.2.1 Mouth rinsing

Two approaches have been developed to protect the enamel surface. The first is aimed at strengthening enamel and reducing acid solubility, that is, the use of topical fluoride agents during and after orthodontic treatment. The second involves the use of materials that protect the tooth surface around and below the orthodontic attachment with a protective coating [5].

In another study, mouthwashes containing 250 ppm fluoride twice a day were used to provide remineralization of the initial lesions on the approximal surfaces to patients undergoing orthodontic treatment. It has been reported that this method significantly increases remineralization [46].

Thuy et al. Lari, on the other hand, reported that the remineralization amount of solutions containing fluorine increased the effect of each other when used together with strontium (Sr) [47]. Tange et al. Lari stated in their *in vitro* study on primary teeth that when xylitol and sodium fluoride are used together, they increase the remineralization effects of each other [48].

5.2.2 Increasing enamel resistance using topical fluorides

The use of fluoride agents has been shown to be effective in preventing WSL formation. The use of fluoride in reducing caries; acting as a kind of catalyst that promotes the formation of high-quality hydroxyapatite; by assisting remineralization during pH fluctuations, it acts by inhibiting the glycolysis of plaque bacteria [49]. The cariostatic effect of topical fluoride is mainly based on calcium fluoride (CaF) depending on the formation. Oral hygiene maintenance combined with daily topical fluoride use has been shown to significantly reduce enamel decalcification.

In patients who have received fixed orthodontic treatment, high concentration fluoride application provides remineralization in the superficial layer of enamel, yet it is not effective in the deeper layers. Low-concentration fluoride application is recommended as it allows slower penetration of calcium and fluorine ions from saliva following orthodontic treatment [50].

Applying fluoride polishes to the tooth surface surrounding the bracket to protect the enamel surface from the acid attack has been suggested as another technique to prevent enamel demineralization [51]. A split-mouth design study reported that Ultraseal XT Plus clear sealant provided a significant reduction in enamel demineralization in individuals undergoing fixed orthodontic treatment. After the study, six lesions were observed on the sealant applied surfaces, while 22 lesions were observed on the non-applied surfaces. Of the teeth detected with white spots, 19 lesions (68%)

were found in the maxillary arch, and nine lesions (32%) were found in the mandibular arch. The highest white spots were seen in maxillary laterals and canines without sealant. It has been stated that this product effectively seals the enamel surfaces adjacent to orthodontic brackets and resists mechanical wear and is recommended for use by clinicians [52].

In a study by Derks et al., it was observed that the use of toothpaste, gel, or these materials containing 1500–5000 ppm fluorine together with chlorhexidine can inhibit demineralization. It was observed that coating the brackets with polymeric material did not have an inhibitory effect on demineralization [53].

5.2.3 Fluoride containing etchant

Thornton (1986) et al. stated that the addition of fluoride to phosphoric acid etch had little or no protective effect in an *in vitro* study. Because it dissolves on the enamel surface and does not show any permanent effect when rinsed [54].

5.2.4 Fluoride containing bonding adhesives

Fluoridated glass ionomer and composite resin materials are used to reduce demineralization [55]. It has shown that glass ionomer cement protects the underlying enamel, as well as around an orthodontic attachment from decalcification. However, it has been shown that the glass ionomer has a weaker bond strength than the composite but the retention is sufficient [56].

5.2.5 Fluoride releasing modules

The study of Marini et al. [57] was carried out by placing an intraoral material that releases 0.04 mg of fluoride per day during the orthodontic treatment. It was observed that caries and white spot lesions did not occur within 6 months. In another study, it was determined that the lesions were reduced by 54% at the end of 4 weeks in those using a high amount of fluorine-containing topical gel (12,500 ppm F) and toothpaste (1450 ppm F), while there was a 44% reduction in those using only toothpaste. However, no statistically significant difference was found [58].

5.3 Teeth whitening

Teeth whitening demineralization is not a therapeutic method, however, if topical fluoride application does not produce the esthetic results desired by the patient after orthodontic treatment, vital teeth whitening should be considered. In white spot lesions, this process would make the lesions less apparent [50].

5.4 Pit and fissure sealers

It has been stated that light-curing pit and fissure sealants applied to the enamel surface adjacent to orthodontic brackets are effective in preventing enamel demineralization without the need for patient compliance. Benham and colleagues reported that micro-abrasion resistant and highly filled flowable composites greatly reduced white spot lesions when applied to pits and fissures [52].

Salar et al. examined 45 extracted third molars by dividing them into three groups. Conventional sealant without fluoride (Group 1), fluoride-releasing sealant

(Group 2), or glass ionomer sealant with high fluoride release (Group 3). According to the results, ProSeal provided increased demineralization inhibition compared with a conventional sealant containing no fluoride, but less than that observed by a glass ionomer sealant [59].

5.5 Argon-laser tooth enamel surface weakening

Argon laser can be used to prevent enamel decalcification by changing the crystal structure of enamel. It has been reported that when argon laser is applied to the enamel surface. Argon laser causes the surface properties of the enamel to change by creating micro-voids that stabilize the ions on the enamel surface during the acid attack. Phosphate, calcium, and fluoride ions in saliva could subsequently precipitate into these cavities, increasing the resistance of tooth enamel to demineralization and increasing mineral uptake from saliva [60].

5.6 Microabrasion

The esthetic appearance of WSL, which has been going on for a long time, can be improved with the microabrasion method. It has been suggested to use the microabrasion technique in the treatment of white spot lesions that occur during dental treatment [61]. Researchers stated that when a mixture of 18% hydrochloric acid, pumice, and glycerin was applied to the tooth surface for 3–5 minutes with an electric toothbrush, mild lesions disappeared completely, while severe lesions reached a satisfactory color. They also stated that the brown-yellow discoloration on the tooth surface disappeared, and smooth enamel surfaces were obtained.

5.7 Amorphous calcium phosphate of casein phosphopeptides

Another material used for the remineralization of decalcifications on the enamel surface is casein phosphopeptide, which is obtained from the milk protein casein. The solution form, which is prepared by dissolving in water, acts by stabilizing calcium and phosphate ions.

In an alkaline medium, casein phosphopeptide combines with calcium phosphate to form CPP-ACP compound. Today, this compound is combined with fluorine ions and used as CPP-ACFP (casein phosphopeptide-amorphous calcium fluoride phosphate) [62].

Researchers working on the remineralization of fluorine and CPP-ACP have shown that toothpaste containing 2% CPP-ACP provides a similar remineralization amount to toothpaste containing 2800 ppm fluoride. In addition to 2% CPP-ACP, it was determined that the best results were obtained in the toothpaste with 1100 ppm fluoride added [63].

In a study, the higher amount of remineralization effect of CPP-ACP applied topically to the initial lesions for 14 days was visualized with an electron microscope, and it was found to be statistically significant [64].

In the study on the remineralization of initial enamel lesions, a 7% reduction in lesion depth was observed when toothpaste containing fluoride (1100 ppm) was applied alone, and a 10% reduction was observed when using toothpaste containing CPP-ACP. It was observed that there was a 13% reduction in lesion depth when toothpaste containing CPP-ACP was applied after the use of fluoridated toothpaste. Since casein is a milk protein, care should be taken in its use in patients with milk allergies [65].

6. Conclusion

White spot lesions could be detected at an early stage with various diagnostic methods, and the formation of lesions could be prevented with appropriate treatments. Studies have shown that none of the caries diagnostic methods developed today is as effective as clinical examination and radiographic examination. It would be more beneficial to use these two diagnostic methods together. In the first months of orthodontic treatment, it is of great importance to evaluate the oral hygiene of patients and to apply preventive measures to stop demineralization. In the treatment of white spot lesions, the factors affecting the formation of the lesions should be eliminated first, and patient education and information should be emphasized. In the treatment of white spot lesions, it is aimed to occur remineralization in the lower layer of the lesion. For this purpose, improvement of oral hygiene, regulation of diet, calcium, fluoride, milk proteins, laser beams, chemical, and mechanical abrasion methods should be applied. If white spot lesions are not treated, cavitation may occur in the lesions and cause esthetic problems. Effective prevention, diagnosis, and treatment of lesions will minimize caries formation and tooth discoloration and also provide an esthetic smile. The most appropriate, cheapest, and easiest-to-apply treatment method should be preferred for the patient.

Author details

Elif Nadide Akay
Department of Orthodontics, Faculty of Dentistry, Istanbul Medeniyet University, Istanbul, Turkey

*Address all correspondence to: elifnadideakay@gmail.com

References

[1] Sudjalim TR, Woods WM, Manton DJ. Prevention of white spot lesions in orthodontic practice: A contemporary review. Australian Dental Journal. 2006;**51**(4):284-289

[2] Bergstrand F, Twetman S. A review on prevention and treatment of post-orthodontic white spot lesions—Evidence-based methods and emerging technologies. The Open Dentistry Journal. 2011;**5**:158-162

[3] Chadwick BL. Products for prevention during orthodontics. British Journal of Orthodontics. 1994;**21**(4):395-398

[4] Lundström F, Krasse B. *Streptococcus mutans* and lactobacilli frequency in orthodontic patients; the effect of chlorhexidine treatments. European Journal of Orthodontics. 1987;**9**(2): 109-116

[5] Saloum FS, Sondhi A. Preventing enamel decalcification after orthodontic treatment. Journal of the American Dental Association (1939). 1987;**115**(2): 257-261

[6] Murray JJ. The Prevention of Dental Disease. Oxford: Oxford University Press; 1989

[7] Mitchell L. Decalcification during orthodontic treatment with fixed appliances—An overview. British Journal of Orthodontics. 1992;**19**(3):199-205

[8] Buschang PH et al. Incidence of white spot lesions among patients treated with clear aligners and traditional braces. The Angle Orthodontist. 2019;**89**(3):359-364

[9] Albhaisi Z, Al-Khateeb SN, Abu Alhaija ES. Enamel demineralization during clear aligner orthodontic treatment compared with fixed appliance therapy, evaluated with quantitative light-induced fluorescence: A randomized clinical trial. American Journal of Orthodontics and Dentofacial Orthopedics. 2020;**157**(5):594-601

[10] Wiechmann D et al. Lingual appliances reduce the incidence of white spot lesions during orthodontic multibracket treatment. American Journal of Orthodontics and Dentofacial Orthopedics. 2015;**148**(3):414-422

[11] Gwinnett AJ, Ceen RF. Plaque distribution on bonded brackets: A scanning microscope study. American Journal of Orthodontics. 1979;**75**(6): 667-677

[12] Pitts NB. Diagnostic tools and measurements—Impact on appropriate care. Community Dentistry and Oral Epidemiology. 1997;**25**(1):24-35

[13] Available from: http://www.istanbul.edu.trdishekimligiEdergiDHD_C39-3_200509B_G_Efes.pdf

[14] Axelson P. Diagnosis and Risk Detection of Dental Caries. Germany: Quintessence Pub; 2000. pp. 179-247

[15] Lussi A. Comparison of different methods for the diagnosis of fissure caries without cavitation. Caries Research. 1993;**27**(5):409-416

[16] Axelsson, P. Diagnosis and risk prediction of dental caries. Quintessence Pub. Co. 15 October 2000. ISBN-10: 0867153628, ISBN-13: 978-0867153620

[17] Weerheijm KL et al. Clinically undetected occlusal dentine caries: A radiographic comparison. Caries Research. 1992;**26**(4):305-309

[18] Verdonschot EH et al. Effects of digital grey-scale modification on the diagnosis of small approximal carious lesions. Journal of Dentistry. 1992;**20**(1): 44-49

[19] Tam LE, McComb D. Diagnosis of occlusal caries: Part II. Recent diagnostic technologies. Journal of the Canadian Dental Association. 2001;**67**(8): 459-463

[20] Lussi A et al. Performance and reproducibility of a laser fluorescence system for detection of occlusal caries in vitro. Caries Research. 1999;**33**(4): 261-266

[21] Schneiderman A et al. Assessment of dental caries with digital imaging fiber-optic transillumination (DIFOTI): In vitro study. Caries Research. 1997;**31**(2):103-110

[22] Longbottom C et al. Detection of dental decay and its extent using a.c. impedance spectroscopy. Nature Medicine. 1996;**2**(2):235-237

[23] Benedict HC. A note on the fluorescence of teeth in ultra-violet rays. Science. 1928;67(1739):442-442. DOI: 10.1126/science.67.1739.442.a

[24] Angmar-Månsson B, ten Bosch JJ. Quantitative light-induced fluorescence (QLF): A method for assessment of incipient caries lesions. Dento Maxillo Facial Radiology. 2001;**30**(6):298-307

[25] Ng SY et al. Ultrasonic studies of unblemished and artificially demineralized enamel in extracted human teeth: A new method for detecting early caries. Journal of Dentistry. 1988;**16**(5):201-209

[26] Lees S, Barber FE, Lobene RR. Dental enamel: Detection of surface changes by ultrasound. Science. 1970;**169**(3952):1314-1316

[27] Wisth PJ, Nord A. Caries experience in orthodontically treated individuals. The Angle Orthodontist. 1977;**47**(1):59-64

[28] Zachrisson BU. Cause and prevention of injuries to teeth and supporting structures during orthodontic treatment. American Journal of Orthodontics. 1976;**69**(3):285-300

[29] Stratemann MW, Shannon IL. Control of decalcification in orthodontic patients by daily self-administered application of a water-free 0.4 per cent stannous fluoride gel. American Journal of Orthodontics. 1974;**66**(3):273-279

[30] Mizrahi E. Enamel demineralization following orthodontic treatment. American Journal of Orthodontics. 1982;**82**(1):62-67

[31] Gorelick L, Geiger AM, Gwinnett AJ. Incidence of white spot formation after bonding and banding. American Journal of Orthodontics. 1982;**81**(2):93-98

[32] Mizrahi E. Surface distribution of enamel opacities following orthodontic treatment. American Journal of Orthodontics. 1983;**84**(4):323-331

[33] Ogaard B. Prevalence of white spot lesions in 19-year-olds: A study on untreated and orthodontically treated persons 5 years after treatment. American Journal of Orthodontics and Dentofacial Orthopedics. 1989;**96**(5):423-427

[34] Geiger AM et al. The effect of a fluoride program on white spot formation during orthodontic treatment. American Journal of Orthodontics and Dentofacial Orthopedics. 1988;**93**(1):29-37

[35] Durning P, McCabe JF, Gordon PH. A laboratory investigation into cements used to retain orthodontic bands. British Journal of Orthodontics. 1994;**21**(1): 27-32

[36] Boersma JG et al. Caries prevalence measured with QLF after treatment with fixed orthodontic appliances: Influencing factors. Caries Research. 2005;**39**:41-47

[37] Caries-risk assessment and management for infants, children, and adolescents. The Journal of Practical Hygiene. 2004;**13**:19-22

[38] Sengun A et al. Evaluation of the dental plaque pH recovery effect of a xylitol lozenge on patients with fixed orthodontic appliances. The Angle Orthodontist. 2004;**74**(2):240-244

[39] Ogaard B et al. Cariostatic effect and fluoride release from a visible light-curing adhesive for bonding of orthodontic brackets. American Journal of Orthodontics and Dentofacial Orthopedics. 1992;**101**(4):303-307

[40] Doherty UB, Benson PE, Higham SM. Fluoride-releasing elastomeric ligatures assessed with the in situ caries model. European Journal of Orthodontics. 2002;**24**(4):371-378

[41] Trairatvorakul C, Kladkaew S, Songsiripradabboon S. Active management of incipient caries and choice of materials. Journal of Dental Research. 2008;**87**(3):228-232

[42] Boyd RL, Murray P, Robertson PB. Effect of rotary electric toothbrush versus manual toothbrush on periodontal status during orthodontic treatment. American Journal of Orthodontics and Dentofacial Orthopedics. 1989;**96**(4):342-347

[43] Jackson CL. Comparison between electric toothbrushing and manual toothbrushing, with and without oral irrigation, for oral hygiene of orthodontic patients. American Journal of Orthodontics and Dentofacial Orthopedics. 1991;**99**(1):15-20

[44] Williams P et al. A clinical trial of an orthodontic toothbrush. European Journal of Orthodontics. 1987;**9**(4): 295-304

[45] Lundström F, Hamp SE, Nyman S. Systematic plaque control in children undergoing long-term orthodontic treatment. European Journal of Orthodontics. 1980;**2**(1):27-39

[46] Altenburger MJ et al. Remineralization of artificial interproximal carious lesions using a fluoride mouthrinse. American Journal of Dentistry. 2007;**20**(6):385-389

[47] Thuy TT et al. Effect of strontium in combination with fluoride on enamel remineralization in vitro. Archives of Oral Biology. 2008;**53**(11):1017-1022

[48] Tange T et al. The effect of xylitol and fluoride on remineralization for primary tooth enamel caries in vitro. Pediatric Dental Journal. 2004;**14**(1): 55-59

[49] Levine RS. Fluoride and caries prevention: 1. Scientific rationale. Dental Update. 1991;**18**(3):105-6-108-10

[50] Bishara SE, Ostby AW. White spot lesions: Formation, prevention, and treatment. Seminars in Orthodontics. 2008;**14**:174-182

[51] Sonesson M et al. Fluoride varnish for the prevention of white spot lesions during orthodontic treatment with fixed appliances: A randomized controlled trial. European Journal of Orthodontics. 2020;**42**(3):326-330

[52] Benham AW, Campbell PM, Buschang PH. Effectiveness of pit and fissure sealants in reducing white spot lesions during orthodontic treatment. A pilot study. The Angle Orthodontist. 2009;**79**(2):338-345

[53] Derks A et al. Caries-inhibiting effect of preventive measures during orthodontic treatment with fixed appliances. A systematic review. Caries Research. 2004;**38**(5):413-420

[54] Thornton JB et al. The effect of fluoride in phosphoric acid on enamel fluoride uptake and the tensile bond strength of an orthodontic bonding resin. American Journal of Orthodontics and Dentofacial Orthopedics. 1986;**90**(2): 91-101

[55] Valk JWP, Davidson CL. The relevance of controlled fluoride release with bonded orthodontic appliances. Journal of Dentistry. 1987;**15**(6):257-260

[56] Cook PA, Youngson CC. An in vitro study of the bond strength of a glass ionomer cement in the direct bonding of orthodontic brackets. British Journal of Orthodontics. 1988;**15**(4):247-253

[57] Marini I et al. A retentive system for intra-oral fluoride release during orthodontic treatment. European Journal of Orthodontics. 1999;**21**(6):695-701

[58] Marinho VC et al. Fluoride toothpastes for preventing dental caries in children and adolescents. Cochrane Database of Systematic Reviews. 2003;**2003**(1):Cd002278

[59] Salar DV et al. Potential inhibition of demineralization in vitro by fluoride-releasing sealants. Journal of the American Dental Association (1939). 2007;**138**(4):502-506

[60] Miresmaeili A et al. Effect of argon laser on enamel demineralization around orthodontic brackets: An in vitro study. Journal of Dentistry. 2014;**11**(4):411-417

[61] Gelgör IE, Tamer B. A practical approach to white spot lesion removal. World Journal of Orthodontics. 2003;**4**:152-156

[62] Cross KJ, Huq NL, Reynolds EC. Casein phosphopeptides in oral health—Chemistry and clinical applications. Current Pharmaceutical Design. 2007;**13**(8):793-800

[63] Reynolds EC et al. Fluoride and casein phosphopeptide-amorphous calcium phosphate. Journal of Dental Research. 2008;**87**(4):344-348

[64] Pai D et al. Use of laser fluorescence and scanning electron microscope to evaluate remineralization of incipient enamel lesions remineralized by topical application of casein phospho peptide amorphous calcium phosphate (CPP-aCP) containing cream. The Journal of Clinical Pediatric Dentistry. 2008;**32**(3): 201-206

[65] Kumar VL, Itthagarun A, King NM. The effect of casein phosphopeptide-amorphous calcium phosphate on remineralization of artificial caries-like lesions: An in vitro study. Australian Dental Journal. 2008;**53**(1):34-40

Chapter 17

The Dental Implant Maintenance

Gayathri Krishnamoorthy, Aparna I. Narayana and Dhanasekar Balakrishnan

Abstract

As dental implant treatment has become a part of mainstream dental therapy, it is imperative to implement dental implant maintenance guidelines to achieve the long-term success of implant prostheses. Earlier, the success of a dental implant was mainly focused on the surgical phase to achieve good primary stability, with time, this belief has taken a major paradigm shift towards implementing and ensuring a periodic recall and following a maintenance phase for dental implants to achieve long-term success. As the dental team strives to attain and maintain the long-term success of implant prostheses, the patient should also recognize that their contribution towards the success of implant prostheses is also equally indispensable. This chapter highlights the importance of maintaining oral hygiene in implant rehabilitated patients and enumerates the implant maintenance protocol to be followed along with the different in-home and in-office procedures which can be implemented to achieve long-term success of the implant and peri-implant structures.

Keywords: dental implants, oral hygiene, maintenance phase, implant survival, oral health

1. Introduction

The dental implant market value globally is expected to increase at a Compound Annual Growth Rate (CAGR) of 11% from 2021 to 2028 [1]. This increase in demand for dental implant market size could be attributed to the numerous applications of implants along with the patient acceptance for implant prostheses. Despite the multitude of advancements made in surgical and technical fields of implant dentistry, the complications faced are still too high [2]. In an observational study that was conducted to evaluate the patient's perception towards implant treatment and maintenance, it was concluded that most people were made aware of the importance of implant oral hygiene measurements and recall, however, the knowledge about implant-related complications and failures was dissatisfying. Although the patients were instructed about the importance of maintaining oral hygiene around implants, only 40.4% had reported having tried cleaning tools for maintenance [3].

We must acknowledge that implant placement requires a multidisciplinary treatment approach wherein a Maxillofacial surgeon, Prosthodontist, Periodontist, Oral Radiologist, Dental Hygienist, and the patient must work as a team to achieve long-term implant success. Hence, patients are considered as co-therapists in maintaining and achieving long-term implant success [4].

As the ideology of long-term implant success has taken a paradigm shift from attaining primary stability to implementing and ensuring periodic recall and maintenance, it is the responsibility of the dental team to convey the importance of oral hygiene maintenance and regular recall visits to the patients which can help them achieve long-term maintenance health of implant and the peri-implant structures.

Although there is scarce information available in the literature about dental implant maintenance protocols, in this chapter, we intend to compile in toto a detailed description of the various parameters which need to be examined and the measures to be implemented for achieving long-term implant success.

2. Risk factors that contribute to implant failures

The success of a dental implant depends primarily on the level of marginal bone loss, absence of mucosal inflammation, and probing depth. Risk factors that undermine the above criteria for long-term implant success should be explained to the patient and a comprehensive treatment plan must be presented to them. This comprehensive treatment plan must include all recommended dental therapy, possible alternative treatment options, the clinical risk which can be faced during the surgery, and the cost of the treatment. This discussion between the practitioner and the patient will help the patient understand why and how the procedure will be carried out.

Patient-specific risk assessment should include an extensive examination of the candidate and detailed medical and dental history. This will help the practitioner weigh the pre-operative and post-operative risks with implant placement. It is ideal and recommended to classify the implant patients according to their medical condition and associated co-morbidities using the American Society of Anesthesiologists Physical Status Classification System (ASA PS Classification) and co-relate their ASA PS status with the Type of dental treatment (**Table 1**) and their associated risk type (**Table 2**).

Sr. no	Dental treatment	Procedures
1.	Type 1 [5]	Examinations, radiographs, study model impressions, oral hygiene instruction, supra-gingival prophylaxis, simple restorative dentistry
2.	Type 2 [5]	Scaling, root planning, endodontics, simple extractions, curettage, simple gingivectomy, advanced restorative procedures, simple implants(endodontic root forms)
3.	Type 3 [5]	Multiple extractions, gingivectomy, quadrant periosteal reflections, impacted extractions, apicoectomy, plate form implants, multiple root form implants, ridge augmentation, subantral augmentation, unilateral subperiosteal implants
4.	Type 4 [5]	Full arch implants, ramus frame implants, full-arch endosteal implants, orthognathic surgery, autogenous bone augmentation, bilateral subantral augmentation

Table 1.
Type of dental treatments.

ASA PS status	Description	Type of dental treatment				Risk of implant placement
		Type 1	Type 2	Type 3	Type 4	
ASA II [6]	A patient with mild systemic disease who has no functional limitations and well-controlled disease, whose BMI is under 35, is a social drinker or smokes cigarettes, or has well-controlled hypertension	+	Sedation and Stress reduction protocol	IV sedation and stress reduction protocol		Mild
ASA III [6]	A patient with severe systemic disease that is not life-threatening and includes functional limitations caused by the disease, poorly treated hypertension or diabetes, renal failure, morbid obesity, stable angina, or pacemaker.	+	IV sedation Stress reduction protocol Physician	Hospitalization		Moderate
ASA IV [6]	A patient with severe systemic disease that is a constant threat to life that includes functional limitations as a result of severe systemic disease, unstable angina, poorly controlled COPD, symptomatic CHF, recent MI, or stroke less than 3 months prior	+	Postpone all elective surgeries			Severe

Table 2.
Inter-relationship between ASA PS classification, type of dental treatment, and risk of implant placement.

3. Diagnostic parameters to evaluate during implant maintenance protocol

The success of any dental prosthesis begins with its maintenance and recall phase. Similarly, after the implants have been placed in the edentulous region, routine recall, evaluation, radiographs, and maintenance are necessary to achieve its long-term success. It is, therefore, the responsibility of the dental team to understand the etiology, provide appropriate preventive treatment and be well-versed with the maintenance protocol which should be performed at regular intervals that will assist the patient to maintain implant health.

The implant maintenance protocol consists of two phases:

3.1 Phase 1: assessment phase

The dentist will assess the patient's medical condition, analyze the risk factor/s which may pose as an etiology for the implant failure (**Table 3**). Along with the medical condition, the dental history of the patient should also be evaluated as it may provide us with information about the patient's oral hygiene and peri-implant status. It has been documented in multiple studies [37–39] that edentulous patients with high plaque scores before implant placement had experienced more implant failures than those with lower plaque scores. Furthermore, it has also been proven that patients treated for their periodontal conditions are more likely to experience

Sr. no	Systemic risk factors	Influence on implant placement	Contra-indication	References
1.	Neuropsychiatric disorders: Epilepsy, schizophrenia, dementia, Parkinson's disease, Alzheimer's disease, Huntington's disease	a. Difficult to maintain oral hygiene predisposing them to periodontal and soft tissue problems b. Accidental swallow of dental instruments c. Difficult to understand the procedure, follow medical instructions, and provide consent d. Alzheimer's disease has shown an association with peri-implantitis [8].	Absolute	[7, 8]
2.	Recent myocardial infarction or cerebrovascular accident	Can trigger post-ischemia complications like cardiogenic shock, myocardial rupture, pericarditis, or chronic ischemic heart disease as observed in 75% of previous myocardial infarction affected patients.	Absolute	[9, 10]
3.	Valvular prosthesis placement	Can cause prosthetic valve endocarditis as observed in 1–3% of patients	Absolute	[9, 11]
4.	Bleeding disorders and patients under anticoagulants for cardiovascular disorders.	a. Can trigger mild thrombocytopenia which may produce abnormal post-operative bleeding b. Major post-surgical bleeding, spontaneous bleeding of the mucous membrane.	Absolute	[9, 12]
5.	Cancer and chemotherapy	a. May affect osseointegration due to bone vascularity reduction and cause dental implant failure. b. Chemotherapy found to jeopardize bone metabolism. c. Intensive chemotherapy can cause lower bone mineral density and a high risk of bone fracture.	Absolute	[7, 13–15]
6.	Respiratory disease	a. Can cause airway hyperresponsiveness b. Can perpetuate asthma if the dental implant surgery is done in a supine position. c. Local anesthetic to be used cautiously in patients with COPD. d. Vasoconstrictors are an absolute contraindication for COPD patients.	Relative	[7, 16–18]
7.	Liver disorder: decompensated hepatic disorder, cystic fibrosis, liver cirrhosis	a. May cause reduced or trouble in producing coagulation factors. b. Due to reduced platelet count can result in uncontrollable hemorrhage in the surgical site. c. Can result in portal hypertension due to hepatic fibrosis during the surgery	Relative	[7, 19]

Sr. no	Systemic risk factors	Influence on implant placement	Contra-indication	References
8.	Endocrine disorders: diabetes mellitus, thyroid disorders, parathyroid disorders, other hormonal disorders.	a. Delayed wound healing, repressed bone formation, and enhanced bone resorption may be seen around implants in diabetic patients. b. Thyroid storm can be induced due to emotional stress, trauma, and infection in hyperthyroidism patients. c. Patients with hypothyroidism may have abnormal bone metabolism which may increase the risk of implant failure. d. Women going through menopause have a higher incidence of periodontitis and osteoporotic alveolar bone which may lead to delayed healing and difficult to achieve success in dental implantation.	Relative	[7, 20, 21]
9.	Immunosuppression	Several case report studies suggest no relationship between HIV and implant failure. It has been proven safe to place implants in patients with controlled HIV	Relative	[22–25]
10.	Osteoporosis	a. No scientific evidence confirms contraindication or implant failure in patients with primary osteoporosis b. In secondary osteoporosis due to accompanying illness or systemic conditions chances of implant failure is more	Relative	[26]
11.	Smoking	a. Increase of implant failure rate 2.5 times more in smokers compared to non-smokers b. In maxilla the chances of implant failure have been reported to be 18% in smokers as compared to 7% in non-smokers c. Smoking cessation before implant placement appears to improve results	Relative	[27, 28]
12.	Age	Many studies have concluded that age is not a significant factor for implant failure unless associated with a systemic disease that may result in bone loss	Relative	[29]
13.	Interleukin-1 genotype	a. No studies to support co-relation between implant failure and IL-1 genotype b. However, a synergistic effect is present between smoking and IL-1 genotype c. Odds ratio of tooth loss increased to 7.7% when smoking and IL-1 genotype is present as opposed to 2.9% when only smoking is present	Relative	[29]

Sr. no	Systemic risk factors	Influence on implant placement	Contra-indication	References
14.	Medications: bisphosphonates	a. Increased risk of developing osteoradionecrosis of the jaw known as Bisphosphonate-related osteoradionecrosis of the jaw (BRONJ) b. Oral bisphosphonates have been associated with an increased risk of implant failure	Absolute	[30–32]
	Anticancer drugs	May cause bone marrow toxicity, immunosuppression which may result in infection, hemorrhage, mucositis, and pain.	Absolute	[9]
	Anticoagulants	a. Chances of experiencing post-operative bleeding problems have been seen only in patients who take high doses of anticoagulants. b. Risk of developing uncontrolled bleeding or life-threatening bleeding is very low. c. Discontinuing anticoagulant therapy before implant placement may also account for increased probability of thromboembolic events	Relative	[33–36]

Table 3.
Lists the different systemic conditions that can pose as a risk factor for implant placement.

implant complications compared to non-periodontal treated patients [40–42]. Hence, to achieve long-term implant survival and success, patients with a previous history of aggressive periodontitis must undergo Supportive Periodontal Therapy (SPT) and diligently follow the regular maintenance phase and recall visits.

A typical maintenance phase should last for 1 h and should be scheduled every 3 months. The following are the parameters that are evaluated during the assessment phase of the implant maintenance protocol.

3.1.1 Peri-implant diagnostic parameters

The diagnostic parameters used to evaluate and monitor oral implants during the maintenance phase should have high specificity and sensitivity. We shall discuss the various peri-implant diagnostic parameters with modified dental indices that will be used during the assessment phase.

3.1.1.1 Plaque and mucosal assessment

Mombelli et al. [43] and Apse et al. [44] modified the plaque and mucosal assessment indices for peri-implant marginal mucosa and plaque evaluation (**Table 4**).

3.1.1.2 Peri-implant bleeding on probing

Similar to natural teeth conditions, the absence of bleeding on probing around peri-implant mucosa suggests a healthy implant soft tissue. In a study conducted by Lang et al. [45], it was concluded that healthy peri-implant sites were characterized

Score	Peri-implant plaque assessment index	Peri-implant marginal mucosa index
	Mombelli et al. [43]	**Apse et al. [44]**
0	No plaque detected	Normal mucosa
1	Plaque is detected only when a probe is run through the smooth marginal surface of the implant	Minimal inflammation and mucosa color change present with mild edema
2	Plaque can be seen by the naked eye	Moderate inflammation with redness, edema, and glazing
3	Abundance of soft matter detected	Severe inflammation with redness, edema, ulceration, and spontaneous bleeding without probing

Table 4.
Peri-implant plaque and mucosal indices.

by absence of bleeding on probing i.e. 0% whereas peri-implant mucositis reported 67% and peri-implantitis reported 91% of bleeding on probing. To avoid false-positive readings for bleeding on probing, Gerber et al. have recommended a minimum pressure of 0.15 N to be applied during the examination [46].

3.1.1.3 Peri-implant probing depth

Probing is an important and realistic diagnostic indicator for monitoring the peri-implant tissues. The probing force required is around 0.2–0.3 N [47] and should always be measured using a periodontal probe from the mid-aspect of the mesiobuccal, buccal, distobuccal, mesiolingual, lingual, and distolingual surfaces of the implant. Probing depth for an implant having a supraosseous platform with healthy mucosa is around 2–4 mm [48]. If the implant had been placed infrosseoulsy the probing depth may be slightly higher. However, an increase in clinical probing depth associated with bleeding on probing should be viewed as signs of peri-implant disease.

3.1.1.4 Width of peri-implant keratinized mucosa

The influence of keratinized tissue around implants is still a controversial issue as there is no consensus in literature regarding the long-term success of implants and the presence or absence of keratinized tissue. However, numerous studies have been conducted which revealed a relationship between lack of keratinized tissue and plaque accumulation [49–52], bone loss [49, 53], increase in soft-tissue recession [51, 52, 54], bleeding on probing [50–53], and greater gingival inflammation [50–53].

3.1.1.5 Peri-implant sulcus fluid analysis (PISF)

PISF has a substantial amount of biochemical mediators which act as a non – invasive host marker for identifying underlying peri-implant diseases. There have been studies conducted which show a positive correlation with PISF and plaque accumulation [55], degree of peri-implant soft tissue inflammation [55], and also the amount of bone resorption [56].

3.1.1.6 Suppuration

Suppuration is a confirmatory indicator of the disease activity and hence immediate anti-infective therapy is recommended [57].

3.1.2 Evaluation of food impaction around implants

Food impaction is one of the most common risk factors for developing peri-implant diseases [58]. Food impaction around implants can cause bleeding, edema, inflammation, halitosis, bone loss, pocket formation, implant mobility, and finally implant failure. The following is a classification for food impaction given by Chopra et al. [59] which will help us diagnose the cause for food impaction.

Class I: Food impaction present between either an implant supporting crown/fixed dental prosthesis (FDP) and the adjacent natural tooth.

Class II: Food impaction present between either an implant supporting a single crown/FDP and a tooth with caries/faulty restoration/crown/FPD.

Class III: Food impaction present between two adjacent implants with either a single crown/FDP.

Class IV: Food impaction below the pontic of an implant with FDP.

Class V: Food impaction around implant-supported/retained dentures.

Class I–Class V has additional sub-categories based on the etiology of food lodgement [59].

3.1.3 Evaluation of implant mobility

Test for implant mobility is a primary factor for identifying the longevity of implant health. Implant mobility can be tested either by the conventional method or by using automated devices. The conventional method uses two rigid instruments that apply a labiolingual force of 500 g around the implant fixture to test its rigidity. The automated devices currently in use are Periotest and a non-invasive device that works on the principles based on Resonance Frequency Analysis (RFA).

The amplitude of implant mobility can be assessed using the Implant mobility scale given by Misch [60] (**Table 5**).

3.1.4 Occlusal evaluation

Occlusal evaluation must be done at regular intervals. Any deflective or premature contacts that may cause loosening or fracture of abutment screws, implant, or prosthetic failure must be evaluated and corrected. Parafunctional habits if present must be documented and treated accordingly as they may cause rapid bone loss [47].

3.1.5 Crestal bone loss and radiographic evaluation

Loss of crestal bone is a significant indicator of any ongoing peri-implant disease. After the prosthesis delivery, crestal bone loss around implants can be a primary indicator

Scale	Description
0	Absence of clinical mobility in any direction when 500 g force is applied
1	Slight detectable horizontal movement with 500 g force
2	Visible moderate horizontal mobility up to 0.5 mm when a force of 500 g applied
3	Severe horizontal movement of more than 0.5 mm is seen when a force of 500 g applied
4	Moderate to severe horizontal movement along with any visible vertical movement

Table 5.
Clinical implant mobility scale.

of the need for initial preventive therapy. Marginal bone loss of 0 to 0.2 mm after the first year of function is common and acceptable [61–63]. However, a bone loss of 0.5 to 1 mm after the abutment is connected and during the first few years of the prosthesis in function is an indicator of excessive stress at the crestal implant-bone interface [64]. The dentist should evaluate and reduce the cause of stress at the implant-bone interface which could be due to deflective occlusal contacts, cantilever length, or parafunction.

At-home implant care	Types	Description
Brushing [65]	1. Manual 2. Automated/sonic brush 3. Motorized/power brush 4. End tufted brush 5. 5. Tapered rotary brush	a. To be performed twice daily for effective plaque removal around implants. b. Patients should be instructed to follow the BASS technique of brushing. c. To access the interdental or under the implant bar or connector region, a tapered rotary brush can be used. d. Automated/ Sonic brushes are superior to manual brushes in that they effectively remove plaque, provide improved interproximal cleaning without damaging the peri-implant tissue, and can be used by patients with limited dexterity. e. In difficult to access regions especially the posterior area, end tufted brushes or tapered rotary brushes can be used.
Interproximal cleaning aids [65]	1. Floss plastic, braided, satin, woven, yarns, dental tapes, tufted, coated	a. Should be used in a 'shoe-shine rag' fashion. b. Along with the mesial and distal surfaces, the facial and lingual surfaces should also be cleaned using the looping technique for effective debridement. c. Patient should be instructed to place the floss sub-gingivally until resistance is met. d. Dental floss can also be used to deliver antiseptic agents to the implants on daily basis.
	2. Interproximal cleansers: Foam tips, interproximal brushes, disposable wooden picks	a. Chosen based on the size of the interproximal area. b. Caution to be excised in cases where the inter-proximal brush has an exposed metal tip which can damage the peri-implant soft tissue and also the abutment's surface. c. Chemotherapeutic agents can be delivered to the implant surface using the proxy and foam tip interdental brushes.
	3. Water irrigation: Hydro floss, Oracura	a. Water stream should be directed interproximally and horizontally between implants or can cause damage to the peri-implant tissue
Chemotherapeutic agents [65]	Povidone iodine, Chlorhexidine gluconate, lasers, photodynamic therapy, or plant alkaloids	a. Can be used in patients who have recurrent tissue inflammation in the form of rinses, gels, lozenges. b. However, chlorhexidine gluconate has been proven to alter the surface topography of implants, and cause cell cytotoxicity thereby affecting the re-osseointegration potential of implants [66]

Table 6.
At-home oral implant hygiene care aids.

A preventive maintenance appointment should be scheduled every 3 to 4 months and a periapical/ bitewing radiograph should be made every 6 to 8 months. The periapical/ bitewing radiograph must be compared with the baseline radiographs to evaluate the crestal bone changes that have/have not occurred in the early stages of loading.

After 1 year, the previous radiographs must be compared with the recent bitewing radiograph and evaluated for further bone loss. If no changes are observed, a radiographic examination must be scheduled every 3 years, however, if there are noticeable unfavorable changes or crestal bone loss present, a radiographic evaluation must be carried out every 6–8 months along with stress reduction and hygiene maintenance protocol [60].

3.2 Phase 2: hygiene phase

Following the systematic assessment phase arduously performed by the clinician, it is now the responsibility of the patient, a co-therapist, to meticulously and habitually follow the implant oral hygiene protocol instructed by the clinician. After the implant

In-office implant care	Types	Description
Scaling [65]	Scalers made from plasteel (resin); hi-tech plastic; graphite-reinforced nylon etc.	a. Metallic instruments should be avoided as they can scratch, contaminate or produce galvanic reactions at the implant-abutment interface. b. If the prostheses limit the access to manual scalers, sonic or ultrasonic scalers with plastic or graphite-reinforced nylon tips may be used. c. Depending on the sites of deposits, either horizontal, oblique, or vertical short working strokes with light pressure should be used to prevent inadvertent damage to the peri-implant tissues.
Polishing [65]	Non-abrasive polishing pastes like aluminum oxide, tin oxide, APF free prophy paste, and low abrasive dentifrice	a. Coarse abrasive polishing pastes and air polishing of implant components are contraindicated. b. Air polishing may cause chipping of the porcelain or composite material. c. May result in unwanted pitting or surface irregularities on the implant components and cause detachment of soft tissue from the implant surface due to air pressure.
Chemotherapeutic agents [65]	Dentomycin, PerioChip, Atridox, or subgingival irrigation using chemotherapeutic agents.	a. Plastic irrigation tip may be used to introduce the antiseptic agents to the base of the implant sulcus. b. Neutral sodium fluoride may be used instead of other fluorides which may have an acidic pH and thereby alter the implant surface
Intraoral camera [65]		a. Can be used to educate the patient about the effect of their oral hygiene care. b. Based on the outcome of their previous oral care, any changes required can be implemented. This will help the patients to self-analyze their regular oral hygiene methods and motivate them to make necessary changes or continue with the same.

Table 7.
In-office oral implant hygiene care aids.

placement, patients usually have improper oral hygiene practice either due to the fear of damaging the implant or because of overzealous oral health care practice. Hence, as clinicians, it is important to convey both verbally and visually the different oral health care aids that can be practiced safely by the patients to achieve long-term implant success.

The following are the agendas to be covered in the hygiene phase:

Directing the patient to control the underlying medical conditions which may cause peri-implant diseases and gradually implant failure.

Educating the patient about the importance of maintaining implant oral health and recall visits.

Training the patient to use different In-home hygiene products for the maintenance of implant oral health.

Oral implant hygiene methods can be broadly categorized as At-home implant care (**Table 6**) and In-office implant care (**Table 7**).

4. The implant health scale

The success of an implant should not focus on the implant fixture alone but also on the success of the entire implant prosthesis. A natural tooth in the oral cavity is not described as a success or failure, instead, a health scale is used to determine the condition and survival of the tooth.

Similarly, the implant health scale was introduced by James and further modified by Misch in the year 1993 [67, 68]. The Internation Congress of Oral Implantologists (ICOI), in Italy Consensus Conference, Pisa, on 5th October 2007, further modified the James-Misch Implant scale and approved a health scale with four categories for endosteal implants that describe their clinical conditions i.e. implant success, implant survival (satisfactory and compromised), and implant failure [69] (**Table 8**).

Implant quality scale	Clinical conditions	Prognosis	Treatment planning
I. Implant success	a. No pain or tenderness during any function b. 0 mobility c. <2 mm bone loss from initial surgery period d. No history of exudates	Very good to excellent prognosis	Normal maintenance
II. Satisfactory survival	a. No pain on function b. Zero mobility c. 2–4 mm of radiographic bone loss d. No history of exudates	Good to excellent depending on the condition of the crestal bone	a. Evaluate for stresses b. Keep shorter intervals between hygiene evaluation c. Yearly radiographs
III. Compromised survival	a. May have sensitivity during function b. No mobility c. Radiograph shows bone loss of >4 mm (less than ½ of implant body) d. Probing depth of >7 mm e. May have a history of exudate	Good to guarded prognosis depending on the ability to reduce the stresses once surgical corrections have improved the soft and hard tissues health.	a. Evaluate for stresses b. Start with antibiotics, topical chemotherapeutic agents c. Surgical reentry d. Evaluate the prosthesis for change/ addition of a new implant

Implant quality scale	Clinical conditions	Prognosis	Treatment planning
IV. Failure (clinical or absolute)	Any of the following: a. Pain b. Mobility c. Radiographic bone loss of more than ½ length of the implant d. Uncontrolled exudate e. No longer in mouth	Very poor prognosis	a. Whether a clinical or absolute failure, the implant should be removed. b. Sleper implants, surgically removed implants, or exfoliated implants fall under this category.

Table 8.
Dental implant health scale, international congress of oral implantologists, Pisa, Italy consensus conference, 2007.

After the final implant assessment phase, the clinician should categorize the implant health based on the assessed clinical condition of the implants.

5. Conclusion

The immediate outcome of implant dentistry for patients is usually esthetics and function. But long-term implant prosthesis success depends on an array of factors such as implant quality, implant surgery procedure, peri-implant health, implant/prosthesis mobility, pain, exudate, etc.

A systematic review [70] was conducted to evaluate the different implant oral hygiene methods that are available and are in use by the general public and the dental team for the debridement of plaque and maintenance of implant oral health. It was concluded, that the knowledge that exists among the clinicians and the general public about oral hygiene maintenance is concerning natural teeth and no particular protocol or regimen were being followed [70]. Hence, academics and private clinics must start spreading awareness both verbally and visually about the different implant oral hygiene aids which can be used to achieve long-term implant success.

The only elucidation to achieve long-term successful implant prosthesis is frequent maintenance recalls, regular professional and at-home implant hygiene care, as well as treating any peri-implant pathology at its earliest. In this chapter, we have meticulously compiled in toto the dental implant maintenance protocol and hope that the information provided will be helpful for the implant interdisciplinary team to guide the patient, educate them and simultaneously work with them to achieve long-term implant success.

Conflict of interests

The authors declare no conflict of interest.

Author details

Gayathri Krishnamoorthy, Aparna I. Narayana* and Dhanasekar Balakrishnan
Manipal College of Dental Sciences, Manipal Academy of Higher Education,
Manipal, India

*Address all correspondence to: aparna.narayan@manipal.edu

References

[1] Dental Implant Market Size, Share & Trends Analysis Report by Implants Type (Titanium, Zirconium), by Region (North America, Europe, Asia Pacific, Latin America, MEA), and Segment Forecasts [Internet]. 2021-2028. Available from: https://www.grandviewresearch.com/industry-analysis/dental-implants-market

[2] Pjetursson BE, Asgeirsson AG, Zwahlen M, Sailer I. Improvements in implant dentistry over the last decade: Comparison of survival and complication rates in older and newer publications. The International Journal of Oral & Maxillofacial Implants. 2014;**29**:308-324. DOI: 10.11607/jomi.2014 suppl.g5.2

[3] Brunello G, Gervasi M, Ricci S, Tomasi C, Bressan E. Patients' perceptions of implant therapy and maintenance: A questionnaire-based survey. Clinical Oral Implants Research. 2020;**31**(10):917-927. DOI: 10.1111/clr.13634

[4] Garg K, Duarte F, Funari K. Hygeinic maintenance of dental implants. Journal of Practical Hygiene. 1997;**6**(2):13-17

[5] Misch CE. Diagnosis and treatment planning: Medical evaluation. In: Misch CE, editor. Contemporary Implant Dentistry. 3rd ed. St. Louis: Mosby; Elsevier; 2007. pp. 51-102

[6] Doyle DJ, Goyal A, Bansal P, Garmon EH. American Society of anesthesiologists classification. In: StatPearls. Treasure Island (FL):StatPearls Publishing; 2021

[7] Yu H, Zhou A, Liu J, Tang Y, Yuan Q, Man Y, et al. Management of systemic risk factors ahead of dental implant therapy: A beard well lathered is half shaved. Journal of Leukocyte Biology. 2021;**110**(3):591-604. DOI: 10.1002/JLB.6MR0621-760RR

[8] Dominy SS, Lynch C, Ermini F, et al. Porphyromonas gingivalis in Alzheimer's disease brains: Evidence for disease causation and treatment with small-molecule inhibitors. Science Advances. 2019;**5**(1):eaau3333

[9] Hwang D, Wang HL. Medical contraindications to implant therapy: Part I: Absolute contraindications. Implant Dentistry. 2006;**15**(4):353-360. DOI: 10.1097/01.id.0000247855.75691.03

[10] Schoen F. The heart. In: Kumar V, editor. Robbins and Cotran: Pathologic Basis of Disease. 7th ed. St. Louis, MO: Saunders; 2005. pp. 584-586

[11] Chambers H. Infective endocarditis. In: Goldman L, editor. Cecil Textbook of Medicine. 22nd ed. St. Louis, MO: Saunders; 2004. pp. 1795-1796

[12] Weyant RJ. Characteristics associated with the loss and peri-implant tissue health of endosseous dental implants. The International Journal of Oral & Maxillofacial Implants. 1994;**9**:95-102

[13] Eisenschenk A, Witzel C, Lautenbach M, Ekkernkamp A, Weber U, Kuntscher MV. Does chemotherapy impair the bone healing and biomechanical stability of vascularized rib and fibula grafts? Journal of Reconstructive Microsurgery. 2007;**23**(1):35-40

[14] Fan C, Foster BK, Wallace WH, Xian CJ. Pathobiology and prevention of cancer chemotherapy-induced bone growth arrest, bone loss, and osteonecrosis. Current Molecular Medicine. 2011;**11**(2):140-151

[15] Crofton PM. Bone and bone turnover. Endocrine Development. 2009;**15**:77-100

[16] Boulet LP, O'Byrne PM. Asthma and exercise-induced bronchoconstriction in athletes. New England Journal Medicine. 2015;**372**(7):641-648

[17] Harrington N, Prado N, Barry S. Dental treatment in children with asthma—a review. British Dental Journal. 2016;**220**(6):299-302

[18] Devlin J. Patients with chronic obstructive pulmonary disease: Management considerations for the dental team. British Dental Journal. 2014;**217**(5):235-237

[19] Leung DH, Narkewicz MR. Cystic fibrosis-related cirrhosis. Journal of Cystic Fibrosis. 2017;**16**(2):S50-S61

[20] Wu YY, Xiao E, Graves DT. Diabetes mellitus related bone metabolism and periodontal disease. International Journal of Oral Science. 2015;7(2):63-72

[21] Chiha M, Samarasinghe S, Kabaker AS. Thyroid storm: An updated review. Journal of Intensive Care Medicine. 2015;**30**(3):131-140

[22] Rajnay ZW, Hochstetter RL. Immediate placement of an endosseous root-form implant in an HIV-positive patient: Report of a case. The Journal of Periodontology. 1998;**69**:1167-1171

[23] Baron M, Gritsch F, Hansy A-M, Haas R. Implants in an HIV-positive patient: A case report. International Journal of Oral & Maxillofacial Implants. 2004;**19**:425-430

[24] Achong RM, Shetty K, Arribas A, Block MS. Implants in HIV-positive patients: 3 case reports. Journal of Oral and Maxillofacial Surgery. 2006;**64**: 1199-1203

[25] Shetty K, Achong R. Dental implants in the HIV-positive patient – Case report and review of the literature. General Dentistry. 2005;**53**: 434-437

[26] Otomo-Corgel J. Osteoporosis and osteopenia: Implications for periodontal and implant therapy. Periodontology 2000. 2012;**59**:111-139

[27] Wilson TG Jr, Nunn M. The relationship between the interleukin-1 periodontal genotype and implant loss. Initial data. Journal Periodontology. 1999;**70**:724-729

[28] Bain CA, Moy PK. The association between the failure of dental implants and cigarette smoking. The International Journal of Oral & Maxillofacial Implants. 1993;**8**:609-615

[29] Hwang D, Wang HL. Medical contraindications to implant therapy: Part II: Relative contraindications. Implant Dentistry. 2007;**16**(1):13-23. DOI: 10.1097/ID.0b013e31803276c8

[30] Marx RE, Sawatari Y, Fortin M, Broumand V. Bisphosphonate-induced exposed bone (osteonecrosis/osteopetrosis) of the jaws: Risk factors, recognition, prevention, and treatment. Journal of Oral and Maxillofacial Surgery. 2005;**63**:1567-1575

[31] Ruggiero SL, Mehrotra B, Rosenberg TJ, Engroff SL. Osteonecrosis of the jaws associated with the use of bisphosphonates: A review of 63 cases. Journal of Oral and Maxillofacial Surgery. 2004;**62**:527-534

[32] Starck WJ, Epker BN. Failure of osseointegrated dental implants after diphosphonate therapy for osteoporosis: A case report. The International Journal of Oral & Maxillofacial Implants. 1995;**10**:74-78

[33] van Steenberghe D, Quirynen M, Molly L, Jacobs R. Impact of systemic diseases and medication on osseointegration. Periodontology 2000. 2003;**33**:163-171

[34] Beirne OR. Evidence to continue oral anticoagulant therapy for ambulatory oral surgery. Journal of Oral and Maxillofacial Surgery. 2005;**63**:540-545

[35] Madrid C, Sanz M. What influence do anticoagulants have on oral implant therapy? A systematic review. Clinical Oral Implants Research. 2009;**20**(4): 96-106

[36] Froum SJ. Dental Implant Complications: Etiology, Prevention, and Treatment. 2nd ed. United Kingdom: Wiley-Blackwell; 2015

[37] van Steenberghe D, Klinge B, Linden U, et al. Periodontal indices around natural and titanium abutments: A longitudinal multicenter study. The Journal of Periodontology. 1993;**64**:538-541

[38] Ferreira SD, Silva GLM, Costa JE, Cortelli JR, Costa FO. Prevalence and risk variables for peri-implant disease in Brazilian subjects. Journal of Clinical Periodontology. 2006;**33**:929-935

[39] Salvi GE, Aglietta M, Eick S, et al. Reversibility of experimental peri-implant mucositis compared with experimental gingivitis in humans. Clinical Oral Implants Research. 2012;**23**:182-190

[40] Hardt CRE, Grondahl K, Lekholm U, Wennstrom JL. Outcome of implant therapy in relation to experienced loss of periodontal bone support. A retrospective 5-year study. Clinical Oral Implants Research. 2002;**13**:488-494

[41] Karoussis IK, Salvi GE, Heitz-Mayfield LJA, et al. Long-term implant prognosis in patients with and without a history of chronic periodontitis: A 10-year prospective cohort study of the ITIR dental implant system. Clinical Oral Implants Research. 2003;**14**:329-339

[42] Ong CT, Ivanovski S, Needleman IG, et al. Systematic review of implant outcomes in treated periodontitis subjects. Journal of Clinical Periodontology. 2008;**35**:438-462

[43] van Oosten MMAC, Sch¨urch Jr. E, Land NP. The microbiota associated with successful or failing osseointegrated titanium implants. Oral Microbiology and Immunology. 1987;**2**(4):145-151

[44] Apse P, Zarb GA, Schmitt A, Lewis DW. The longitudinal effectiveness of osseointegrated dental implants, The Toronto study: Peri-implant mucosal response. The International Journal of Periodontics & Restorative Dentistry. 1991;**11**(2):95-111

[45] Lang NP, Wetzel AC, Stich H, Caffesse RG. Histologic probe penetration in healthy and inflamed peri-implant tissues. Clinical Oral Implants Research. 1994;**5**(4):191-201

[46] Gerber JA, Tan WC, Balmer TE, Salvi GE, Lang NP. Bleeding on probing and pocket probing depth in relation to probing pressure and mucosal health around oral implants. Clinical Oral Implants Research. 2009;**20**(1):75-78

[47] Humphrey S. Implant maintenance. Dental Clinics of North America. 2006;**50**(3):463-478

[48] Lang NP, Berglundh T, Heitz-Mayfield LJ, Pjetursson BE, Salvi GE, Sanz M. Consensus statements and recommended clinical procedures regarding implant survival and complications. The International Journal

of Oral & Maxillofacial Implants. 2004;**19**:150-154

[49] Bouri A Jr, Bissada N, Al-Zahrani MS, Fadoul F, Nounen I. Width of keratinized gingiva and the health status of the supporting tissues around dental implants. The International Journal of Oral & Maxillofacial Implants. 2008; **23**(2):323-326

[50] Chung DM, Oh TJ, Shotwell JL, Misch CE, Wang HL. Significance of keratinized mucosa in maintenance of dental implants with different surfaces. Journal of Periodontology. 2006;**77**(8):1410-1420

[51] Schrott AR, Jimenez M, Hwang JW, Fiorellini J, Weber HP. Five-year evaluation of the influence of keratinized mucosa on peri-implant soft-tissue health and stability around implants supporting full-arch mandibular fixed prostheses. Clinical Oral Implants Research. 2009;**20**(10):1170-1177

[52] Adibrad M, Shahabuei M, Sahabi M. Significance of the width of keratinized mucosa on the health status of the supporting tissue around implants supporting overdentures. The Journal of Oral Implantology. 2009;**35**(5):232-237

[53] Ross-Jansaker AM, Renvert H, Lindahl C, Renvert S. Nine-to fourteen-year follow-up of implant treatment. Part III: Factors associated with peri-implant lesions. Journal of Clinical Periodontology. 2006;**33**(4):296-301

[54] Zigdon H, Machtei EE. The dimensions of keratinized mucosa around implants affect clinical and immunological parameters. Clinical Oral Implants Research. 2008;**19**(4): 387-392

[55] Niimi A, Ueda M. Crevicular fluid in the osseointegrated implant sulcus: A pilot study. The International Journal of Oral & Maxillofacial Implants. 1995;**10**(4):434-436

[56] Behneke N, Behneke B, D'Hoedt B, Wagner W. Hard and soft tissue reactions to ITI screw implants: 3-year longitudinal results of a prospective study. The International Journal of Oral & Maxillofacial Implants. 1997;**12**(6) :749-757

[57] Klinge M, Hultin M, Berglundh T. Peri-implantitis. Dental Clinics of North America. 2005;**49**(3):661-676

[58] Bidra AS. Nonsurgical management of inflammatory periimplant disease caused by food impaction: A clinical report. The Journal of Prosthetic Dentistry. 2014;**111**:96-100

[59] Chopra A, Sivaraman K, Narayan AI, Balakrishnan D. Etiology and classification of food impaction around implants and implant-retained prosthesis. Clinical Implant Dentistry and Related Research. 2019;**21**(2): 391-397. DOI: 10.1111/cid.12716

[60] Misch E. In: Misch CE, editor. An Implant is not a Tooth: A Comparison of Periodontal Indices in Contemporary Implant Dentistry. 3rd ed. Mosby: Elsevier; 2007. pp. 1055-1072

[61] van Steenberghe D, Lekholm U, Bolender C, Folmer T, Henry P, Herrmann I, et al. Applicability of osseointegrated oral implants in the rehabilitation of partial edentulism: A prospective multicenter study on 558 fixtures. The International Journal of Oral & Maxillofacial Implants. 1990;**5**(3):272-281

[62] Adell R, Lekholm U, Rockler B, Brånemark PI. A 15-year study of osseointegrated implants in the treatment of the edentulous jaw.

International Journal of Oral Surgery. 1981;**10**(6):387-416. DOI: 10.1016/s0300-9785(81)80077-4

[63] Cox JF, Zarb GA. The longitudinal clinical efficacy of osseointegrated dental implants: A 3-year report. The International Journal of Oral & Maxillofacial Implants. 1987;**2**(2):91-100

[64] Oh TJ, Yoon J, Misch CE, Wang HL. The causes of early implant bone loss: Myth or science? The Journal of Periodontology. 2002;**73**(3):322-333. DOI: 10.1902/jop.2002.73.3.322

[65] Gulati M, Govila V, Anand V, Anand B. Implant maintenance: A clinical update. International Scholarly Research Notices. 2014;**2014**:908534. DOI: 10.1155/2014/908534

[66] Krishnamoorthy G, Narayana A, Balkrishnanan D. Chlorhexidine for the treatment of peri-implantitis- is it a benison? Journal of Long-Term Effects of Medical Implants. DOI: 10.1615/JLongTermEffMedImplants.2021039510

[67] Misch CE. The implant quality scale: A clinical assessment of the health disease continuum. Oral Health. 1998;**15**:15-25

[68] Misch CE. Implant success or failure: Clinical assessment in implant dentistry. In: Misch CE, editor. Contemporary Implant Dentistry. St. Louis, MO. Elsevier; 1993. pp. 33-66

[69] Misch CE, Perel ML, Wang HL, Sammartino G, Galindo-Moreno P, Trisi P, et al. Implant success, survival, and failure: The International Congress of Oral Implantologists (ICOI) Pisa Consensus Conference. Implant Dentistry. 2007;**17**(1):5-15. DOI: 10.1097/ID.0b013e3181676059

[70] Louropoulou A, Slot DE, Van der Weijden F. Mechanical self-performed oral hygiene of implant supported restorations: A systematic review. The Journal of Evidence-Based Dental Practice. 2014;**14**(60):9.e1. DOI: 10.1016/j.jebdp.2014.03.008

Chapter 18

Herbs and Oral Health

Zuhair S. Natto

Abstract

Herbal medicine has long been used to prevent and control disease, and it can minimize the potential side effects of chemical products. However, side effects from herbs do exist. Most of the challenges with herbal medicine revolves around inadequate information about the effect of herbs in the oral cavity, the mechanism of action, and potential side effects. There are several herbs described in this chapter have anti-inflammatory, anti-bacterial, anti-viral, anti-fungal in oral micro-organisms. It includes aloe vera, ginger, clove, cinnamon, garlic, neem, miswak, turmeric, tulsi, green tea, chamomile, fenugreek, anise plant, peppermint, bloodroot, caraway, eucalyptus, phyllanthus emblica, black seed, myrrh, rosemary, sage, and thyme; some may act as an alternative management option to current treatments for oral conditions such as caries prevention, gingivitis, periodontitis, oral burn, ulcers and inflammation, after extraction, dry mouth, pain reduction, anesthesia, intracanal medications, ill-fitting dentures, peri-implant mucositis and peri-implantitis. It can be used in several forms such as mouthwashes, toothpastes, topical agents or local drug delivery devices. However, more research is needed to understand their mechanisms and potential side effects.

Keywords: bacterial plaque, herbs, oral health, gingiva, periodontal disease, caries

1. Introduction

Herbs is defined as "any plants that lack the woody tissue characteristic of shrubs or trees" [1–7]. Several herbs have shown positive effects against a variety of inflammatory medical problems, such as dysphagia, gastric ulcers, wound healing, and sore throat. It is the core component of the complementary and alternative medicine (CAM) [1–7]. It has been used to manage blood problems and eliminate waste, stimulate body and blood circulation, minimize irritation [1–7]. It has several forms such as tablets, syrups, or it can be used externally as a dressings, or topical application [1–7].

Herbs could have a potential beneficial effect in the dental field, such as with gum swelling, specifically, and in oral healthcare overall. However, few studies have scientifically reviewed these topics. In this chapter, the most common herbal supplements that can be used in dentistry (i.e., neem, ginger, clove, aloe vera, eucalyptus, garlic, miswak, turmeric, tulsi, charcoal, and cinnamon) are reviewed. Evidence-based findings will be presented to support or refute the use of these agents in oral care.

2. Most common herbs used in dentistry

2.1 Aloe Vera

Aloe vera is effective in periodontal disease conditions [1]. It is available in several forms, such as a mouthwash, toothpaste, or gel [1]. In a recent systematic review, aloe vera as a mouthwash was effective in all included studies in reducing plaque and gingival inflammation (**Table 1**, [2]). Moreover, aloe vera had no or very minimal side effects compared to other chemical mouthwashes [2]. It has a strong detoxifying agent, a neuro-sedative properties and immune booster [1, 2]. It can act as a mercury scavenger and antioxidant. It accerlated healing after surgical extraction including the third molar [1, 2].

Aloe vera toothpaste is another form that is effective on periodontal index and gingival scores and that can be used as an alternative to traditional toothpaste [3]. Aloe vera gel has inhibitory activities on some cariogenic organisms (*Streptococcus mutans*) [4], such as periodontopathic (*Aggregatibacter actinomycetemcomitans, Porphyromonas gingivalis*) and an opportunistic periodontopathogen (*Bacteroides fragilis*) [4]. It can be used as intracanal medicaments against *Enterococcus faecalis* (**Table 1**, [5]). It can be used to manage antiviral infection such as herpes simplex and herpes zoster, or as an antifungal agent against *candida albicans* [3–5].

There are several other uses for aloe vera such as aid in chemical burns, dry sockets, relief of aphthous ulcers, canker sores, lichen planus, pemphigus, desquamative gingivitis, migratory glossititis, and burning mouth syndrome [1–5]. It can helps in reducing the information related to ill-fitting dentures [1–5]. It can also be used in peri-implant mucositis and peri-implantitis [1–5].

2.2 Ginger

Ginger, which is scientifically named *Zingiber officinale roscoe*, can be used as a pain killer and is as effective as ibuprofen [6]. It can be used as an alternative for ibuprofen [6]. Combined with non-surgical periodontal therapy in chronic periodontitis cases among the type 2 diabetes population, ginger can help [7]. The reducing colony forming unit (CFUs/uL) of *S. mutans* is comparable to other oral rinses, such as chlorhexidine, and is also effective against *Lactobacillus* (**Table 1**).

Ginger may be a promising anti-cariogenic against *Streptococcus mutans* and *Streptococcus sobrinus* [7]. It contains phenolic compounds such as gingerol and shogaol, hydrocarbons, and oleoresins. These compounds have been investigated and shown to be effective anti-inflammatory, anti-bacterial, and antioxidant agents in oral microorganisms, which can help in disease prevention [8]. Moreover, ginger can help to reduce costs and side effects, and can introduce a safe inhibitory agent compared to conventional mouthwash [9]. It can be used also as an intracanal dressing, and in cases with recurrent apthous stomatitis and denture stomatitis [6–8]. However, it can lead to gastrointestinal irritation, heartburn, or diarrhea [6–8]. It can interfere with warfarin and inhibit platelet aggregation [6–8].

2.3 Clove

The principal phenolic components of clove, which is known scientifically as *Syzygium aromatic (S. aromatic)*, are volatile oil, eugenol, and eugenyl acetate. It has some physical properties that have an adverse effect on surface roughness and

Herbs	Main dental use	Main oral targeted organism
Aloe vera	Periodontal index, gingival scores, inhibitory activities on some organisms, intracanal Medicaments, oral medicine, after extraction, ill fitting denture, around implants complications.	*Streptococcus mutans, Aggregatibacter actinomycetemcomitans, Porphyromonas gingivalis, Bacteroides fragilis, Enterococcus faecalis*
Ginger	Pain killer, anti-inflammatory, anti-bacterial, intracanal dressing, recurrent apthous stomatitis and denture stomatitis	*Streptococcus mutans, Streptococcus sobrinus, Lactobacillus*
Clove	Inhibit the decalcification and promote the remineralization, topical agent, anti-bacterial	*S. mutans, Porphyromonas gingivalis, Prevotella intermedia, Candida albicans, Herpes Simplex virus 1 and 2*
Cinnamon	Endodontic irrigate solution, antimicrobial properties against cariogenic bacteria and fungicidal activity .	*E. faecalis, Candida tropicalis and Candida glabatra*
Garlic	Inhibition of the growth of the periodontal pathogens, Endodontic irrigate solution.	*Aggregatibacter actinomycetemcomitans, P. gingivalis, Fusobacterium nucleatum, Streptococcus mutans and Lactobacillus acidophilus*
Neem	Endodontic irrigation soluation, antiviral, antibacterial, antisclerotic and antiinflammatory properties. A local drug delivery system, inhibition of oral epithelial cell carcinoma.	*E. faecalis, P. gingivalis, S. mutans, S. faecalis, S. salivarius, S. mitis, and S. sanguis*
Miswak	Reduction of plaque, bacterial oral germs, prevent cavities, halitosis. Dentifrice, chronic periodontitis, mouthwash,remineralization effects, anti-cariogenic, whitening properties, and orthodontic chain preservation.	*Porphyromonas gingivalis and Herpes simplex virus-1.*
Turmeric	Antibacterial, antitumor, antioxidant, anti-inflammatory and analgesic properties. Mouth rinse, erythematous halo, ulcer size, and pain, oral submucous fibrosis	*Aggregatibacter actinomycetemcomitans, Porphyromonas gingivalis, and Tannerella forsythia.*
Tulsi	Antimicrobial agents. Toothpaste or mouthwash	*A. actinomycetemcomitans, P. gingivalis and P. intermedia*
Green tea	Antibacterial properties. Minimize bone loss in periodontal disease cases, mouth rinse, local drug delivery, and chewing gum.	*Streptococcus mutans, Streptococcus sobrin, P. gingivalis and P. melaninogenicus.*
Chamomile	Anti-inflammatory property, mouth rinse for gingivitis and periodontal disease, management of burning mouth syndrome, irrigant solution.	*Porphyromonas gingivalis*
Fenugreek	Gingival index, plaque index, bleeding on probing, pocket depth, and clinical attachment levels.	
Anise plant	Antibacterial properties, mouth rinse, increase healing process	*E. corrodens and Prevotella spp.*
Peppermint	Toothpaste or mouth rinse, antibiofilm properties. Topical analgesic and reduces pain. Treatment of gingivitis, periodontitis, oral mucosa of viral, bacterial, fungal and protozoal etiology. Decrease the treatment time, faster tissue regeneration, faster relieved pain and swelling, and improved the patients' quality of life. Mouthwash.	*Streptococcus mutans*

Herbs	Main dental use	Main oral targeted organism
Bloodroot	Periodontal disease, toothpaste or other oral hygiene products.	*P. gingivalis.*
Carawa	Mouth wash in gingivitis or periodontal disease. Flavor component in toothpaste and mouthwash products.	*Fusobacterium nucleatum,* early and late bacterial colonizers .
Eucalyptus	Anti-bacterial, antibiotics and oral infections prevention, dissolve root canal sealer	*A. actinomycetemcomitans and P. gingivalis, Streptococcus mutans, Lactobacillus acidophilus*
Phyllanthus emblica	Antimicrobial, antioxidant, antiresorptive and antiinflammatory activity. Locally delivered gel	Group of bacteria
Black seed	Suppresses pro-inflammatory cytokines, anti-bacterial, and decrease oral halitosis.	*Porphyromonas gingivalis, A. actinomycetemcomitans and Prevotella intermedia, S. mutans, Enterobacter cloacae, Streptococcus oralis, Streptococcus anginosus, Staphylococcus epidermide.*
Myrrh	Antimicrobial properties, immune enhancer. Topical or a mouth wash, manage pharyngitis, tonsillitis, gum swelling, aphthous ulcers, intramucosal wounds, gingivitis and ulcers. Anti-inflammatory activity such as IL-1β, IL-6, and TNF-α.	*Streptococcus mutans, Lactobacillus spp, Porphyromonas gingivalis, A. actinomycetemcomitans, Treponema denticola, and Tannerella forsythia*
Rosemary	Antioxidant, antibacterial, antifungal, anticancer.	*Staphylococcus aureus, Staphylococcus albus, Vibrio cholerae and Escherichia coli*
Sage	Mouthwash or gargle, sore throat, gingivitis, antibacterial, antifungal.	*Streptococcus mutans, Lactobacillus rhamnosus, Actinomyces viscosus, Candida albicans*
Thyme	Spasmodic, whooping cough, oral herpes, chronic candidiasis and halitosis.	*S. aureus, E. coli, C. albicans Streptococcus mutans*

Table 1.
The most common herbs used in dentistry and the dental application.

hardness, as well as transverse strength [10–13]. A high dose of clove oil can cause serious problems, such as sore throat, vomiting, toxicity, damage to the kidney and liver, epilepsy, and difficulty breathing. In small doses, it can inhibit decalcification and promotes remineralization (**Table 1**, [14]). It can be used as a topical agent, as a benzocaine before needle insertion, and has similar pain scores [15]. The crude extract of *S. aromaticum* (clove) has shown inhibitory activity against periodontal oral pathogens, including *S. mutans* (**Table 1**, [16]).

Other potential dental uses include antibacterial activity against *Porphyromonas gingivalis and Prevotella intermedia* [13]. It minimize several cytokines and factors such as IL-6, COX-2 and TNF-α. It has antifungal activity against *Candida albicans* [10–16], and antiviral activity against *Herpes Simplex virus 1 and 2* [10–16]. It can be used as mouthwashes, toothpastes, topical agents and local drug delivery devices [10–16]. Clove and its components are generally considered as "safe". However, it has been demonstrated as a cytotoxic agent towards fibroblasts and endothelial cells in vitro studies [10–16]. Moreover, hepatotoxicity, generalized seizures and disseminated intravascular coagulopathy has been reported as severe side effects [10–16]. Other potential side effects include skin irritation, ulcer formation, contact dermatitis, tissue necrosis, and delayed healing [10–16].

2.4 Cinnamon

Cinnamon is commonly referred to *Cinnamon Zeylanicum* or *Cinnamon cassia*. It can be used as an endodontic irrigant to minimize the *E. faecalis*, which is comparable to 3% of sodium hypochlorite [17]. Cinnamon has good antimicrobial properties against cariogenic bacteria such as *S. mutans* and *Lactobacillus casei* [18], as well as fungicidal activity against *Candida tropicalis* and *Candida glabatra* (**Table 1**, [18]).

Chewing gum containing cinnamon may help in the management of halitosis cases by minimizing volatile sulfur compounds inside the oral cavity [19]. The toothpaste that contained *Cinnamomum zeylanicum* showed anti-bacterial activity against periodontal pathogens (**Table 1**, [20]). It can be used in the dental unit water lines, which minimized bacterial count [21].

There are potential side effects such as tooth discoloration with high exposure to cinnamon [17–21], allergic reaction such as swelling, inflammation, burning, soreness of the mouth and lips [17–21].

2.5 Garlic

Several in vitro studies found that the inhibition of the growth of the periodontal pathogens can happen with the aqueous extract, allicin [22], and diallyl sulfide of garlic [23]. The targeted pathogens are *Aggregatibacter actinomycetemcomitans*, *P. gingivalis*, and *Fusobacterium nucleatum* (**Table 1**, [24]).

When used as an irrigant, it is an effective, safe, and natural product, and is comparable to sodium hypochlorite after using it for a period of 12 months following root canals of primary molars [25]. The maximum zone of inhibition against cariogenic bacteria, such as *Streptococcus mutans* and *Lactobacillus acidophilus*, was in hard neck garlic extract, followed by chlorhexidine mouthwash [26]. The methanolic component of garlic had no anti-bacterial effects on *S. aureus* and *P. aeruginosa* [27].

Unpleasant breath or body odor is the most common side effects of garlic use [22–27]. Other side effects include heartburn, burning in a mouth or throat [22–27]. Patients need medical advice before garlic use if he/she is taking the following medications: acetaminophen; birth control pills; or warfarin [22–27].

2.6 Neem

Neem is scientifically known as *Azadirachta indica* and can be used as an endodontic irrigation solution to minimize the *E. faecalis*, which is comparable to 3% of sodium hypochlorite [17]. It has antiviral, anti-bacterial (*S. mutans, S. faecalis, S. salivarius, S. mitis, and S. sanguis)*, anti-sclerotic, and anti-inflammatory properties. A local drug delivery system using 10% neem oil chip statistically reduced *P. gingivalis* and all clinical parameters in periodontal-diseased patients (**Table 1**, [28]).

The highly pure neem leaf extract has proven potential inhibition of oral epithelial cell carcinoma through downregulation of intra tumor pro inflammatory pathways [29]. However, it was less effective in plaque scores reduction among orthodontic patients compared to *Salvadora persica* miswak-based mouthwash [30]. It has Anti-candidial activity against *C. albicans,* and it inhibits *S. mutans* and *E. faecalis* which cause root canal failure in endodontic procedure [17, 28–30].

2.7 Miswak

Salvadora persicahas have potential benefits in reduction of plaque, bacterial oral germs, cavity prevention, and halitosis [31]. It contains high amounts of calcium, chloride, phosphate, and thiocyanate, which, as a consequence, can affect saliva and oral health [32]. When used in the dentifrice, it can lead to significant reduction in plaque index scores compared to conventional dentifrice [33]. The miswak raw extract is effective against *Porphyromonas gingivalis* and *herpes simplex virus-1* in chronic periodontitis patients (**Table 1**, [34]).

The mouthwash form has been investigated as an effective method for plaque reduction [35]. It can also be used as a chewing gum, mouthwash, and chewing stick [31–35]. It has remineralization effects following dental caries. Miswak can accelerate the wound healing after oral/periodontal surgery or extraction. It has potential anti-cariogenic, whitening properties and orthodontic chain preservation [35].

2.8 Turmeric

Curcumin (Turmeric) has shown anti-bacterial, anti-tumor, antioxidant, anti-inflammatory, and analgesic properties [36]. It can be used as a topical application, mouthwash, subgingival irrigant or local drug delivery system to treat periodontal diseases, with equivalent or even higher efficacy compared with chlorhexidine in periodontopathic bacteria reduction such as *Aggregatibacter actinomycetemcomitans, Porphyromonas gingivalis*, and *Tannerella forsythia* (**Table 1**, [36]).

The extract gel can be used as a treatment for erythematous areas, ulcers, and pain [37]. It can help in cases with oral submucous fibrosis, leukoplakia, lichen planus and it gave better results compared with the systemic form alone, or antioxidants (**Table 1**). It has anticancer activity as well [36, 37].

Although it considered safe, it may cause gastric irritation, nausea, diarrhea, allergic reaction, and interfering with blood-clot formation [36, 37].

2.9 Tulsi

Tulsi is released in several metabolites found in these plants, which have antimicrobial agents. It can be used in toothpaste or mouthwash [38]. It is similar to chlorhexidine in its antimicrobial property, and as an alternative in patients who cannot use chlorhexidine [39]. Tulsi extracts have antimicrobial activity against *A. actinomycetemcomitans, P. gingivalis*, and *P. intermedia*, with different inhibition zones (**Table 1**, [40]).

2.10 Green tea

Green tea and its principal compound (*flavonoid epigallocatechin-3-gallate*) are responsible for protective effects against several diseases and has anti-bacterial properties [41]. They can minimize bone loss in osteoporosis and periodontal disease cases by inducing apoptotic cell death of osteoclasts and osteoclasts-like cells (**Table 1**, [41]).

Green tea extract rich in epigallocatechin gallate minimizes alveolar bone loss in rats with periodontal disease [42]. It can be used in different forms, such as mouthwash, local drug delivery, and chewing gum. It has catechins that is anti-bacterial against *Streptococcus mutans*, *Streptococcus sobrin*, *P. gingivalis*, and *P. melaninogenicus* (**Table 1**, [42]).

2.11 Chamomile

Chamomile, known as *Matricaria recutita*, contains volatile oils, flavonoids, apigenin, luteolin, and quercetin [43]. It has an anti-inflammatory property that is as effective as a mouthwash for gingivitis and periodontal disease. There was a zone of inhibition when tested against *P. gingivalis* (**Table 1**, [44]). However, eucalyptus oil was the most effective, followed by tea tree oil, chamomile oil, and turmeric oil [45]. It can be used in management of burning mouth syndrome cases and as an irrigate solution (**Table 1**, [46]). It can be used topically in the treatment of eczema [43–46]. In fact, a randomized clinical trial found it to be equivalent to hydrocortisone cream [43–46]. However, it can cause allergic reactions which included bronchial constriction and skin reactions [43]. It is controversial to use with a pregnant women since it caused a newborn death in a single case report.

2.12 Fenugreek

There was a significant reduction in several parameters, such as gingival index, plaque index, bleeding on probing, pocket depth, and clinical attachment levels, when fenugreek was used clinically (**Table 1**, [47]). It has antibacterial activity against S. mutans, biofilm formation and acid production [47]. It was able to increase the salivary pH up to 7.83 and decreased the demineralization of the tooth's outer surface [47]. Fenugreek is considered unsafe to use during pregnancy, breastfeeding and for children. Do not use this product without medical advice if you are pregnant [47]. It can interact with blood sugar levels and cause hypoglycemia), or cause bleeding/blood clotting disorders [47].

2.13 Anise Plant

Anise has potent anti-bacterial properties due to the presence of anethole [43]. It has a strong effect against *Staphylococcus aureus*, as well as some gram-positive and gram-negative microorganisms. In the oral cavity, it works on anaerobic and facultative aerobic periodontal bacteria such as *E. corrodens* and *Prevotella spp* (**Table 1**, [43]). When used as a mouthwash, it was comparable to chlorhexidine in reducing bleeding on probing and increasing the healing process [43]. Anise is likely safe for most adults [43].

2.14 Peppermint

Mentha piperita can be used in a toothpaste or mouthwash, which showed anti-biofilm properties against *Streptococcus mutans* and dental plaque (**Table 1**, [48]). It can be used topically as an analgesic and to reduce pain. It can also reduce a toothache [48]. It showed antimicrobial, analgesic, anti-inflammatory, immunomodulatory, and astringent properties. It can be used in treatment of gingivitis, periodontitis, and oral mucosa of viral, bacterial, fungal, and protozoal etiology (**Table 1**). It can lead to a decrease in treatment time, faster tissue regeneration, faster relieved pain and swelling, and improved quality of life for the patients. It has also been used as a mouthwash [48]. It can be used safely in most of the cases [48]. However, it may interfere with iron absorption [48]. It can cause burning and gastrointestinal distresses in some cases. It is contraindicated in patients with chronic heartburn, severe liver damage, gallbladder inflammation or obstruction [48], and peppermint oil should be avoided in any facial application on children and infants [48].

2.15 Bloodroot

Bloodroot is an alkaloid known as *Sanguinaria canadensis*. It has been used for periodontal disease due to its ability to inhibit the growth of oral bacteria such as *P. gingivalis* (**Table 1**, [43]). It's available in toothpaste or as other oral hygiene products, and it is safe in long-term use. However, a recent report found that dental preparations with bloodroot may be associated with leukoplakia which is a precancerous lesion [43]. It is contraindicated in children, pregnant or lactating women [43]. The overdose can lead to stomachache, diarrhea, visual impairment, glaucoma, miscarriage, paralysis, and heart disease [43].

2.16 Caraway

The main components of *Carum carvi* are carvone and limonene. It can be used as a mouthwash in gingivitis or periodontal disease (**Table 1**, [43]). It can also be used as a flavor component in toothpaste and mouthwash products. It can target *Fusobacterium nucleatum* and early- and late-bacterial colonizers on tooth surfaces [43]. However, it should not be used in children under 2 years old because it may be cause irritation to the skin and mucous membranes [43].

2.17 Eucalyptus

Eucalyptus is effective against *A. actinomycetemcomitans* and *P. gingivalis* (**Table 1**). It can be used as a promising alternative to antibiotics and oral infections prevention [49]. It can stimulate the innate cell-mediated immune response, tumor chemotherapy [50]. Eucalyptus oil has the ability to dissolve root canal sealer (**Table 1**, [51]). It has anti cariogenic activity against *Streptococcus mutans* and *Lactobacillus acidophilus* [49–51]. There are several potential side effects associated with the use of Eucalyptus such as: allergy, rashes, burning sensation, drowsiness, difficulty in breathing, cardiovascular collapse and multi-organ failure due to substantial ingestion of eucalyptus mouthwash [49–51].

2.18 Phyllanthus Emblica

Emblica officinalis has several properties, such as cytoprotective, antimicrobial, antioxidant, anti-resorptive, and anti-inflammatory activity. It can be used as a locally delivered gel and as an adjunct to scaling and root planning, which will reduce the periodontal inflammation in chronic periodontitis cases compared with scaling alone [52]. It can reduce all strains of yeasts stick in the buccal epithelial cells compared with normal saline solution [53]. It can be used a mouthwash to treat mouth ulcers, and aphthous [52, 53]. It is the best remedy for scurvy due to vitamin C contents and pain reliefs [52, 53]. Even though Phyllanthus has been used as traditional medicine for long term, side effects may include stomach upset and diarrhea [52, 53]. It should be avoided in children, pregnant women, breastfeeding mothers, and patients with Wilson's disease [52, 53]. It can inhibit blood clotting and should not be used plavix (clopidogrel) because it increased bleeding [52, 53].

2.19 Black seed

Miracle herb, or *Nigella sativa*, can reduce nitric oxide levels and inhibit pro-inflammatory cytokines such as IL-1b, IL-6, TNF-α, IFN-c, and PGE2. It can also increase the anti-inflammatory IL-10 [54, 55]. It works against *Porphyromonas gingivalis*, *A. actinomycetemcomitans*, and *Prevotella intermedia* (**Table 1**). It also decreases oral halitosis [54–58]. The black seed were found to have a bactericidal effect surface inhibition against *S. mutans* [54–58]. It can be used as an intracanal antisepsis in root canal therapy due to its activity against *Enterobacter cloacae*, *Streptococcus oralis*, *Streptococcus anginosus*, and *Staphylococcus epidermides* [54–58]. It has beneficial effects on oral ulcerations, oral mucositis, bone and wound healing after extraction or surgery [54–58].

2.20 Myrrh

Commiphora molm has three components: the resin, the gum, and the volatile oil. It has antimicrobial properties and immune enhancer [59–61]. It can be used as a topical or a mouth wash to manage pharyngitis, tonsillitis, gingivitis and ulcers with 2–3 times per day [59–61]. There is no known side effects with its used [62–65]. It works against caries bacteria such as *Streptococcus mutans* and *Lactobacillus spp*, and periodontal disease microbes such as *Porphyromonas gingivalis*, *A. actinomycetemcomitans*, *Treponema denticola, and Tannerella forsythia* (**Table 1**, [62–65]). It has anti-inflammatory activity through proinflammatory cytokines reduction such as IL-1β, IL-6, and TNF-α [66]. It can be used in cases with gum swelling, aphthous ulcers, and intramucosal wounds [62–66]. It can lead to significant reduction in plaque and gingival inflations compared with 0.2% Chlorhexidine Gluconate mouthwash [64].

2.21 Rosemary

Rosmarinus officinalisy has antioxidant activity and effective as an antibacterial and antifungal agents [43]. It can inhabit cancer development in animal studies [43]. It works against *Staphylococcus aureus, Staphylococcus albus, Vibrio cholerae and Escherichia coli* (**Table 1**, [43]). However, it should be avoided during pregnancy to minimize the risk of abortion [43]. It can lead to iron deficiency in same cases as well [43].

2.22 Sage

The main components of *Salvia officinalis* are alpha and beta-thujone, rosmarinic acid, camphor, tannins, flavonoids, and cineole [43]. It can be used as mouthwash or gargle several times to treat a sore throat and gingivitis [43]. It has antibacterial (*Streptococcus mutans, Lactobacillus rhamnosus, and Actinomyces viscosus*), and antifungal (*Candida albicans*) (**Table 1**, [43]). The long term used can increased heart rate, caused mental confusion and convulsions [43]. It should be avoided during pregnancy and cases with fever [43].

2.23 Thyme

Thymus vulgaris is one of the most commonly recommended herbs in Europe in spasmodic and whooping cough [43]. It can be used to treat oral herpes, chronic candidiasis and halitosis [43]. It targeted *S. aureus, E. coli and C. albicans* [43]. Patients with orthodontic brackets can used it as varnish to reduce *Streptococcus mutans* near the bracket (**Table 1**, [43]).

3. Conclusions

Herbal medicine can be beneficial in the dental field in dental caries, periodontal disease, candida and viral infection, oral ulcers and lesions. It has several advantages such as easy accessibility, natural products, low cost and toxicity, and faster healing time. However, it can lead to serious problems if used inappropriately. Therefore, a physician consultation is required before any dental use to avoid any potential complications or drug interaction, and a deeper investigation, preclinically and clinically, is needed before official herbal medicine use is highly recommended.

Conflict of interest

The authors declare no conflict of interest.

Author details

Zuhair S. Natto
Faculty of Dentistry, Department of Dental Public Health, King Abdulaziz University, Jeddah, Saudi Arabia

*Address all correspondence to: znatto@kau.edu.sa

References

[1] Fulzele P, Baliga S, Thosar N, Pradhan D. Evaluation of aloe vera gel as a storage medium in maintaining the viability of periodontal ligament cells-an in vitro study. The Journal of Clinical Pediatric Dentistry. 2016;**40**(1):49-52. DOI: 10.17796/1053-4628-40.1.49

[2] Al-Maweri SA, Nassani MZ, Alaizari N, Kalakonda B, Al-Shamiri HM, Alhajj MN, et al. Efficacy of aloe vera mouthwash versus chlorhexidine on plaque and gingivitis: A systematic review. International Journal of Dental Hygiene. 2020;**18**(1):44-51. DOI: 10.1111/idh.12393

[3] Sayar F, Farahmand AH, Rezazadeh M. Clinical efficacy of aloe vera toothpaste on periodontal parameters of patients with gingivitis-a randomized, controlled, single-masked clinical trial. The Journal of Contemporary Dental Practice. 2021;**22**(3):242-247

[4] Fani M, Kohanteb J. Inhibitory activity of aloe vera gel on some clinically isolated cariogenic and periodontopathic bacteria. Journal of Oral Science. 2012;**54**(1):15-21. DOI: 10.2334/josnusd.54.15

[5] Ghasemi N, Behnezhad M, Asgharzadeh M, Zeinalzadeh E, Kafil HS. Antibacterial properties of aloe vera on intracanal medicaments against Enterococcus faecalis biofilm at different stages of development. International Journal of Dentistry. 2020;**2020**:8855277. DOI: 10.1155/2020/8855277

[6] Rayati F, Hajmanouchehri F, Najafi E. Comparison of anti-inflammatory and analgesic effects of ginger powder and ibuprofen in postsurgical pain model: A randomized, double-blind, case-control clinical trial. Dental Research Journal. 2017;**14**(1):1-7. DOI: 10.4103/1735-3327.201135

[7] Zare Javid A, Bazyar H, Gholinezhad H, Rahimlou M, Rashidi H, Salehi P, et al. The effects of ginger supplementation on inflammatory, antioxidant, and periodontal parameters in type 2 diabetes mellitus patients with chronic periodontitis under non-surgical periodontal therapy. A double-blind, placebo-controlled trial. Diabetes, Metabolic Syndrome and Obesity: Targets and Therapy. 2019;**12**:1751-1761. DOI: 10.2147/DMSO.S214333

[8] Rashmi KJ, Tiwari R. Pharmacotherapeutic properties of ginger and its use in diseases of the oral cavity: A narrative review. Journal of Advanced Oral Research. 2016;7:1-6

[9] Shrimathi S, Kemparaj U, Umesh S, Karuppaiah M, Pandian P, Krishnaveni A. Comparative evaluation of cocoa bean husk, ginger and chlorhexidine mouth washes in the reduction of steptococcus mutans and lactobacillus count in saliva: A randomized controlled trial. Cureus. 2019;**11**(6):e4968. DOI: 10.7759/cureus.4968

[10] Reisbick MH, Brodsky JF. Strength parameters of composite resins. The Journal of Prosthetic Dentistry. 1971;**26**(2):178-185. DOI: 10.1016/0022-3913(71)90050-3

[11] Grajower R, Hirschfeld Z, Zalkind M. Compatibility of a composite resin with pulp insulating materials. A scanning electron microscope study. The Journal of Prosthetic Dentistry. 1974;**32**(1):70-77. DOI: 10.1016/0022-3913(74)90101-2

[12] Millstein PL, Nathanson D. Effect of eugenol and eugenol cements on cured composite resin. The Journal of Prosthetic Dentistry. 1983;**50**(2):211-215. DOI: 10.1016/0022-3913(83)90016-1

[13] Paige H, Hirsch SM, Gelb MN. Effects of temporary cements on crown-to-composite resin core bond strength. The Journal of Prosthetic Dentistry. 1986;**55**(1):49-52. DOI: 10.1016/0022-3913(86)90072-7

[14] Marya CM, Satija G, Avinash J, Nagpal R, Kapoor R, Ahmad A. In vitro inhibitory effect of clove essential oil and its two active principles on tooth decalcification by apple juice. International Journal of Dentistry. 2012;**2012**:759618. DOI: 10.1155/2012/759618

[15] Alqareer A, Alyahya A, Andersson L. The effect of clove and benzocaine versus placebo as topical anesthetics. Journal of Dentistry. 2006;**34**(10):747-750. DOI: 10.1016/j.jdent.2006.01.009

[16] Uju DE, Obioma NP. Anticariogenic potentials of clove, tobacco and bitter kola. Asian Pacific Journal of Tropical Medicine. 2011;**4**(10):814-818. DOI: 10.1016/S1995-7645(11)60200-9

[17] Panchal V, Gurunathan D, Muralidharan NP. Comparison of antibacterial efficacy of cinnamon extract, neem extract as irrigant and sodium hypochlorite against Enterococcus fecalis: An in vitro study. Indian Journal of Dental Research. 2020;**31**(1):124-128. DOI: 10.4103/ijdr.IJDR_177_18

[18] Wiwattanarattanabut K, Choonharuangdej S, Srithavaj T. In vitro anti-cariogenic plaque effects of essential oils extracted from culinary herbs. Journal of Clinical and Diagnostic Research. 2017;**11**:DC30-DC35. DOI: 10.7860/JCDR/2017/28327.10668

[19] Zhu M, Carvalho R, Scher A, Wu CD. Short-term germ-killing effect of sugar-sweetened cinnamon chewing gum on salivary anaerobes associated with halitosis. The Journal of Clinical Dentistry. 2011;**22**(1):23-26

[20] Saquib SA, AlQahtani NA, Ahmad I, Kader MA, Al Shahrani SS, Asiri EA. Evaluation and comparison of antibacterial efficacy of herbal extracts in combination with antibiotics on periodontal pathobionts: An in vitro microbiological study. Antibiotics. 2019;**8**(3):89. DOI: 10.3390/antibiotics8030089

[21] Mamajiwala AS, Sethi KS, Raut CP, Karde PA, Khedkar SU. Comparative evaluation of chlorhexidine and cinnamon extract used in dental unit waterlines to reduce bacterial load in aerosols during ultrasonic scaling. Indian Journal of Dental Research. 2018;**29**(6):749-754. DOI: 10.4103/ijdr.IJDR_571_17

[22] Bakri IM, Douglas CW. Inhibitory effect of garlic extract on oral bacteria. Archives of Oral Biology. 2005;**50**:645-651. DOI: 10.1016/j.archoralbio.2004.12.002

[23] Bachrach G, Jamil A, Naor R, Tal G, Ludmer Z, Steinberg D. Garlic allicin as a potential agent for controlling oral pathogens. Journal of Medicinal Food. 2011;**14**:1338-1343. DOI: 10.1089/jmf.2010.0165

[24] Velliyagounder K, Ganeshnarayan K, Velusamy SK, Fine DH. In vitro efficacy of diallyl sulfides against the periodontopathogen Aggregatibacter actinomycetemcomitans. Antimicrobial Agents and Chemotherapy. 2012;**56**:2397-2407. DOI: 10.1128/AAC.00020-12

[25] Elheeny AAH. Allium sativum extract as an irrigant in pulpectomy of primary molars: A 12-month short-term evaluation. Clinical and Experimental Dental Research. 2019;**5**(4):420-426. DOI: 10.1002/cre2.197

[26] Kshirsagar MM, Dodamani AS, Karibasappa GN, Vishwakarma PK, Vathar JB, Sonawane KR, et al. Antibacterial activity of garlic extract on cariogenic bacteria: An in vitro study. Ayu. 2018;**39**(3):165-168. DOI: 10.4103/ayu.AYU_193_16

[27] Momeni R, Hosseini Z, Aghamolaei T, Ghanbarnejad A. Determinants factors to pap smear screening among married women in a city of South Iran: Applying the BASNEF model. BMC Women's Health. 2020;**20**(1):237. DOI: 10.1186/s12905-020-01102-6

[28] Vennila K, Elanchezhiyan S, Ilavarasu S. Efficacy of 10% whole Azadirachta indica (neem) chip as an adjunct to scaling and root planning in chronic periodontitis: A clinical and microbiological study. Indian Journal of Dental Research. 2016;**27**(1):15-21. DOI: 10.4103/0970-9290.179808

[29] Morris J, Gonzales CB, De La Chapa JJ, Cabang AB, Fountzilas C, Patel M, et al. The highly pure neem leaf extract, SCNE, inhibits tumorigenesis in oral squamous cell carcinoma via disruption of pro-tumor inflammatory cytokines and cell Signaling. Frontiers in Oncology. 2019;**9**:890. DOI: 10.3389/fonc.2019.00890

[30] Niazi FH, Kamran MA, Naseem M, AlShahrani I, Fraz TR, Hosein M. Anti-plaque efficacy of herbal mouthwashes compared to synthetic mouthwashes in patients undergoing orthodontic treatment: A randomised controlled trial. Oral Health & Preventive Dentistry. 2018;**16**(5):409-416. DOI: 10.3290/j.ohpd.a40983

[31] Ahmad H. Biological activities of Salvadora persica L. (Meswak). Medicinal & Aromatic Plants. 2017;**2**:129. DOI: 10.4172/2167-0412.1000129

[32] Kaur S, Abdul Jalil R, Akmar SL. The immediate term effect of chewing commercially available Meswak (Salvadora Persica) on levels of calcium, chloride, phosphate and thiocyanate in whole saliva. Annals of Dentistry. 2004;**11**(1):51-59. DOI: 10.22452/adum.vol11no1.8

[33] Gupta P, Agarwal N, Anup N, Manujunath BC, Bhalla A. Evaluating the anti-plaque efficacy of meswak (Salvadora persica) containing dentifrice: A triple blind controlled trial. Journal of Pharmacy & Bioallied Sciences. 2012;**4**(4):282-285. DOI: 10.4103/0975-7406.103238

[34] Sekar S, Jacob S, Suthanthiran TK, Dhasthaheer S, Vikraman S, Kaliappan K. Characterization and formulation of Miswak film for the treatment of chronic periodontitis: An in vitro study. Journal of Pharmacy & Bioallied Sciences. 2020;**12**(Suppl 1):S199-S203. DOI: 10.4103/jpbs.JPBS_59_20

[35] Nordin A, Bin Saim A, Ramli R, Abdul Hamid A, Mohd Nasri NW, Bt Hj Idrus R. Miswak and oral health: An evidence-based review. Saudi Journal of Biological Sciences. 2020;**27**(7):1801-1810. DOI: 10.1016/j.sjbs.2020.05.020

[36] Forouzanfar F, Forouzanfar A, Sathyapalan T, Orafai HM, Sahebkar A. Curcumin for the management of periodontal diseases: A review. Current Pharmaceutical Design. 2020;**26**(34):4277-4284. DOI: 10.2174/1381612826666200513112607

[37] Nurdiana N, Krishnasamy S. Effect of two percent turmeric extract gel on minor recurrent aphthous stomatitis. Padjadjaran Journal of Dentistry. 2016;**28**(1):1-6. DOI: 10.24198/pjd.vol28no1.13503

[38] Lolayekar NV, Kadkhodayan SS. Estimation of salivary pH and viability of

Streptococcus mutans on chewing of tulsi leaves in children. Journal of the Indian Society of Pedodontics and Preventive Dentistry. 2019;**37**(1):87-91. DOI: 10.4103/JISPPD.JISPPD_91_17

[39] Ahmed SV, Reddy CS, Kudlure SM, Gomasani S. Effect of tulsi extract and honey mouthrinses on salivary Streptococcus mutans count in comparison with 0.2% of chlorhexidine: A randomized controlled trial. Journal of Indian Association of Public Health Dentistry. 2017;**15**(4):306-311. DOI: 10.4103/jiaphd.jiaphd_55_17

[40] Mallikarjun S, Rao A, Rajesh G, Shenoy R, Pai M. Antimicrobial efficacy of tulsi leaf (Ocimum sanctum) extract on periodontal pathogens: An in vitro study. Journal of Indian Society of Periodontology. 2016;**20**(2):145-150. DOI: 10.4103/0972-124X.175177

[41] Vargas-Sanchez PK, Pitol DL, de Sousa LG, Beloti MM, Rosa AL, Rossi AC, et al. Green tea extract rich in epigallocatechin gallate impairs alveolar bone loss in ovariectomized rats with experimental periodontal disease. International Journal of Experimental Pathology. 2020;**101**(6):277-288. DOI: 10.1111/iep.12379

[42] Venkateswara B, Sirisha K, Chava VK. Green tea extract for periodontal health. Journal of Indian Society of Periodontology. 2011;**15**(1): 18-22. DOI: 10.4103/0972-124X.82258

[43] Taheri JB, Azimi S, Rafieian N, Zanjani HA. Herbs in dentistry. International Dental Journal. 2011;**61**(6):287-296. DOI: 10.1111/j.1875-595X.2011.00064.x

[44] Hans VM, Grover HS, Deswal H, Agarwal P. Antimicrobial efficacy of various essential oils at varying concentrations against Periopathogen Porphyromonas gingivalis. Journal of Clinical and Diagnostic Research. 2016;**10**(9):ZC16-ZC19

[45] Aitken-Saavedra J, Chaves Tarquinio SB, De Oliveira da Rosa WL, Fernandes da Silva A, Almeida Machado BM, Santos Castro I, et al. Effect of a homemade salivary substitute prepared using chamomile (Matricaria chamomilla L.) flower and flax (Linum usitatissimum L.) seed to relieve primary burning mouth syndrome: A preliminary report. Journal of Alternative and Complementary Medicine. 2020;**26**(9): 799-806. DOI: 10.1089/acm.2019.0478

[46] Venkataram V, Gokhale ST, Kenchappa M, Nagarajappa R. Effectiveness of chamomile (Matricaria recutita L.), MTAD and sodium hypochlorite irrigants on smear layer. European Archives of Paediatric Dentistry. 2013;**14**(4):247-252. DOI: 10.1007/s40368-013-0062-3

[47] Sundaram G, Ramakrishnan T, Parthasarathy H, Raja M, Raj S. Fenugreek, diabetes, and periodontal disease: A cross-link of sorts! Journal of Indian Society of Periodontology. 2018;**22**(2):122-126. DOI: 10.4103/jisp.jisp_322_17

[48] Ashrafi B, Rashidipour M, Marzban A, Soroush S, Azadpour M, Delfani S, et al. Mentha piperita essential oils loaded in a chitosan nanogel with inhibitory effect on biofilm formation against *S. mutans* on the dental surface. Carbohydrate Polymers. 2019;**212**:142-149. DOI: 10.1016/j.carbpol.2019.02.018

[49] Bankur PK, Mathew M, Almalki SA, Jalaluddin M, Jayanti I, Durgaraju M. An in vitro evaluation of antibacterial efficacy of various concentration of eucalyptus globulus leaf extract on periodontal pathogens. The Journal of

Contemporary Dental Practice. 2019;**20**(9):1041-1044

[50] Yap PS, Lim SH, Hu CP, Yiap BC. Combination of essential oils and antibiotics reduce antibiotic resistance in plasmid-conferred multidrug resistant bacteria. Phytomedicine. 2013;**20**(8-9): 710-713. DOI: 10.1016/j.phymed.2013. 02.013

[51] Yadav HK, Yadav RK, Chandra A, Thakkar RR. The effectiveness of eucalyptus oil, orange oil, and xylene in dissolving different endodontic sealers. Journal of Conservative Dentistry. 2016;**19**(4):332-337. DOI: 10.4103/ 0972-0707.186447

[52] Grover S, Tewari S, Sharma RK, Singh G, Yadav A, Naula SC. Effect of subgingivally delivered 10% emblica officinalis gel as an adjunct to scaling and root planning in the treatment of chronic periodontitis - a randomized placebo-controlled clinical trial. Phytotherapy Research. 2016;**30**(6):956-962. DOI: 10.1002/ptr.5600

[53] Thaweboon B, Thaweboon S. Effect of Phyllanthus emblica Linn. On candida adhesion to oral epithelium and denture acrylic. Asian Pacific Journal of Tropical Medicine. 2011;**4**(1):41-45. DOI: 10.1016/ S1995-7645(11)60029-1

[54] Mekhemar M, Hassan Y, Dörfer C. Nigella sativa and thymoquinone: A natural blessing for periodontal therapy. Antioxidants. 2020;**9**(12):1260. DOI: 10.3390/antiox9121260

[55] Tada A, Nakayama-Imaohji H, Yamasaki H, Elahi M, Nagao T, Yagi H, et al. Effect of thymoquinone on fusobacterium nucleatum-associated biofilm and inflammation. Molecular Medicine Reports. 2020;**22**(2):643-650. DOI: 10.3892/mmr.2020.11136

[56] ALHarthi SSY, Natto ZS, Midle JB, Gyurko R, O'Neill R, Steffensen B. Association between time since quitting smoking and periodontitis in former smokers in the National Health and Nutrition Examination Surveys (NHANES) 2009 to 2012. Journal of Periodontology. 2019;**90**(1):16-25. DOI: 10.1002/JPER.18-0183

[57] Alshaeri HK, Natto ZS. A contemporary look at COVID-19 medications: Available and potentially effective drugs. European Review for Medical and Pharmacological Sciences. 2020;**24**(17):9188-9195. DOI: 10.26355/ eurrev_202009_22870

[58] Alshaeri HK, Alasmari MM, Natto ZS, Pino-Figueroa A. Effects of annona muricata extract on triple-negative breast cancer cells mediated through EGFR signaling. Cancer Management and Research. 2020;**12**:12519-12526. DOI: 10.2147/ CMAR.S278647

[59] Shalaby MA, Hammouda AA. Analgesic, anti-inflammatory and anti-hyperlipidemic activities of commiphora molmol extract (myrrh). Journal of Intercultural Ethnopharmacology. 2014; **3**(2):56-62

[60] El Ashry ES, Rashed N, Salama OM, Saleh A. Components, therapeutic value and uses of myrrh. Pharmazie. 2003;**58**(3):163-168

[61] Mansour G, Ouda S, Shaker A, Abdallah HM. Clinical efficacy of new aloe vera and myrrh-based oral mucoadhesive gels in the management of minor recurrent aphthous stomatitis: A randomized, double-blind, vehicle-controlled study. Journal of Oral Pathology & Medicine. 2014;**43**(6): 405-409

[62] Al-Mobeeriek A. Effects of myrrh on intra-oral mucosal wounds compared with tetracycline and chlorhexidine-based mouthwashes. Clinical, Cosmetic and Investigational Dentistry. 2011;**3**:53-58

[63] Almekhlafi STA, Alwossabi AM, Awadth N, Thabet AA, Algaadari Z. Antimicrobial activity of Yemeni myrrh mouthwash. Journal of Chemical and Pharmaceutical Research. 2014;**6**(5): 1006-1013

[64] Kariuki HMAH, Wagaiyu EG. Effect of a natural extract toothpaste on the bacteria colonies of initial dental plaque colonizers. IOSR Journal of Dental and Medical Sciences. 2017;**16**(9):13-21

[65] Bassiouny G, Al-Barrak H. The anti-plaque effect of miswak and myrrh mouthwashes versus chlorhexidine in the treatment of chronic gingivitis; A comparative clinical trial. Medical Science. 2014;**9**(33):32-37

[66] Min-Sun Kim G-SB, Park K-C, et al. Myrrh inhibits LPS-induced inflammatory response and protects from cecal ligation and puncture-induced sepsis. Evidence-based Complementary and Alternative Medicine. 2012;**2012**:11

Chapter 19

The Contrasting Effects between Caffeine and Theobromine on Crystallization: How the Non-fluoride Dentifrice Was Developed

Tetsuo Nakamoto, Alexander U. Falster and William B. Simmons Jr

Abstract

Caffeine and theobromine are members of the xanthine family. Coffee and soft drinks contain caffeine, whereas, in cacao, theobromine is the main ingredient. The mineral contents of the tooth which sucked the caffeine-containing dam's milk were decreased. To determine if caffeine would affect enamel, dams were fed with a caffeine and pups were killed and first and second molars were extracted. Enamel was exposed to the acid solution and dissolved minerals from the enamel were measured. Calcium, phosphorus and magnesium from the first molars of the caffeine group were significantly dissolved. To determine why minerals were released, enamel was separated. The crystallite size of the enamel from the caffeine group showed decreased. If the pups with the same dietary regimen, but given a cariogenic diet, the caffeine group should show a higher incidence of dental caries. The caffeine group revealed higher caries scores. An in vitro experiment to grow apatite crystals was conducted, adding the various members of the xanthine. Theobromine produced larger crystal sizes than caffeine. Theobromine was added to the maternal diet. Dissolution experiments revealed that these minerals were far less dissolved. Comparative studies of the various parameters between theobromine and fluoride were conducted. Theobromine was superior to fluoride in every aspect.

Keywords: caffeine, crystallization, developing teeth, fluoride, growth and development, non-fluoride dentifrice, theobromine

1. Introduction

Caffeine (1,3,7-trimethylxanthine) is the substance most frequently consumed in our daily life. For example, coffee, most of the soft drinks and over-the-counter medications contain caffeine [1]. On the other hand, cocoa contains theobromine (3,7-dimethylxanthine). The main source of theobromine which is daily consumed by humans from childhood to adult is chocolate. Cocoa produces no adverse effect, in normal dosage [2]. These two similar families of xanthine, but the opposite properties on the crystal formation of the hydroxylapatite (HAP) of the teeth were discovered accidentally. Fluoride is the only known chemical that affected the HAP of the enamel by converting it to fluorohydroxylapatite.

In the dental community, fluoride has been used not only as the main ingredient of dentifrice but is also used in many others. However, recently fluoride was designated as one of the developmental neurotoxicants as more adverse effects of fluoride are revealed [3]. Although besides the developmental neurotoxicants, fluoride is also known to affect the pineal gland [4] and thyroid gland [5] and there is even some evidence between bone disease and fluoride exposure [6].

In addition, there are many reports [7–12] that infants, newborns and young children were exposed to fluoride and fluorosis among them is common. Unfortunately, in dentistry, fluorosis was mainly considered as an esthetic problem to which no more serious consideration is paid attention. Recently, it was proposed that fluoride exposure in early life may become a root cause of the disease in later life [13].

Pups' teeth were affected by the sucking milk of lactating dams which were given a caffeine-containing diet [14]. (In each animal experiment described, we obtained the permission to use the animals from the animal care committee at the LSU Health Sciences Center.) Then, eventually, non-fluoride dentifrices were developed.

2. The effect of caffeine on enamel

2.1 Dissolution studies

Further studies were conducted to determine whether the effects of caffeine come from either enamel or dentin, or both. If certain effects come from enamel, it would be an extremely interesting phenomenon, because the only chemical known to affect the HAP of the enamel is fluoride. In addition, any changes in the HAP on the enamel by caffeine might be linked to possible incidences of future dental caries.

Using the method described [15] on how to study the enamel surface of the teeth which were affected by the nutritional deficiency, the condition of the enamel was studied. The samples from the first or second molars were obtained at postnatal day 22 which is the end of lactation. The teeth were exposed to weak acid for 80 minutes and four fractions were collected at 20 minutes intervals. The experimental procedures were described in detail [16, 17]. The enamel surface of secondary electron photomicrographs are shown in the control (**Figure 1**) and caffeine group (**Figure 2**).

The apparent effects of crystallization by caffeine on the enamel of first molars where calcium, phosphorus and magnesium were released more of the teeth in the caffeine exposed offspring (**Table 1**). The first molars showed a statistically significant amount of dissolution in the caffeine group of the respective ions measured for 80 minutes compared to the non-caffeine control group [16].

On the other hand, there is no significant difference between caffeine and the control group in each mineral dissolved in the second molars.

This difference in the caffeine's effects between first and second molars can be explained as follows. The first stage of development is called the hyperplastic growth period which is primarily an increase of DNA of the organ. Synthesis of DNA and cell division at first take place rapidly [18], but thereafter, slow down. Further tissue growth can occur by cytoplasmic enlargement.

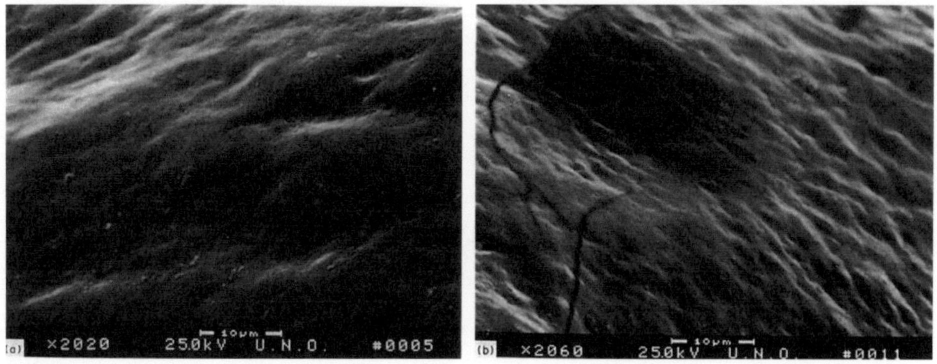

Figure 1.
Left: Before acid exposure in the control. Right: 80 minutes after the acid exposure.

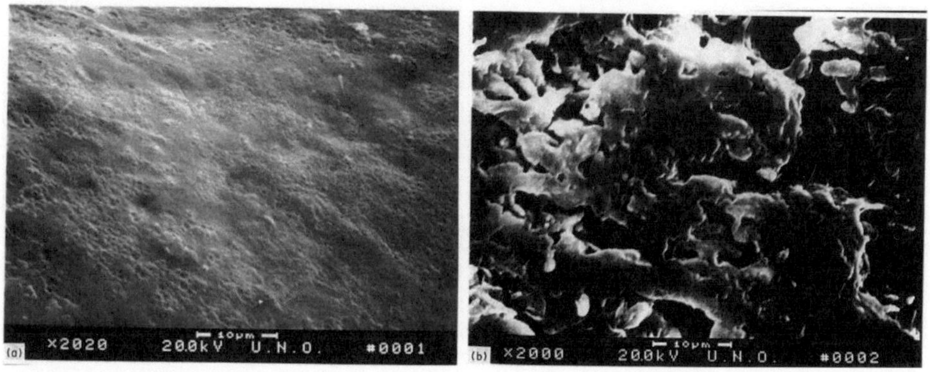

Figure 2.
Left: Before acid exposure of the caffeine group. Right: 80 minutes after the acid exposure.

The measured DNA content as an index of cell number distinguishes growth by an increase of cell number (hyperplasia). Cell division eventually ceases will be seen to determine when the organ is no longer vulnerable to nutritional stress. If nutritional stress, such as caffeine exposure in the early part of life were applied hyperplastic growth period, the organ or body would never recover to the original condition. Therefore, this period is called a critical growth period.

The second stage is a gradual decrease in cell number and a slow increase of cell size in the organ. The third stage is primarily an increase in cell size, which is called the hypertrophic growth period. If the nutritional stress were applied in this period, organ or animal grows back normally, provided that enough nutrition is given [19, 20].

During the period of growth and development, the critical period of growth is the most important concept. For example, the huge increase of DNA in the brain occurs primarily during gestation and early lactation period whereas an increase of the DNA of the heart continues until adulthood [21]. This indicates that the critical period of growth is different among the organs, therefore, the effects of the nutritional stress on each organ is different, depending upon when the stress is applied.

Likewise, caffeine exposures for the growing period were different between the first and second molars, indicating that the critical period of growth during caffeine exposure was different between the first and second molars. First molars are affected

	First molar			Second molar	
	Control	**Caffeine**		**Control**	**Caffeine**
			20 min		
Ca	5.23 ± 0.33	8.63 ± 1.07*		7.45 ± 1.29	7.36 ± 0.86
P	2.67 ± 0.36	5.66 ± 1.07*		4.09 ± 0.98	4.41 ± 0.89
Mg	0.20 ± 0.02	0.44 ± 0.07*		0.28 ± 0.04	0.31 ± 0.04
			40 min		
Ca	10.74 ± 1.17	16.83 ± 1.10*		13.59 ± 1.15	13.63 ± 0.92
P	7.34 ± 0.77	12.49 ± 1.40*		10.03 ± 1.45	8.68 ± 0.95
Mg	0.39 ± 0.06	0.72 ± 0.06*		0.45 ± 0.04	0.55 ± 0.05
			60 min		
Ca	12.36 ± 1.22	18.19 ± 1.12*		14.68 ± 1.15	14.85 ± 1.19
P	8.03 ± 0.78	14.72 ± 1.98*		10.47 ± 1.15	10.42 ± 0.97
Mg	0.43 ± 0.04	0.74 ± 0.06*		0.49 ± 0.03	0.55 ± 0.05
			80 min		
Ca	13.68 ± 1.30	19.64 ± 1.19*		15.21 ± 1.22	15.94 ± 0.91
P	9.39 ± 0.91	18.12 ± 2.62*		11.05 ± 1.10	12.88 ± 1.80
Mg	0.42 ± 0.04	0.71 ± 0.05*		043 ± 0.05	052 ± 005

*Each value is an average of seven determinations. *Significantly different from the control at $P < 0.05$.*

Table 1.
Mean amount of minerals dissolved from first or second molars during each time interval (μg/four first or second molars; mean ± SEM).

by caffeine intake by the offspring during this period. Therefore, the experiments were conducted only using the first molars.

2.2 Crystallization studies of HAP

To find out what is happening to the enamel of the first molars, samples that were not used in the studies were powered and enamel was separated from dentin [22]. Then a pure enamel sample was run for 4 hours on a Gandolfi X-ray powder camera. Also, various other aspects of the samples were studied in detail [17].

The filmstrip run on the Gandolfi camera recorded more diffuse lines for the samples of the caffeine group compared to the control (**Figure 3**).

X-ray diffraction analysis on enamel samples by the Gandolfi X-ray camera showed the caffeine supplementation in the maternal diet affected mineralization of enamel, as broader lines indicated smaller crystallites of enamel. Smaller crystallites increase susceptibility to dissolution.

This explains why the caffeine group of the teeth showed the higher dissolution of each ion from the surface of enamel throughout the experimental period [16].

2.3 Cariogenic studies

Because the teeth were affected by caffeine it is natural to make a simple assumption, that is, is it possible to produce in vivo dental caries in the caffeine group [16].

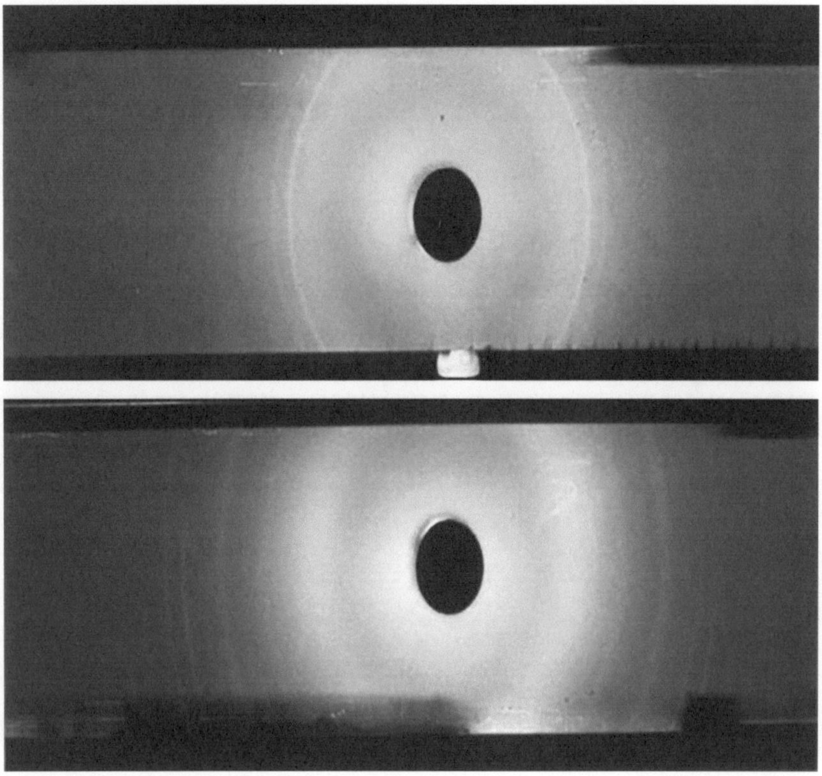

Figure 3.
Top: control. Bottom: caffeine group.

Thus, the experiment was conducted by raising the offspring the same way as above. At weanling on postnatal day 22, offspring were fed the cariogenic diet until day 50 (a total of 28 days) to see whether the caffeine group show a response in dental caries using the methods described [23]. The caffeine group showed significantly higher caries scores than that of the non-caffeine control ($P < 0.05$) (3.36 ± 0.33 versus 2.65 ± 0.22) (mean ± SEM) [24].

Therefore, the hypothesis turned to be true as is shown in **Figures 4** and 5. The amount of caffeine that was added to the maternal diet was 2 mg/100 g bodyweight of the dam. The equivalent comparison between the caffeine in the rat and human is based on metabolic body weight ($kg^{0.75}$) [25]. (Metabolic rates are expressed in terms of metabolic body size—i.e., $kg^{0.75}$, the point at which the dependence on different body sizes disappears.) The human caffeine intake is comparable with slightly more than two cups of coffee daily.

This is the normal amount of caffeine consumed by humans. Although extrapolation from rat data to human dental caries incidence requires extreme caution, nevertheless present data indicate that caffeine exposure during the early growth period impairs the structure of the enamel crystal formation of the developing teeth. Particularly, it may require attention where the offspring born from a pregnant woman who habitually consumes caffeine-containing soft drinks and/or coffee drinkers may develop teeth that are prone to dental caries of the offspring in the future. It seems clear that caffeine exposure during the critical growth period affects the amelogenesis of the enamel, affecting the crystal size of the HAP during mineralization.

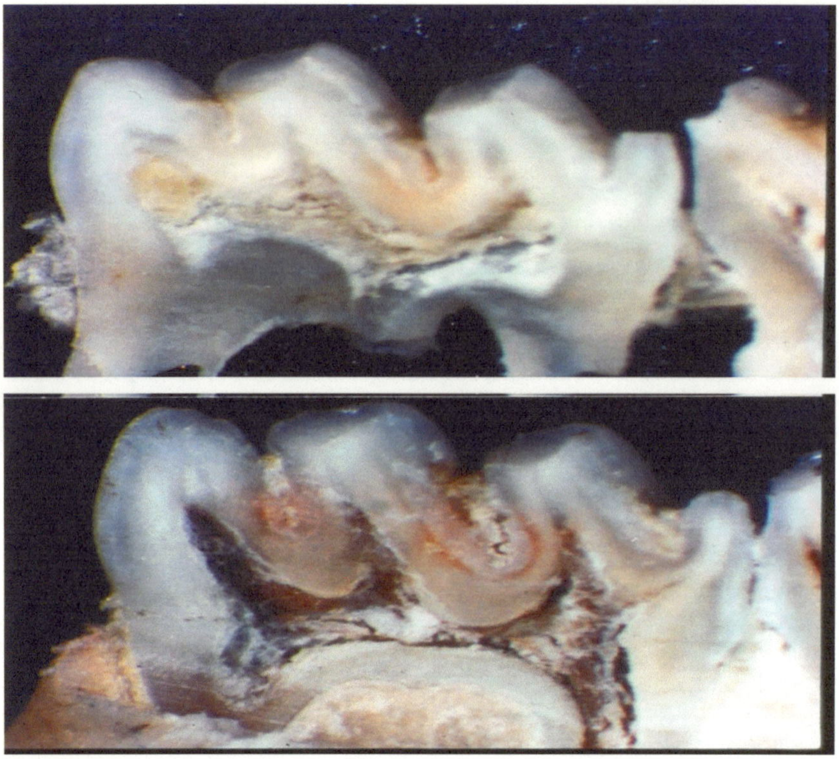

Figure 4.
Molar of the control at day 50 stained with 0.06% murexide in 70% ethanol for 16 hours (top), the caffeine group (bottom).

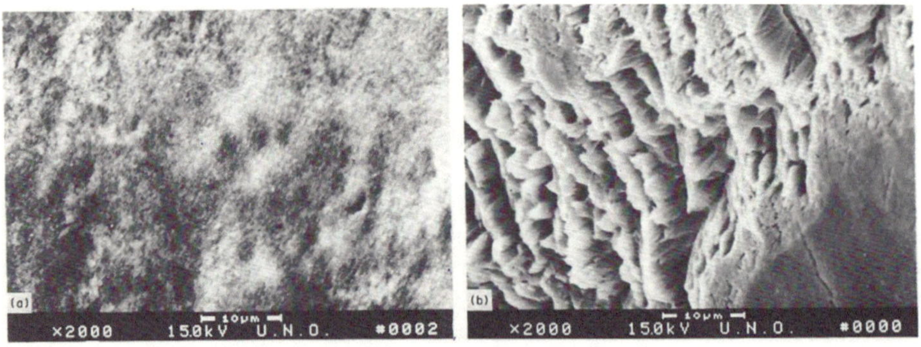

Figure 5.
Secondary electron image of control at day 50 (left) and the caffeine group (right).

3. In vitro study for other xanthine family members

3.1 HAP formation

A series of caffeine studies on crystallization research required more than several years. Thus, a simple in vitro study was conducted to see whether other xanthine family members could reveal if any, other different crystallization value(s) from caffeine.

All the solutions contained 0.01 molar $CaCl_2$ and Na_3PO_4. Several sets of experiments were conducted with the addition of each of methylxanthine at low concentrations, 50 mg, and 200 mg/L. The effect of the xanthine compounds was compared with a control solution containing $CaCl_2$ and Na_3PO_4 only. Solutions were mixed at 25°C, and pH adjusted to 9–9.5 with 0.1 molar NaOH and left to crystallize for 20 days. The crystalline was washed five times with distilled water and prepared for X-ray diffraction (**Figure 6**).

All the data from the various members of the xanthine family on the effects of crystallization were already reported [26, 27].

To our surprise, the value of theobromine was much lower than caffeine. Specifically, 1-methylxanthine values were lower than the caffeine group but not as low as the theobromine group.

Caffeine (small crystal size) and theobromine (large crystal size) with the lack of one position of the methyl group, crystal size was opposite. Therefore, it should be further investigated how the methyl position 1 alone can influence the crystallization.

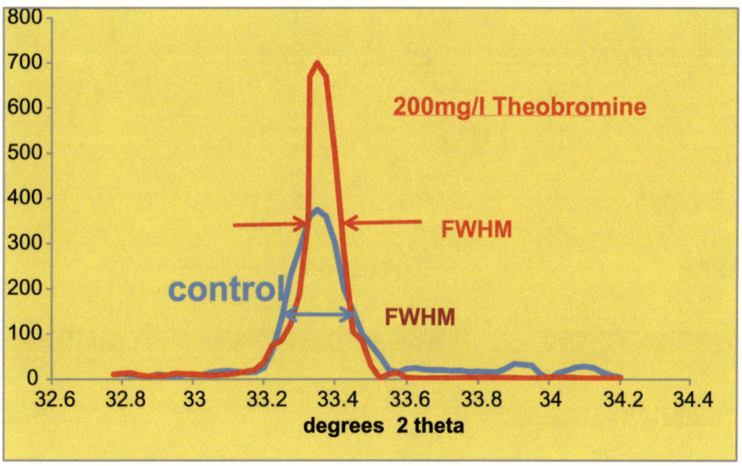

Figure 6.
The (300) reflection was scanned to investigate crystallinity. FWHM (full width-half maximum peak height) divided by maximum peak height (FWHM/M) and for the (300) reflection is given in **Table 2.**

FWHM/M of apatite grown in vitro		
Additive	**mg/L**	**FWHM/M**
Control	0	0.75
Caffeine	200	1.00
Caffeine	50	0.90
Theobromine	200	0.15
Theobromine	50	0.19
1-methylxanthine	200	0.60
1-methylxanthine	50	0.68
Lower values of the ratio indicate better crystal size.		

Table 2.
Hydroxylapatite which was grown in vitro of three xanthine families, caffeine, theobromine and 1-methylxanthine are shown.

The crystal size of position 1 alone did not have much effect on the crystal size. See the chemical formulae (**Figure** 7).

The crystal size of the theobromine group taken by an electron microscope was shown below and the size was four times bigger than that of the control group (**Figure** 8).

3.2 Theobromine and oral application

Theobromine and caffeine contents of the average commercial sweet chocolates are approximately 8:1 ratio [28]. The half-life of theobromine and caffeine is different and that of theobromine is longer than caffeine.

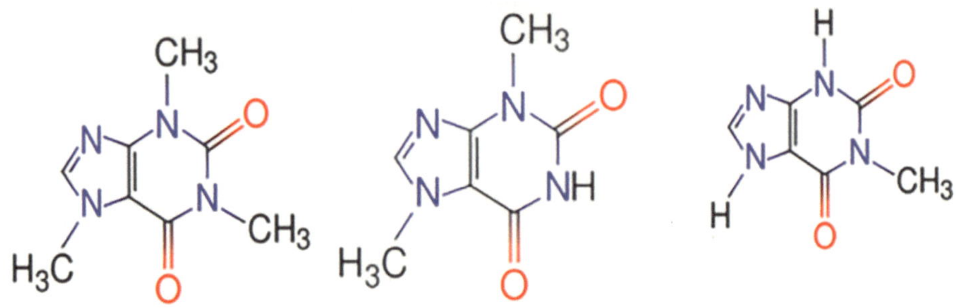

Caffeine

1,3,7-trimethyxanthine

Theobromine

3,7-dimethyxanthine

1- methylxanthine

Figure 7.
The chemical formula of three xanthines.

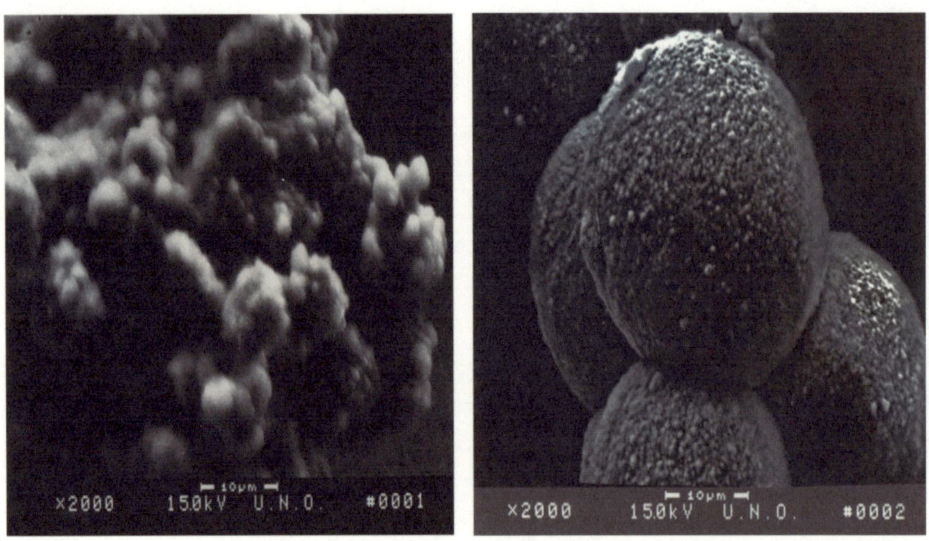

Figure 8.
(Left) Theobromine group: 200 mg/L, Crystal size: 2 μm. (Right) Control group: Crystal size: 0.5 μm.

The inhibitory effect of cocoa which contains theobromine on plaque accumulation and cariostatic activity has been suggested [29]. However, its anticaries activity is not strong enough to suppress significantly cariogenic activity [30]. On the other hand, the addition of a water-soluble extract of cacao powder significantly reduced caries scores in specific pathogen-free rats infected with *Streptococcus sobrinus* 6715 [31]. Theobromine-based dentifrice had the added benefits of increasing the salivary pH and decreasing the *S. mutans* levels [32].

4. In vivo study exposed theobromine

4.1 In vivo crystallization studies

The amount of theobromine added to the maternal diet in the study was 1 mg/100 g body weight. If this amount is converted by the metabolic body weight ($kg^{0.75}$) [25], this corresponds approximately to slightly more than one to three bars of 1 oz milk chocolate for a 65 kg human. After raising the offspring fed with a maternal diet containing theobromine, molars were extracted and studied the following aspects.

4.1.1 X-ray diffractometry

A consistent relationship of higher crystallinity, i.e., larger crystallites, in the whole molars from the rats exposed to theobromine, compared to the control and/or caffeine group was observed in the X-ray diffractometry [27].

4.1.2 Microprobe analysis

Calcium and phosphorus concentrations were determined in the enamel of molars extracted from theobromine exposed rats or control rats by an “ARL-SEMQ”™ electron

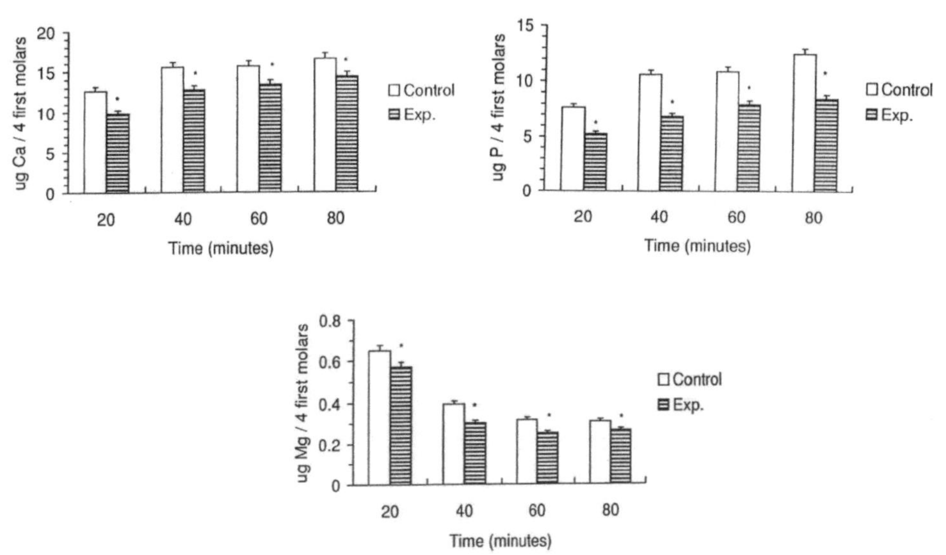

Figure 9.
*Calcium (upper left), phosphorus (upper right) and magnesium (bottom) theobromine group were significantly * (P < 0.05) less than the control.*

microprobe analysis. The instrument was operated at an acceleration potential of 15 kV and a beam current of 1.0×10^{-7} A. Fluorapatite from Cerro de Mercado, Mexico, was used as a standard. The results obtained are shown in our previous report [26, 27].

This study was conducted to see whether the composition of crystallites of the enamel formed by theobromine is different from the control group. The overall content of CaO and P_2O_5 appears to be comparable within the expected margin of error. This suggests that the composition of crystallites of the enamel between control and experimental groups are the same.

4.2 Dissolution studies

The same experimental procedures, as was in the caffeine study [16], were conducted. The molars from the offspring whose dams were fed with the diet supplemented with theobromine were extracted. The dissolution studies were done. The result showed decreased dissolution (Ca, P, and Mg) of the ions from this group due to the larger crystal size (**Figure 9**) [27].

5. Comparison of theobromine and fluoride

5.1 Microhardness test

The unique roles of theobromine were accidentally discovered during the caffeine study. Because previously only fluoride has been known to affect the enamel, the next steps were to investigate the comparative studies between theobromine and fluoride on the effects of the enamel in a similar environment using the in vitro system.

If remineralization occurs, then the increased enamel is associated with increased microhardness [33]. The microhardness test was conducted using theobromine [34]. An in vitro study confirmed that theobromine increased the microhardness of the enamel [35–37].

The enamel of human teeth with varying concentrations of theobromine vs. sodium fluoride vs. control groups (distilled water) was performed. Scanning electron microscopy (SEM) and Knoop Microhardness Testing (NMT) were conducted. A Knoop microhardness instrument was used. Knoop Microhardness tests were performed every day for a period of 8 days on each sample and the data were recorded. Day 1 represents the baseline hardness.

On day 8, it was not tested to avoid interfering with the surface of the tooth before taking the scanning electron photomicrographs. The hardness data are shown at the end of the 8th day and the results were published [26]. **Figure 10** shows SEM photomicrographs of the enamel of control, fluoride and theobromine.

In general, the teeth that were coated with theobromine appeared to be cleaner, smooth and excellent mineralization was observed under the electron microscope especially when compared with control group teeth.

5.2 Acid dissolution study

Samples were covered with small uniformly cut circles of double-stick tape.

The tooth was covered in nail polish and the tape was removed to expose a fairly uniform enamel surface on each tooth.

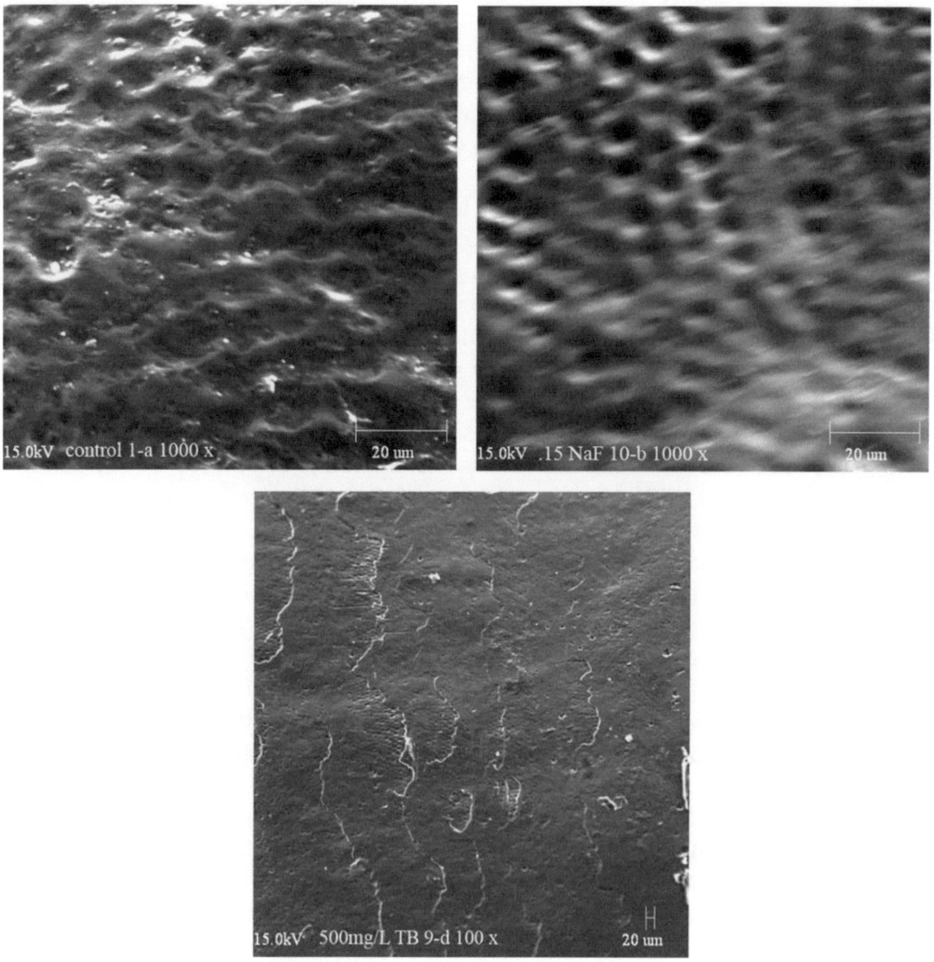

Figure 10.
Upper left: control group. Upper right: 0.15% w/v fluoride ion. Bottom: theobromine group: 500 mg/L.

Each tooth was immersed in either 0.15% w/v fluoride ion solution or theobromine 100 mg/L solution for 30 minutes. Then, each tooth was exposed to a 0.001 N HCl acid solution for 10 minutes to determine how much calcium is released from the enamel. The amount calcium (ppm) released from the surface of the enamel in the F-0.15% was an average of 0.930 whereas theobromine-100 mg was 0.848. The fluoride group of teeth released 9.66% more calcium compared to the theobromine group, suggesting that the pre-exposures by theobromine solution is more effective to make the enamel surface of teeth more resistant than fluoride solution. Theobromine is reported as an effective remineralizing agent [38].

5.3 Clinical hypersensitivity studies with either theobromine or fluoride-containing toothpastes

Hypersensitivity is a short and sharp pain arising from exposed dentin by an external stimulus [39]. The prevalence of hypersensitivity varies [40]. The therapeutic approach is to occlude dentin tubules [41].

Clinical studies were conducted in four different samples. The detail of the experimental design has been already described [26, 42]. Importantly theobromine-based toothpaste has shown that the hypersensitivity disappeared within a week [42]. On the other hand, fluoride-based toothpastes indicated practically no effects to alleviate sensitivity without much occlusion on the dentinal tubes during this experimental period of 1 week.

5.4 Preventive effect of dental caries by theobromine

A study using an established in vitro caries pH cycling model [43] was conducted [44]. Treatment with theobromine results in resistance to acid attack. A recent study has shown that theobromine gel had more effective remineralizing potential than fluoride gel [45].

In the oral environment, remineralization and demineralization are happening constantly. The hardness test conducted on the enamel surface [26] clearly showed that theobromine was much more effective than fluoride. However, in another study using pH cycling method, theobromine does not appear to offer any anti-caries benefits [46]. Applied theobromine to the demineralized enamel surface caused recrystallization and increased surface microhardness.

Crystallite size is the main factor that controls the dissolution of HAP. Small crystallites have a much higher surface area/volume ratio compared to larger crystallites. Dissolution is more rapid on smaller crystallites than on larger ones. Thus, larger crystallites of HAP in the enamel resist dissolution under cariogenic conditions better than smaller ones.

From the comparative studies between theobromine and fluoride each parameter measured indicated that theobromine is superior to fluoride. Recently, a clinical study on the evaluation of the anticaries activity of either theobromine or fluoride-based toothpaste against *plaque S. mutans* in children of age group from 6 to 9 years was conducted [47]. It was concluded that theobromine-based toothpaste is beneficial as a safe anti-cariogenic agent. Furthermore, theobromine showed more antimicrobial effects against *S. mutans*, *Lactobacillus acidophilus*, and *Enterococcus faecalis* in the in vitro study. Theobromine showed greater zones of inhibition than other commercially available fluoridated children's toothpastes [48].

In addition, a recent in vitro study indicated that theobromine is an effective cariostatic agent and a safe alternative to fluoride in preventive dental care [36, 49]. The theobromine group is superior compared to the fluoride group in each parameter studied.

6. How did Ancient Mayans embed round jade inlays?

In ancient times in the Mayan culture, cocoa was used only among the wealthy and even until recently, in certain countries, cocoa was used to exchange wealth. What is surprising about the skull is that jade was embedded as an inlay into each tooth (**Figure 11**), which required drilling the enamel surface of the tooth.

However, drilling the precise hole to embed the jade would have been difficult if not impossible. It seems that somehow after placing the jade into each tooth, they must have had the knowledge to fix the jade within the hole.

A simple experiment was conducted by us [26] to determine how ancient Mayan knew the unique role of cocoa 1100 years ago. We have experimented with the knowledge obtained in the past years with theobromine. One can see the study presented in the previous report [26]. Thus, the mystery of how ancient Mayan placed jade in the front teeth was solved. We know now that theobromine which was extracted from cocoa was used to fill the marginal space around the jade and initiate mineralization to fix the jade

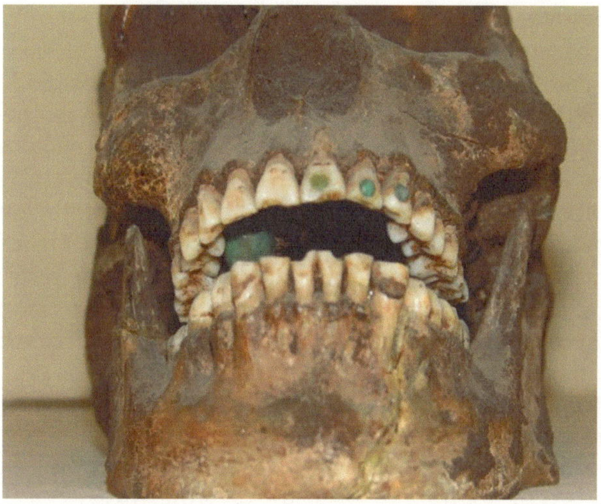

Figure 11.
Mayan skull was reported to be 1100 years old. Note that Jades were embedded.

insert on the teeth. These results are strong evidence that ancient Mayans knew the role of theobromine in cocoa on the mineralization of hard tissue over 1100 years ago.

It is also interesting to note that the strong and unusually heavy-looking mandible of this skull supports the finding that theobromine also plays a role in the growth and development of bones [27]:

7. Why the present finding of the role of theobromine is so revolutionary?

7.1 Adverse effects of fluoride

In the past, fluoride is the one that was solely used in the dental profession to prevent dental caries and added to most of the toothpaste. In addition, fluoride has been used a high amount of varnish solution [50] and glass-ionomer cement [51].

Fluoride has been described as the same category of alcohol, nicotine, and lead and advised to avoid them during pregnancy [52]. Fluorosis [53, 54] is very common.

Maternal exposure to fluoride during pregnancy was associated with lower IQ scores in children aged from 3 to 4 years [55]. This is the first report describing the possible effects of lower IQ scores of offspring as a result of maternal fluoride intake. Previously, numerous studies associated with fluoride exposures and lower IQ scores of children were already reported. This phenomenon was observed despite the parents' education and family income in China [56], India [57] and Taiwan [58]. Cognitive alterations in children born from exposed mothers to fluoride could start in early prenatal stages of life and appear later at school age; and likely continue into adulthood [59].

One of the neurodevelopmental disabilities is autism [60] and the decreased secretion of melatonin from the pineal gland alters circadian rhythms and sleep patterns [61].

Another interesting aspect is the relationship between caffeine-containing drinks and fluoride. The higher fluorosis severity was associated with soft drinks and coffee consumption, as most soft drinks contain caffeine [62]. This was explained that the presence of fluoride would remain longer due to the ingestion of caffeine-containing beverages [63].

7.2 Fluoride exposures in early life

A 6 oz. container of 1500 ppm fluoride toothpastes contains 254.7 mg of fluoride. A one-year-old (8.14 kg) child ingesting less than one-fifth of the contents of the container would possibly exceed a toxic dose [9]. It has been well known that coronary heart disease and related disorders such as stokes, diabetes and hypertension may originate during fetal development [64]. As further examples, overfeeding of newborns tend to lead to obesity in later adult life. Caffeine exposures during the gestation and lactation periods appeared reduced locomotive activity in the later ages of animals [65]. By the undernourishment in utero, intrauterine programming during this period could contribute to the risk of osteoporotic fractures in later life [66]. "Programming phenomena" in the body of early life [67] is explained as nutritional stress during the critical period of growth that causes permanent or long-term changes in the structure or function of the organ.

Unfortunately, certain areas of the U.S. have an incidence of fluorosis of about 70% [54] to 80% [53] in children. These examples stipulate very high incidences of possible fluoride's effects on growing children.

Consider each step. Fluorosis of teeth is a result of the effect of fluoride on ameloblasts cells. The other parts of the organs as well could have been affected by this chemical. Excess fluoride exposures have already been known to cause various diseases described above.

The exposure of fluoride must be not only the excess dose of fluoride but also the duration of exposure and timing [52] such as the critical growth period as explained. Fluorosis has been reported to be associated with the lower performance of neuropsychological tests [68]. Developmental enamel defect is twice as frequently with mental retardation [52]. However, there are not many studies that investigated the relationship between fluorosis in teeth and systemic diseases at the same time. For example, is the incidence of fluorosis related to specific diseases? To answer this question, there is a need for close clinical cooperation between dentistry and medicine in future studies of fluoride.

Patients with fluorosis may develop certain diseases in later life. The growth and development of organs or bodies on the surface could have been minor. However, genetic influences could have already occurred, possibly resulting in a slight alteration of structure or function at the cellular levels [67].

Despite little difference in average levels of tooth decay between fluoridated and unfluoridated water of the same country [69], there are still areas in the US where water is fluoridated and water fluoridation may add a small amount of fluoride into the bodies.

In the body, continuous formation and breakdown have been happening throughout the life cycle. If the periods of the formation far exceed breakdown such as the rapid growth period, minor changes of cellular levels might not appear readily. When the period of breakdown is exceeded in the later stages of life, diseases associated with fluoride exposures in early life could become a root cause of disease in later life [13].

We do not know at this time what kind of diseases, if any, might appear in later life by fluoride exposures in early life. However, early nutritional stresses on the developing fetus cause various diseases [64–66]. The current concept on the number of fluoride exposures in early life and root causes of disease in the future is not an unrealistic hypothesis. If this were proven to be true by future epidemiological studies and/or even one could argue "do we need to wait until such time". The time might have come now to reexamine the routine use of fluoride in dental practice from a fundamental aspect.

7.3 Development of non-fluoride dentifrice

During the study of caffeine on the effects of developing teeth, we have accidentally discovered that one of the xanthine family, theobromine, showed the opposite effects from caffeine on the crystallization of hydroxylapatite (HAP). Theobromine combined with calcium and phosphorus which is called "rennou" was added to accelerate the crystal formation of non-fluoride dentifrice.

Cacao contains theobromine. Chocolate which comes from cacao has been consumed without any ill effects by humans in the past. Cacao has an interesting history. In 1753, Swedish taxonomer Carl Linnaeus named the cacao plant "theo-broma" which translates to "food of gods". He was a believer in the power of cacao. Ancient Mayans at least 1100 years ago already knew the unique roles of cacao on crystallization and possibly used it to fix jade inside of the enamel. The specific characteristics of theobromine led to the formation of fluoride-free toothpastes.

Theobromine-based dentifrice is revolutionary. This is because space travel in our future, military or even camping where the water supply is most often limited, it is not needed to rinse the mouth with water or just spit after brushing teeth. However, most importantly, even if one swallows it, there are no adverse effects. Theobromine

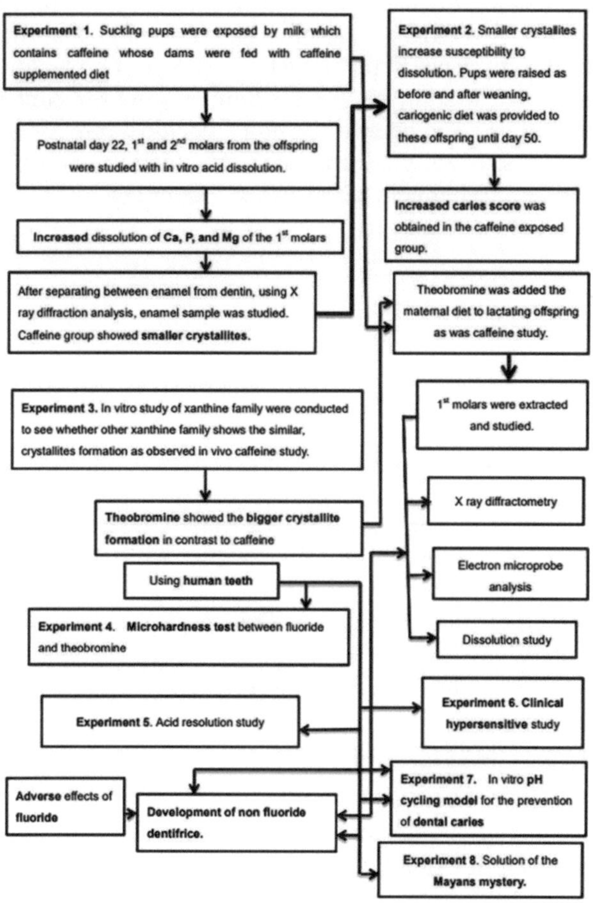

Figure 12.
The flow chart shows how non-fluoride dentifrice was developed.

changes the crystallization dynamics of apatite group species, resulting in fewer and larger crystallites. It likely interacts with ions being deposited at the growing HAP crystal surface. Thus, the ratio of surface area versus volume of the crystals is lowered and dissolution is not as rapid or pronounced as in smaller crystals.

In conclusion, non-fluoride-based dentifrice was introduced for the replacement of fluoride-based toothpastes. Further studies of theobromine-based dentifrice have to be examined as a reliable alternative of the safe replacement of fluoride-based dentifrice. This requires vigorous basic and clinical studies by scientists and clinicians.

So far, all the evidence presented shows that the theobromine is superior to that of fluoride and most importantly, the use of theobromine is safe. The current development of non-fluoride dentifrice is most timely. The flow chart in **Figure 12** was added to summarize the development of this non-fluoride dentifrice.

Acknowledgements

Some of the comparative studies between theobromine and fluoride was conducted by Mr. Arman Sadeghpour as part of his Ph.D. dissertation under the strict guidance of Drs Tetsuo Nakamoto, and William B. Simmons Jr. and Mr. Alexander U. Falster. The authors met Mr. Joseph Fuselier who was organizing a biotechnology group interested in the New Orleans area after Hurricane Katrina, August, 2005. He has much-needed experience in the industrial aspects of biotechnology. Mr. R. Jantzen Hubbard and a little later, Ms. Natalie Borchers and Mr. Andrew Lisle Fuselier joined the group to develop and operate the non-fluoride toothpaste, now known to be chocolate toothpastes. The authors appreciate Ms. Julie Schiavo, librarian at LSU Health Sciences Center, for her help with various references.

Author details

Tetsuo Nakamoto[1,2*], Alexander U. Falster[3] and William B. Simmons Jr [2,3]

1 Department of Physiology, Louisiana State University Health Sciences Center New Orleans, New Orleans, LA, USA

2 Theodent, The Bioinnovation Center, New Orleans, LA, USA

3 Maine Mineral and Gem Museum, Bethel, ME, USA

*Address all correspondence to: tnakam@lsuhsc.edu

References

[1] Grahams DM. Caffeine—Its identity, dietary sources, intake and biological effects. Nutrition Reviews. 1978;**36**:97-102

[2] Tarka SM, Zoumas BI, Gans JH. Short-term effects of graded levels of theobromine in laboratory rodents. Toxicology and Applied Pharmacology. 1979;**49**:127-149

[3] Grandjean P, Landrigan PJ. Neurobehavioural effects of developmental toxicity. Lancet Neurology. 2014;**13**:330-338

[4] Luke J. Fluoride deposition in the aged human pineal gland. Caries Research. 2001;**35**:125-128

[5] Susheela AK, Bhatnagar M, Vig K, Mondal NK. Excess fluoride ingestion and thyroid hormone derangements in children living in Delhi, India. Fluoride. 2005;**38**:98-108

[6] Sandhu R, Lal H, Kundu ZS, Kharb S. Serum fluoride and sialic acid levels in osteosarcoma. Biological Trace Element Research. 2011;**144**:1-5. DOI: 10.1007/s12011009-8382-1

[7] Wiatrowski E, Kramer L, Osis D, Spencer H. Dietary fluoride intake of infants. Pediatrics. 1975;**55**:517-522

[8] Naccache H, Simard PL, Trahan L, Brodeur JM, Demers M, Lachapelle D, et al. Factors affecting the ingestion of fluoride dentifrice by children. Journal of Public Health Dentistry. 1992;**52**:222-226

[9] Schulman JD, Wells LM. Acute fluoride toxicity from ingesting home-use dental products in children, birth to 6 years of age. Journal of Public Health Dentistry. 1997;**57**:150-158

[10] Levy SM, Warren JJ, Davis CS, Kirchner L, Kanellis MJ, Wefel JS. Patterns of fluoride intake from birth to 36 months. Journal of Public Health Dentistry. 2001;**61**:70-77

[11] Erdal S, Buchanan S. A quantitative look at fluorosis, fluoride exposure, and intake in children using a health risk assessment approach. Environmental Health Perspectives. 2005;**113**:111-117. DOI: 10.1289/ehp.7077

[12] Zero DT. Dentifrices, mouthwashes, and remineralization/caries arrestment strategies. BMC Oral Health. 2006;**6**(Suppl 1):S9. DOI: 10.1186/1472-6831-6S1-S9

[13] Nakamoto T, Rawls HR. Fluoride exposure in early life as the possible root causes of disease in later life. The Journal of Clinical Pediatric Dentistry. 2018;**42**(5):1-5. DOI: 10.17796/1053-4625-42.5.1

[14] Nakamoto T, Shaye R, Mallek HM. Effects of maternal caffeine intake on the growth of tooth germs in protein-energy malnourished neonates. Archives of Oral Biology. 1985;**30**:105-109

[15] Aponte-Merced L, Navia JM. Pre-eruptive protein-energy malnutrition and acid solubility of rat molar enamel surface. Archives of Oral Biology. 1980;**25**:701-705

[16] Hashimoto K, Joseph F Jr, Falster AU, Simmons WB Jr, Nakamoto T. Effects of maternal caffeine intake during lactation on molar enamel surfaces in new-born rats. Archives of Oral Biology. 1992;**37**:105-109

[17] Falster AU, Hashimoto K, Nakamoto T, Simmons WB Jr. Physical examination of caffeine's effects on the

enamel surface of first molar in new-born rats. Archives of Oral Biology. 1992;**37**:111-118

[18] Miller SA. Protein metabolism during growth and development. In: Munro HN, editor. Mammalian Protein Metabolism. Vol. Volume III. New York, London: Academic Press; 1969. pp. 183-233

[19] Enesco M, Leblond CP. Increase in cell number as a factor in the growth of the organs and tissues of the young male rat. Journal of Embryology and Experimental Morphology. 1962;**10**: 530-562

[20] Goss RJ. Hypertrophy versus hyperplasia. How much organs can grow depends on whether their functional units increase in size or in number. Science. 1966;**53**:1615-1620

[21] Winick M, Noble A. Quantitative changes in DNA, RNA, and protein during prenatal and postnatal growth in the rat. Developmental Biology. 1965;**12**:451-466

[22] Manly S, Hodge HC. Density and refractive index studies of dental hard tissue-method for separation and determination of purity. Journal of Dental Research. 1939;**18**:133-141

[23] Keyes PH. Dental caries in the molar teeth of rats. II. A methods for diagnosis and scoring several types of lesions simultaneously. Journal of Dental Research. 1958;**37**:1088-1099

[24] Nakamoto T, Cheuk SL, Yoshino S, Falster AU, Simmons WB Jr. Cariogenic effect of caffeine intake during lactation on first molars of newborn rats. Archives of Oral Biology. 1993;**38**:919-922

[25] Kleiber M. Body size and metabolic rate. In: The Fire of Life: An Introduction to Animal Energetics. New Jersey; 1961. pp. 177-216

[26] Nakamoto T, Falster AU, Simmons WB Jr. Theobromine: A safe and effective alternative for fluoride in dentifrices. Journal of Caffeine Research. 2016;**6**:1-9. DOI: 10.1089/jcr.2015.0023

[27] Nakamoto T, Simmons WB Jr, Falster AU. Products of apatite-forming-systems. 1999 Issued; Patent Number 5:919,426

[28] Zoumas BL, Kreiser WR, Martin RA. Theobromine and caffeine content of chocolate products. Journal of Food Science. 1980;**45**:314-316

[29] Paolino VJ, Kashket S. Inhibition by cocoa extracts of biosynthesis of extracellular polysaccharide by human oral bacteria. Archives of Oral Biology. 1985;**30**:359-363

[30] Ooshima T, Osaka Y, Sasaki H, Osawa K, Yasuda H, Matsumoto M. Cariostatic activity of cacao mass extract. Archives of Oral Biology. 2000;**45**:805-808

[31] Ito K, Nakamura Y, Tokunaga T, Iijima D, Fukushima K. Anti-cariogenic properties of a water-soluble extract from cacao. Bioscience, Biotechnology, and Biochemistry. 2003;**67**:2567-2573

[32] Durhan MA, Ozsalih S, Gokkaya B, Kulan PY, Kargul B. Caries preventive effects of theobromine containing toothpaste on early childhood caries: Preliminary results. Acta Stomatologica Croatica. 2021;**55**(1):19-28. DOI: 10.15644/asc55/1/3

[33] ten Cade JM, Arends J. Remineralization of artificial enamel lesions in vitro. II. Determination of activation energy and reaction order. Caries Research. 1978;**12**:213-222

[34] Kargul B, Ozcan M, Peker S, Nakamoto T, Simmons WB Jr, Falster AU.

Evaluation of human enamel surfaces treated with theobromine: A pilot study. Oral Health & Preventive Dentistry. 2012;**10**:275-282

[35] Gundogar DU, Keskin G, Cinar C. Comparison of fluoride and the novel anti-caries agent theobromine on initial enamel caries: An in vitro study. Fluoride. 2019;**52**:456-466

[36] Shawky RM, Khattab NM, Yassa MK. Evaluation of the remineralizing effect of theobromine and fluoride using scanning electron microscope. Egyptian Dental Journal. 2021;**67**:119-126

[37] Sulistianingsih I, Hidayat O. The remineralization potential of cocoa bean extract (*Theobroma cacao*) to increase the enamel microhardness. Padjadjaran Journal of Dentistry. 2017;**29**(2):107-112

[38] Taneja V, Nekkanti S, GuptaK HJ. Remineralization potential of theobromine on artificial carious lesions. Journal of International Society of Preventive and Community Dentistry. 2019;**9**:576-583

[39] Canadian Advisory Board on Dentin Hypersensitivity. Consensus-based recommendations for the diagnosis and management of dentin hypersensitivity. Journal of the Canadian Dental Association. 2003;**69**:221-226

[40] Splieth CH, Tachou A. Epidemiology of dentin hypersensitivity. Clinical Oral Investigations. 2013;**17**(Suppl 1):S3-S8

[41] Schmidlin PR, Sahrmann P. Current management of dentin hypersensitivity. Clinical Oral Investigations. 2013;**17** (Suppl1):S55-S59. DOI: 10.1007/s00784-012-0912-0

[42] Amaechi BT, Mathews SM, Mensinkai PK. Effect of theobromine-containing toothpaste on dentin tubule occlusion in situ. Clinical Oral Investigations. 2015;**19**:109-116. DOI: 10.1007/s00784-014-1226-1

[43] White DJ. Reactivity of fluoride dentifrices with artificial caries I. Effects on early lesions: F uptake, surface hardening and remineralization. Caries Research. 1987;**21**:126-114

[44] Amaechi BT, Porteous N, Ramalingam K, Mensinkai PK, Ccahuana Vasquez RA, Sadeghpour A, et al. Remineralization of artificial enamel lesions by theobromine. Caries Research. 2013;**47**:399-405. DOI: 10.1159/000348589

[45] Elsherbini MS. Assessment of remineralization potential of theobromine and sodium fluoride gels on artificial caries like lesions. Brazilian Dental Science. 2020;**23**:1-11. DOI: 10.14295/bds.2020.v23i3.1975

[46] Lipper F. The effects of fluoride, strontium, theobromine and their combination on caries lesion rehardning and fluoridation. Archives of Oral Biology. 2017;**80**:217-221

[47] Ranju MB, Girish MS, Prashanth S. Comparative evaluation of antimicrobial efficacy of theobromine toothpaste and a low-fluoridated toothpaste against *Plaque Streptococcus mutans* in children. World Journal of Dentistry. 2018;**9**:215-219

[48] Lakshmi A, Vishnurekha C, Baghkomeh RN. Effect of theobromine in antimicrobial activity: An in vitro study. Dental Research Journal. 2019;**16**:76-80

[49] Farhad F, Kazemi S, Bijani A, Pasdar N. Efficacy of theobromine and sodium fluoride solutions for remineralization of initial enamel caries lesions. Frontiers in Dentistry. 2021;**18**:10-17

[50] Laila AI, Dehailan L, Martinez-Mier EA, Lippert F. The effect of fluoride varnishes on caries lesions: An in vitro investigation. Clinical Oral Investigations. 2016;**20**(7):1655-1662. DOI: 10.1007/s00784-015-1648-4

[51] Sidhu SK, Nicholson JW. A review of glass-ionomer cements for clinical dentistry. Journal of Functional Biomaterials. 2016;7:16. DOI: 10.3390/jfb7030016

[52] MacArthur JD. Prenatal fluoride and autism. Townsend Letter. 2016;**393**:49-55

[53] Lalumandier JA, Rozier RG. The prevalence and risk factors of fluorosis among patients in a pediatric dental practice. Pediatric Dentistry. 1995;**17**:19-25

[54] Morgan L, Allres D, Tavares M, Bellinger D, Needleman H. Investigation of the possible associations between fluorosis, fluoride exposure, and childhood behavior problems. Pediatric Dentistry. 1998;**20**:244-252

[55] Green R, Lanphear B, Hornung R, Flora D, Martinez-Mier EA, Neufeld R, et al. Association between maternal fluoride exposure during pregnancy and IQ scores in offspring in Canada. Journal of American Medical Association Pediatrics. 2019;**173**:940-948. DOI: 10.1001/jamapediatrics.2019.1729

[56] Xiang Q, Liang Y, Chen L, Wang C, Chen B, Chen X, et al. Effect of fluoride in drinking water on children's intelligence. Fluoride. 2003;**36**:84-94

[57] Sebastian ST, Sunitha S. A cross-sectional study to assess the intelligence quotient (IQ) of school going children aged 10-12 years in villages of Mysore district, India with different fluoride levels. Journal of the Indian Society of Pedodontics and Preventive Dentistry. 2015;**33**:307-311

[58] Lung SC, Hsiao PK, Chiang KM. Fluoride concentrations in three types of commercially packed tea drinks in Taiwan. Journal of Exposure Analysis and Environmental Epidemiology. 2003;**13**:66-73

[59] Valdez Jimenez I, Guzman L, Cervantes Flores M, Costilla-Salazar R, Calderon Hernandez J, Alcaraz Contreras Y, et al. In utero exposure to fluoride and cognitive development delay in infant. Neurotoxicology. 2017;**59**:65-70. DOI: 10.1016/j.neuro.2016.12.011

[60] Blaylock RL. Excitotoxicity: A possible central mechanism in fluoride neurotoxicity. Fluoride. 2004;**37**:301-314

[61] Malin AJ, Bose S, Busgang SA, Gennings C, Thorpy M, Wright RO, et al. Fluoride exposure and sleep patterns among older adolescents in the United States: A cross-sectional study of NHANES 2015-2016. Environmental Health. 2019;**18**:106. DOI: 10.1186/s12940-019-0546-7

[62] Perez-Perez N, Torres-Mendoza N, Borges-Yanez A, Irigoyen-Camacho ME. Dental fluorosis: Concentration of fluoride in drinking water and consumption of bottled beverages in school children. Journal of Clinical Pediatric Dentistry. 2014;**38**:338-344

[63] Chan JT, Qui CC, Whitford GM, Weatherred JG. Influence of coffee on fluoride metabolism in rats. Proceedings of the Society for Experimental Biology and Medicine. 1990;**194**:43-47

[64] Barker DJP. The Fetal Origins of Adult Disease. In Proceeding: Royal Society. London: Biological Society; 1995;**262**:37-43.

[65] Hughes RN, Beveraidge IJ. Behavioral effects of exposure to caffeine during gestation, lactation or both. Neurotoxicology and Teratology. 1991;**13**:641-647

[66] Cooper C, Javaid MK, Taylor P, Walker-Bone K, Dennison E, Arden N. The fetal origins of osteoporotic fracture. Calcified Tissue International. 2002;**70**:391-394

[67] Lucas A. Programming by early nutrition in man. In: Bock GR, Whelan J, editors. The Childhood Environment and Adult Disease. New Jersey; 1991. pp. 38-55

[68] Choi A, Zhang Y, Sun G, Bellinger DC, Wang K, Yang XJ, et al. Association of lifetime exposure to fluoride and cognitive functions in Chinese children: A pilot study. Neurotoxicology and Teratology. 2015;**47**:96-101. DOI: 10.1016/j.ntt2014.11.001

[69] Diesendorf M. Have the benefits of water fluoridation been overestimated? International Clinical Nutrition Review. 1990;**10**:292-303

Chapter 20

Empirical Study on Medical Information and Communication Technology System in Dentistry in Southeast Asia

Ichiro Nakajima, Ken-ichiro Ejima, Yoshinori Arai, Kunihito Matsumoto, Kazuya Honda, Hirofumi Aboshi, Marina Hamaguchi, Akao Lyvongsa, Bounnhong Sidaphone, Somphone Phanthavong, Chanthavisao Phanthanalay and Souksavanh Vongsa

Abstract

In the field of dentistry, diagnoses based on data obtained using medical imaging modalities such as digital panoramic radiography and cone beam computed tomography (CBCT) have been widely recommended for advanced dental care. In Lao People's Democratic Republic (Laos), there are place where advanced dental imaging devices are available in only one university dental hospital. The establishment of an information and communication technology (ICT) system has been expected as telemedicine system, for sharing medical imaging data among medical institutions in Laos. Recently, regional medical cooperation using telemedicine has been developed in Japan, and medical imaging data have been provided and shared among medical institutions, by using a mobile tablet terminal application. Therefore, we have carried out the empirical research on the telemedicine system with the university in Laos. The technologies and research results from our project will be presented in this chapter.

Keywords: osteoporosis, medical ICT, cone beam CT, teleradiology, Lao People's Democratic Republic

1. Introduction

Telemedicine has great potential to address some challenges faced by both developed and developing countries in providing accessible, cost-effective, high-quality health care services [1]. It has been developed by such information and communication technologies (ICTs) in medical fields (medical ICT) [2–8]. However, there are few studies on the effect of ICT on dentistry in areas with low medical supply from a long-term perspective. To build sustainable health care as set forth by the United Nations, it is necessary to conduct and present a case study on the role of ICT in medical care.

Therefore, this chapter reports the results of an international joint project that medical ICT was effective on clinical introduction of the digital imaging system in dentistry in Laos. The report of this project activity will state the importance of continuing human resource development in the field of international health care in the long term.

2. Medical ICT in telemedicine

ICTs have great potential to address some challenges faced by both developed and developing countries in providing accessible, cost effective, high-quality health care services [1]. Based on expertise, telemedicine uses medical ICTs to overcome geographical barriers and increase access to health care services. In Japan, at a broad level, telemedicine is divided into two types [9].

2.1 Telemedicine for patients

Medical treatment is provided to patients by the physician in charge. A patient at home interacts with the physician in charge located in a remote medical facility through the video telephone system. Simultaneously, based on the transmitted information, the physician in charge determines the physical and mental condition of the patient and the patient's medical treatment. This type of telemedicine is sometimes referred to as "telecare." "Telenursing" is an example of this type, where a nurse performs a key role and aids patients in home care.

2.2 Telemedicine between health care providers

This telemedicine is conducted primarily between the physician in charge and medical specialist and is referred to as "narrow sense telemedicine."

Besides, it is mainly classified into teleradiology, telepathology, teledermatology, and telepsychiatry. In WHO report, each field is defined as follows.

- Teleradiology is the use of ICT to transmit digital radiological images (e.g., X-ray images) from one location to another for the interpretation and/or consultation.

- Telepathology is the use of ICT to transmit digitized pathological results (e.g., microscopic images of cells) for interpretation and/or consultation.

- Teledermatology is the use of ICT to transmit medical information concerning skin conditions (e.g., skin tumors) for interpretation and/or consultation.

- Telepsychiatry is the use of ICT for psychiatric evaluations and/or consultation via video and telephony.

Of the four fields of telemedicine that were highlighted in the survey, teleradiology has the highest rate of established service provision. Teleradiology is built on the medical ICT system of diagnostic imaging studies from one location to another for conferences or consultations.

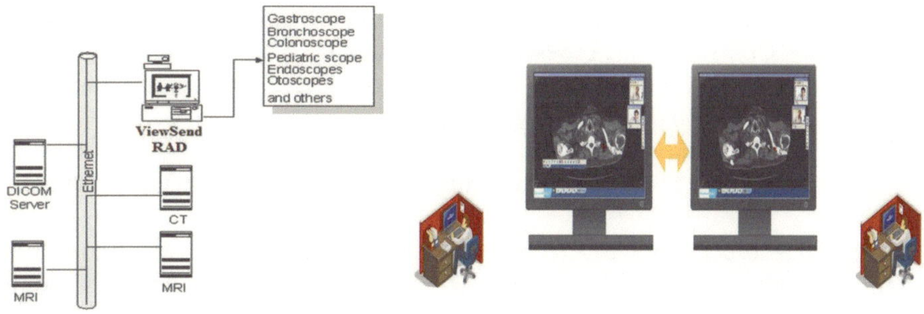

Figure 1.
Rapid application development system (RAD) developed by ViewSend ICT. ViewSendRAD provides a real-time 3-in-1 telemedsolution for telemedicine, tele-radiology, and videoconferencing. This product is designed to be a real-time software solution –collaboration, consultation, or training. These functions were advantageous to sharing information and deepening understanding of imaging data in the joint research.

In Japan, the teleradiology system is well used to support underserviced hospitals in the depopulated area to have timely access to a radiologist. Recent telemedicine research has developed the system that integrates functions of telemedicine and video conference (**Figure 1**).

3. Digital image processing of dent-maxillofacial radiographs

Digital panoramic radiography (DPR) and cone-beam-type of computed tomography (CBCT) were developed and patented by Nihon University School of Dentistry in the late 1980s and 1990s, respectively [10] (**Figure 2**). These technologies were transferred to Morita Corporation (Kyoto).

Regarding CBCT, Nihon University School of Dentistry obtained the Kinki Bureau of International Trade and Industry Regional New Industry Creation Technology Development Subsidy (1997–1999) to develop a commercial machine and pharmaceutical approval in 2001. CBCT allows three-dimensional diagnostic imaging of the teeth and inner ear. The National Health Insurance has covered it since 2012 in Japan, and since then, it has become an essential diagnostic imaging in dental care. Presently, CBCT machines are available at a rate of 1 per 10,000 people in Japan. We have installed the Veraviewepocs R100, a model of CBCT, at the University of Health

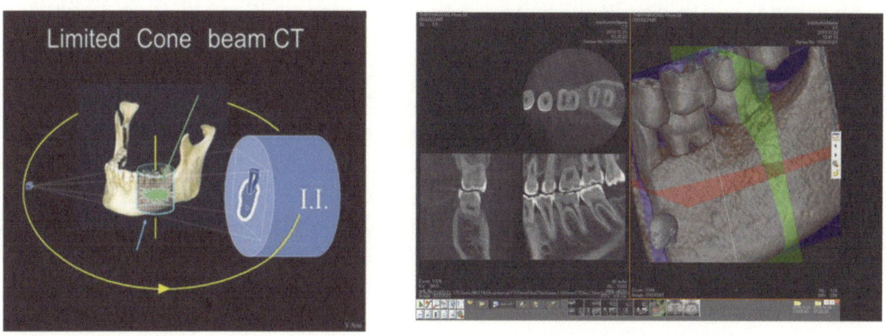

Figure 2.
Schematic diagram of the CBCT device used in this study. Left: measurement principle. Right: maxillofacial tomographic image. These figures are taken from Ref. [10].

Sciences (UHS). Veraviewepocs R100 can be used to perform panoramic tomography and CBCT. This CBCT has four types of fields of view (FOV): diameter of 4 cm and height of 4 cm, 4 cm × 8 cm, 8 cm × 8 cm and 10 cm× 8 cm. The optimal size of FOV was selected according to the purpose of diagnosis.

When FOV with a diameter of 4 cm and height of 4 cm is used, its dose is several times that of panoramic tomography but only approximately 1/100 that of conventional CT.

The spatial resolution of CBCT is calculated via the modulation transfer function using the wire method. It was as good as >10% at 2.0-line pair/mm. It was few times higher than that of conventional CT.

As described above, this device was characterized by low radiation dose and high resolution. It was optimized for dental practice. Currently, it has been further improved and provides detailed views of very fine anatomical structures in the head and neck, such as the temporal bone, paranasal sinus, eye sockets, jaw, and skull base. Consequently, it can be used for ENT (ear, nose, and throat) and plastic surgery, and all dental indications.

4. Digital medical imaging in Laos

Lao People's Democratic Republic (hereinafter referred to as Laos) is an Association of Southeast Asian Nations member country with a population of approximately 6.49 million (as of 2019) in a land area (approximately 240,000 km^2) equivalent to Japan's mainland [11]. There are 429 dentists in Laos. Among these, 153 have dental clinics in Vientiane city, and 72 work in the UHS (as of 2019). Compared to neighboring countries, there are scarce medical personnel and resources, causing delay of home medical care system for the elderly population.

Currently, as life expectancy increases, the needs for dentistry for the elderly population have become apparent (i.e., oral tumors, and periodontal disease) in the world [12]. Diagnostic imaging is becoming essential in the field of dentistry from the viewpoint of medical safety.

The DPR and the CBCT images have been widely used for diagnosing diseases in the complex maxillofacial area and have become indispensable for safe and secure medical care in the dental field [13, 14]. However, in Laos, DPR and CBCT are expensive, so only one pair of DPR and CBT devices are installed at the University of Health Sciences (UHS), which is the only medical university in the country. Thus, there has been an unsolved problem in the effective utilizing of the digital medical imaging devices in community medicine in Laos.

The establishment of medical ICT system has been expected to solve these problems of sharing digital imaging data among medical institutes.

Recently, regional medical cooperation using medical ICT has been developed in Japan [15, 16], and medical imaging data have been provided and shared using a mobile tablet terminal application among medical institutions [17]. Therefore, we were inspired to take advantage of medical ICT to solve the inconvenient situation of the CBCT in Laos, as the joint research project between Nihon University and UHS (Duration 2011–2020).

The outline of the project is as follows.

- Purpose: Our project aims to provide DPR and CBCT images to dentists by constructing the medical ICT network using smartphones and tablet type terminals (data terminal equipment) from UHS in Vientiane city.

- Based on the sustainability of effective utilization of this medical ICT, likewise, we have developed an approach of sharing information on digital medical imaging among dentist in Laos.

- Significance: Our project is important to demonstrate the accessibility of providing and sharing image data information between different medical institutions using medical ICT in Laos. As a result, the foundation of a medical ICT system utilizing data terminal equipment will be established in the Southeast Asian region, and a model for building the spread and deployment of Japanese-style medical care overseas will be created.

- Contents: We conducted technical training on medical ICT using data terminal equipment for university faculty members and then examine the problems and solutions to diagnostic situations based on medical ICT with them in Laos. Furthermore, we verify the economic effects of medical ICT in the country in collaboration with local dental institutions.

From the perspective of sustainability in the application of dental diagnostic imaging in Laos, we decided to gradually start technology transfer to clinical dentists through joint research among researchers. Our project started from the stage of clinical research as the first phase to empirical research as the second phase, utilizing the medical ICT system.

In this joint research project, we first trained clinical researchers for digital image on maxillofacial radiology in Laos. In the next stage, we supported researchers to create an environment where they could train radiology professionals.

5. Diagnostic imaging research (first phase)

5.1 Research purpose

Clinical research planning was conducted to clarify changes in the development and aging of the jawbone of Lao people by digital imaging via telemedicine. The research theme was a morphological study on the cortical bone of the mandible in Lao people, using digital panoramic images.

Osteoporosis is a major public health problem confronting both developed and developing countries [18, 19]. Osteoporosis can affect both children and adults and is especially detected in postmenopausal women. The typical clinical presentation of osteoporosis is the radiographic detection of bone fractures, largely in the absence of causative trauma. These fractures occur due to a reduction in bone mineral density and general reduction in bone mass. Osteoporosis is usually diagnosed by measuring bone mineral density of the spine or femur. Dual energy X-ray absorptiometry (DXA) is recommended for precise diagnosis of low bone mass. No DXA equipment is currently available in Laos. Recently, it has been reported that mandibular cortical bone thickness is associated with bone mineral density and can be an effective indicator for the diagnosis of bone litigation. Therefore, we are conducting joint research to create a standard mandibular cortical wide (MCW) in Laos. Our diagnostic imaging study aimed to establish the diagnosis technology for osteoporosis using digital imaging of the jawbone. To proceed with this study, an ICT system for diagnostic imaging between Japan and Laos was required.

5.2 Utilized ICT system

In most countries, such a medical ICT system has been developed with Picture Archiving and Communication System and enterprise communication in teleradiology fields.

We have already installed the teleradiology system (View Send ICT, Tokyo) between Japan and Laos (**Figure 3**). The definition of a network with built security complied with the Japanese Ministry of Health, Labour and Welfare "Guidelines for Security Management of Medical Information Systems" using Virtual Private Network encryption. We designed a system that does not cause information leakage. Under these research conditions, we conducted clinical research on dental imaging.

5.3 Outline of research projects

A conference was held in real time between researchers in Japan and Laos by sharing image information and using a TV monitor, utilizing the medical ICT function. Researchers shared information on morphological measurement of the teeth and jawbones on images (**Figure 4**).

In 2015, as part of a quality assessment of our teleradiology collaboration, Matsumoto et al. [20] evaluated the validity of patient information gathered during teleradiology, panoramic imaging technique at the Lao PDR UHS, and ability of Laotian oral and maxillofacial radiologists to interpret images and detect temporomandibular joint (TMJ) abnormalities [20]. A total of 2446 joints from 1223 radiographs were evaluated for TMJ abnormalities to compare the image interpretation abilities of Laotian and Japanese radiologists. They reported that the kappa coefficient was 0.836 for the comparison of the judgments of the two observers in detecting TMJ abnormalities on radiographs ($P < 0.01$), which was considered very good agreement. Based on these results, we started research on osteoporosis between Japan and Laos using digital imaging data as materials.

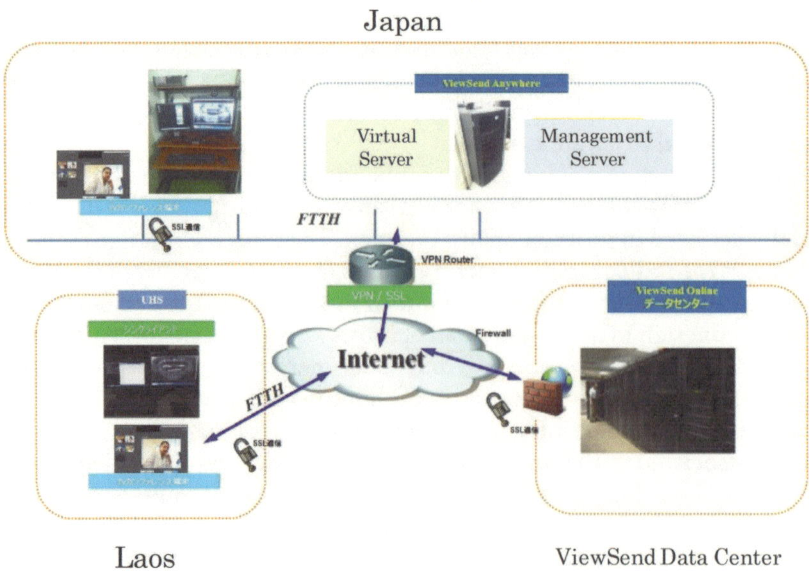

Figure 3.
Network overview of teleradiology in the first phase.

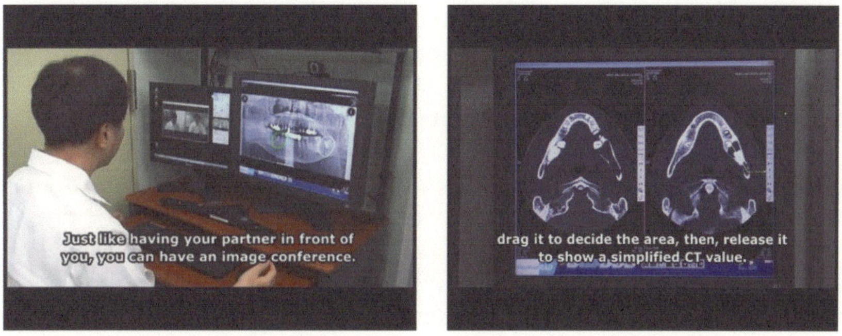

Figure 4.
Diagnostic imaging using medical ICT.

In the same year, Sisounthone et al. also established the average MCW in 519 Laotian subjects (age, 7–79 years; mean, 38.21 years) [21] (**Figure 5**). According to these results, the average MCW showed significant differences between all age groups. The average MCW in the youngest age group of 7–19 years was 2.90 ± 0.81 mm (range, 1.50–5.80), which was higher than the data obtained for the 4–6 years age group in this study. They also described a statistically significant sexual dimorphism in overall average MCW. In summary, the MCW of Laotian children aged 4–6 years increases slightly, but changes were more significant following adolescence.

In 2018, Souksavanh et al. established MCW standards for Laotian preschool children (4–6 years) at Vientiane [22]. According to their study, MCW increased slightly with increasing age but had no significant difference between age groups.

Moreover, the positive correlation between MCW and height was significant, but no significant correlation was noted between MCW and weight, suggesting that MCW in this period is not a useful indicator for the diagnosis of osteogenesis in children. They concluded that further studies were needed to examine if other panoramic radio morphometric indices could be more relevant in children.

In this way, the introduction of the medical ICT system has been shown to be effective tool in promoting international joint research in the field of medical imaging, indicating the possibility of effective calibration of image reading among dentists in Laos.

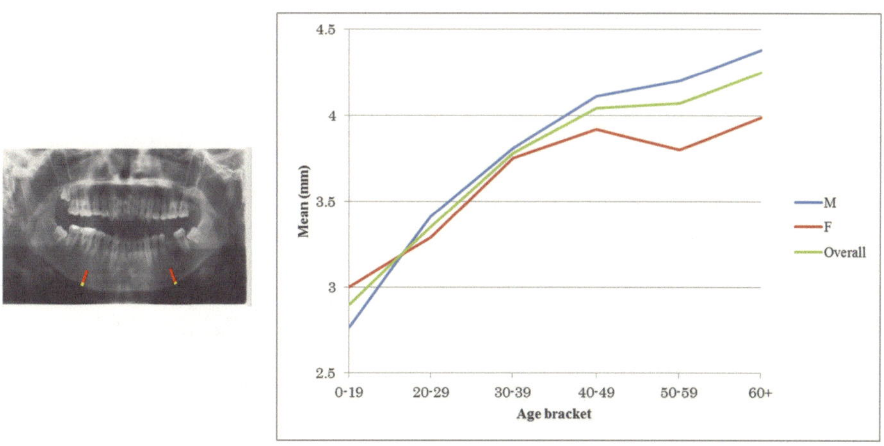

Figure 5.
Changing in MCW in Laotian people. Left: measurement of MCW. Yellow bars indicate MCW. Right: Changing of MCW in Lao people. These figures are taken from Ref. [21].

6. Clinical training for diagnostic imaging utilizing medical ICT (second phase)

6.1 Purpose of educational development

After previous research achievements, the foundation for clinical research using dentistry images was formed in Laos. We determined that the diagnostic imaging technique was shared between Japan and Laos, based on research achievements. As the second step, the educational system was developed to support the diagnostic imaging technique utilizing telemedicine for dentists in Laos.

The purposes of the medical ICT systems in the second phase were as follows.

- To determine the symptoms of stomatognathic lesions on digital images accurately.
- To operate medical ICT equipment correctly.
- To explain the symptoms to the patient using digital images adequately.

6.2 Utilized telemedicine system

Medical ICT is known to be developed to the point where image data can be shared with mobile tablet terminals/smartphones that use data terminal devices.

Recently, many studies confirmed the effect of tablet terminals in medical education. The use of mobile tablet terminals has an impact on how medical residents approach medical education, clinical practice, and patient education [23, 24]. The educational tool may be useful in collecting data on mobile tablet terminals used by other graduate medical education programs.

In 2018, as a clinical training tool, therefore, we adopted new ICT system, using the mobile tablet (View Send ICT, Tokyo). This system allows dentists to receive image data from a university hospital on a mobile tablet terminal in Vientiane city. This system created an environment in which the dentist who requested the diagnosis could view the image data anywhere in the city (**Figure 6**).

6.3 Project activities

The workshop was held with the Laotian collaborators who participated in the first phase as the main members. The purpose of the workshop was to transfer the techniques of digital image reading and telemedicine operation for faculty members.

A total of 72 faculty members enrolled in the digital medical imaging class in the Faculty of Dentistry, UHS (hereinafter referred to as the Faculty of Dentistry). Following the lecture of radiology, a hands-on seminar on medical ICT was held (**Figure 7**). In the seminar, the digital panoramic images were sent and downloaded as teaching materials from the medical image database of the Faculty of Dentistry of the UHS to the tablet terminal (iPad®), and the participants will be informed about the operative method of diagnostic imaging. Participants had the training of reading images using tablet terminal. Ten clinically experienced dentists were selected from the seminar participants. The dentist requests the dental radiology room of the Faculty of Dentistry to perform image examination by DPR or CBCT for the patient,

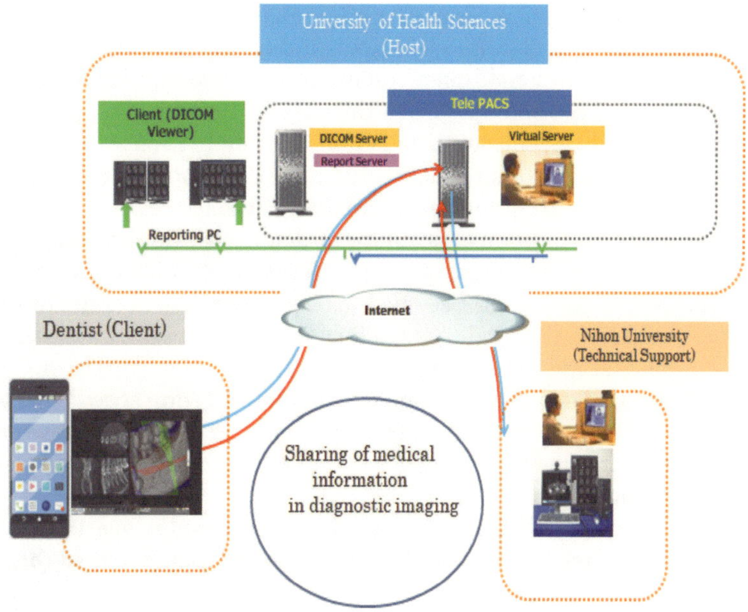

Figure 6.
Overview of the medical ICT system in phase 2.

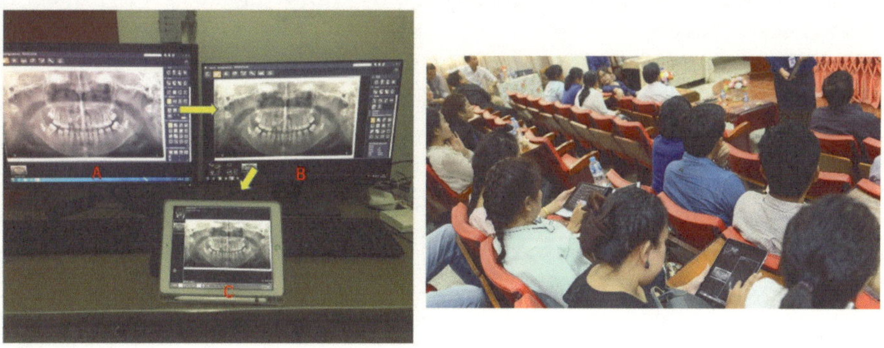

Figure 7.
Medical ICT system using the tablet terminal. Left: Digital image data (A) are transferred through PC server (B) to the tablet terminal (C). Right: Workshop for dentists (teachers).

and always shares the image data with the tablet terminal. The dentist explained regarding oral diseases to the patient with a tablet terminal. The demonstration experiment period was 90 days.

6.4 Effect of clinical training

A total of 171 medical ICTs were used in all clinical departments in 3 months (66 actual days excluding holidays). Of these, the numbers of requests for CBCT and DPR imaging were 126 and 45, respectively. Medical ICT has been used in approximately 700 cases (January 2021). The average daily medical ICT utilization rate for all clinical departments was 2.6 cases/day. For example, in the case of dental hospitals of Nihon University, telemedicine is used approximately 10 cases a month. Because of the difference in medical conditions in Japan and Laos, it is not possible to simply compare them, but the number of telemedicine cases in Laos tended to be larger. These results suggested the possibility that the use of DPR and CBCT in university hospitals has a positive effect on access to dental imaging in Laos. After this 90-day test period, we interviewed 10 hospital faculty members about the advantages and problems of telemedicine using the questionnaire (**Table 1**).

Respondents listed three points, "accuracy of diagnosis", "improvement in patient satisfaction", and "increase in the number of patients" as the effect of using telemedicine. The evaluation of medical ICT seemed to be positive. Use of tablet terminals may promote the sharing of digital medical imaging data between university hospital and dentists or dentists and patients, in the dental fields.

However, they pointed out three problems, "communication speed", "image accuracy", and "complexity of operations and the system". The reasons of these problems were the internet environment (low capacity) and operation of the mobile tablet terminal (inexperienced).

All respondents answered "Yes, I think so very much" for the question on the usefulness of telemedicine in their country. They seemed to understand the need for telemedicine through clinical training.

Given these results, we continued discussions to improve the problems of medical ICT in the hospital. As a result of the discussion, we were able to agree on problem extraction and countermeasures (**Figure 8**). As a future development, we will support the spread of digital medical imaging diagnosis by improving medical ICT under the plan-do-check-act cycle.

Question 1 Which is the effect of using telemedicine?	**Case**
a. Accuracy in diagnosis	6
b. Increase in number of patients	2
c. Improvement in patient satisfaction	5
d. Others ()	0
e. No change	0
Question 2 What are the problems to be solved in telemedicine system?	
a. Image data accuracy	2
b. Communication speed	6
c. Operation and system complexity	2
d. Number of imaging cases	0
e. No problem	0
Question 3 Do you think this telemedicine service is useful in Laos?	
a. Yes, I think so very much	10
b. Yes, I think so	0
c. No, I do not think so	0
d. No, I do not think at all	0

Table 1.
Advantages and problems of telemedicine.

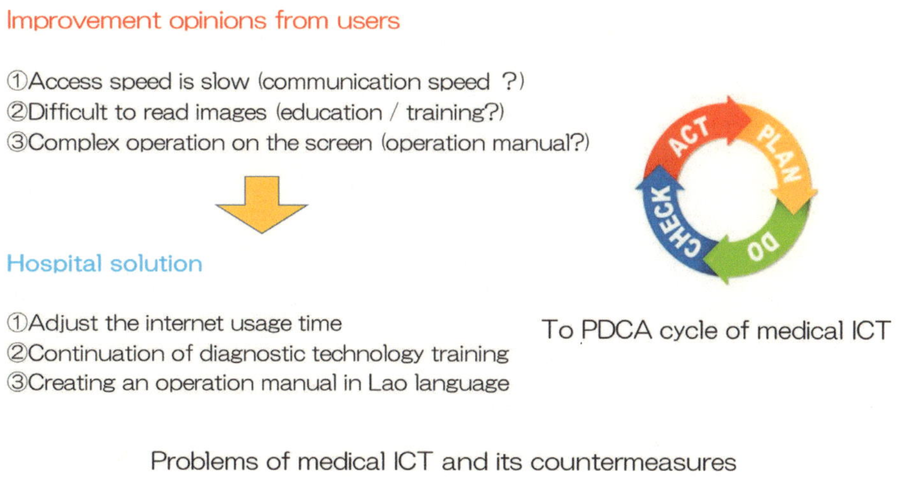

Figure 8.
Improvement of medical ICT system based on opinions from faculty members.

Outcome of this project that lasts 10 years suggest an importance to share the common goal of training specialists under the international collaboration.

For the introduction of medical ICT in community medicine, it is necessary to further examine the clinical evidence. As the further step, we will continue to develop the network of teleradiology in order to contribute sustainable oral health in Laos.

7. Conclusions

The results of our project show that information sharing of dental images by tablet terminals is effective in Laos. In this project, both Laotians and Japanese shared the common goal of training specialists. We concluded that teleradiology can usefully improve dental services in Laos.

Acknowledgements

This work has received funding from the Nihon University Chairman of the Board of Trustees Grant and the Nihon University President Grant Initiative.

Conflict of interest

The authors declare no conflict of interest.

Notes/thanks/other declarations

We would like to thank Mr. Kenei Shie, President of ViewSend ICT for providing technical support for the activities of this research project for more than 10 years.

Author details

Ichiro Nakajima[1*], Ken-ichiro Ejima[2], Yoshinori Arai[2], Kunihito Matsumoto[2], Kazuya Honda[2], Hirofumi Aboshi[3], Marina Hamaguchi[4], Akao Lyvongsa[5], Bounnhong Sidaphone[5], Somphone Phanthavong[6], Chanthavisao Phanthanalay[6] and Souksavanh Vongsa[7]

1 Department of Community Dentistry, Nihon University School of Dentistry, Tokyo, Japan

2 Department of Oral and Maxillofacial Radiology, Nihon University School of Dentistry, Tokyo, Japan

3 Department of Legal Medicine, Nihon University School of Dentistry, Tokyo, Japan

4 Department of Haematology and Rheumatology, Nihon University School of Medicine, Tokyo, Japan

5 Faculty of Dentistry, Department of Oral Surgery, University of Health Sciences, Vientiane, Lao People's Democratic Republic

6 Faculty of Dentistry, Department of Restorative Dentistry, University of Health Sciences, Vientiane, Lao People's Democratic Republic

7 Faculty of Dentistry, Department of Basic Sciences in Dentistry, University of Health Sciences, Vientiane, Lao People's Democratic Republic

*Address all correspondence to: nakajima.ichirou@nihon-u.ac.jp

References

[1] WHO Publications. Telemedicine opportunities and developments in member state. Report on the second global survey on eHealth Global Observatory for eHealth series—Volume 2 [internet]. 2021. Available from: https://www.afro.who.int/publications/telemedicine-opportunities-and-developments-member-state [Accessed: 21 September 2021]

[2] Toda H, Yoshimura K, Yanashima K, Hamaguchi M, Nakajima I, Otsuka Y, Uehara S, Katsuragi H, Shinohara K, Vongsa S, Sathathone D, Prabouasane K, Somsamouth B, Takei M. Prototype of a medical and dietary record system cloud to support diabetic patient care in Lao. In: Proceedings of IEEE International the 14th Symposium on Medical Information Communication; 20-22 May 2020; Nara: IEEE; 2020. pp. 1-4

[3] Rouleau G, Gagnon MP, Côté J, Payne-Gagnon J, Hudson E, Dubois CA. Impacts of information and communication technologies on nursing care: An overview of systematic reviews. Journal of Internet Research. 2017;**19**(4):e122. DOI: 10.2196/jmir.6686

[4] Deserno TM, Dugas M, Löbe M, Stausberg J. A topical collection on ICT for Health Science Research – EFMI Special Topic Conference. EFMI STC 2019 on ICT for Health Science Research. Journal of Medical Systems. 2021;**45**:e70. DOI: 10.1007/s10916-021-01739-2

[5] Zonneveld M, Patomella AH, Asaba E, Guidetti S. The use of information and communication technology in healthcare to improve participation in everyday life: A scoping review. Disability and Rehabilitation. 2020;**42**(23):3416-3423. DOI: 10.1080/09638288.2019.1592246

[6] Mihailovic B, Miladinovic M, Vujicic B. Telemedicine in dentistry (teledentistry). In: Graschew G, Roelofs TA, editors. Advances in Telemedicine: Applications in Various Medical Disciplines and Geographical Regions. Europe: InTech; 2010. pp. 215-230. DOI: 10.5772/14352

[7] Knott NJ. The use of information and communication technology (ICT) in dentistry. British Dental Journal. 2013;**214**(4):151-153. DOI: 10.1038/sj.bdj.2013.157

[8] Estai M, Kruger E, Tennant M. Role of telemedicine and mid-level dental providers in expanding dental-care access: Potential application in rural Australia. International Dental Journal. 2016;**66**:195-200. DOI: 10.1111/idj.12217

[9] Telemedicine in Japan[Internet]. 2013. Available from: http://jtta.umin.jp/pdf/telemedicine/telemedicine_in_japan_20131015-2_en.pdf [Accessed: 21 September 2021]

[10] Arai Y, Tammisalo E, Iwai K, Hashimoto K, Shinoda K. Development of a compact computed tomographic apparatus for dental use. Dento Maxillo Facial Radiology. 1999;**28**(4):245-248. DOI: 10.1038/sj/dmfr/4600448

[11] Japan International Corporation Agency: The study on power network system master plan in Lao people's democratic republic final report [Internet]. 2020. Available from: https://openjicareport.jica.go.jp/pdf/12328027_01.pdf [Accessed: 21 September 2021]

[12] Gil-Montoya JA, Ferreira de Mello AL, Barrios R, Gonzalez-Moles MA, Bravo M. Oral health in the elderly patient and its impact on general well-being:

A nonsystematic review. Clinical Interventions in Aging. 2015;**10**:461-467. DOI: 10.2147/CIA.S54630

[13] Truhlar RS, Morris HF, Ochi S. A review of panoramic radiography and its potential use in implant dentistry. Implant Dentistry. 1993;**2**(2):122-130. DOI: 10.1097/00008505-199305000-00010

[14] Kiljunen T, Kaasalainen T, Suomalainen A, Kortesniemi M. Dental cone beam CT: A review. Physica Medica. 2015;**31**(8):844-860. DOI: 10.1016/j.ejmp.2015.09.004

[15] Nakamura T. The development of medical networks through ICT in Japan. Networks and Communication Studies. 2016;**21**(2007):363-380. DOI: 10.4000/netcom.2256

[16] Ito J, Edirippulige S, Aono T, Armfield NR. The use of telemedicine for delivering healthcare in Japan: Systematic review of literature published in Japanese and English languages. Journal of Telemedicine and Telecare. 2017;**23**(10):828-834. DOI: 10.1177/1357633X17732801

[17] Takao H, Sakai K, Mitsumura H, Komatsu T, Yuki I, Takeshita K, et al. A smartphone application as a telemedicine tool for stroke care management. Neurologia Medico-Chirurgica. 2021;**61**(4):260-267. DOI: org/10.2176/nmc.oa.2020-0302

[18] National Institutes of Health Osteoporosis and Related Bone Diseases [Internet]. 2019. Available from: https://www.bones.nih.gov/ [Accessed: 21 September 2021]

[19] Taguchi A, Sanada M, Krall E, Nakamoto T, Ohtsuka M, Suei Y, et al. Relationship between dental panoramic radiographic findings and biochemical markers of bone turnover. Journal of Bone and Mineral Research. 2003;**18**(9):1689-1694. DOI: 10.1359/jbmr.2003.18.9.1689

[20] Matsumoto K, Vongsa S, Nakajima I, Ejima K, Kohinata K, Suzuki T, et al. Assessment of quality and interpretation of panoramic radiographs obtained in the Lao People's Democratic Republic as part of a teleradiology collaboration with Japan. Journal of Oral Science. 2015;**57**(3):235-239. DOI: org/10.2334/josnusd.57.235

[21] Sisounthone J, Ejima K, Nakajima I, Honda K, Hosono S, Vongsa S, et al. Application of telemedicine to assess mandibular cortical width on panoramic images of dental patients in the Lao People's Democratic Republic. Oral Radiology. 2015;**31**(3):155-159. DOI: 10.1007/s11282-015-0198-4

[22] Vongsa S, Aboshi H, Ejima K, Sidaphone B, Lyvongsa A, Ngonephady S, et al. Mandibular cortical width on panoramic images of children in the Lao People's Democratic Republic. Journal of Hard Tissue Biology. 2018;**27**(1):23-28. DOI: org/10.2485/jhtb.27.23

[23] Dupaix J, Chen JJ, Chun MB, Belcher GF, Cheng Y, Atkinson R. The effect of mobile tablet computer (iPad) Implementation on Graduate Medical Education at a Multi-specialty Residency Institution. Hawaii Journal of Medicine & Public Health. 2016;**75**(7):190-195

[24] Archibald D, Macdonald CJ, Plante J, Hogue RJ, Fiallos J. Residents' and preceptors' perceptions of the use of the iPad for clinical teaching in a family medicine residency program. BMC Medical Education. 2014;**14**:e174. DOI: 10.1186/1472-6920-14-174